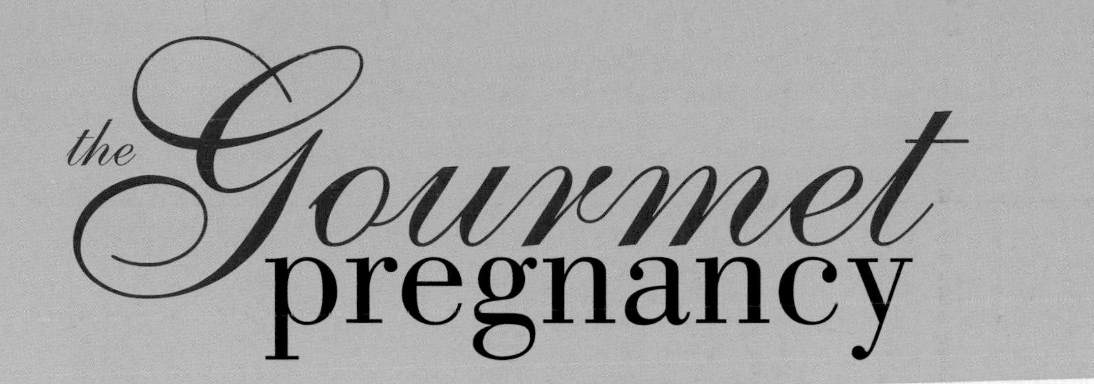

the Gourmet pregnancy

LEAH DOUGLAS

PHOTOGRAPHY BY
MICHAEL DOUGLAS

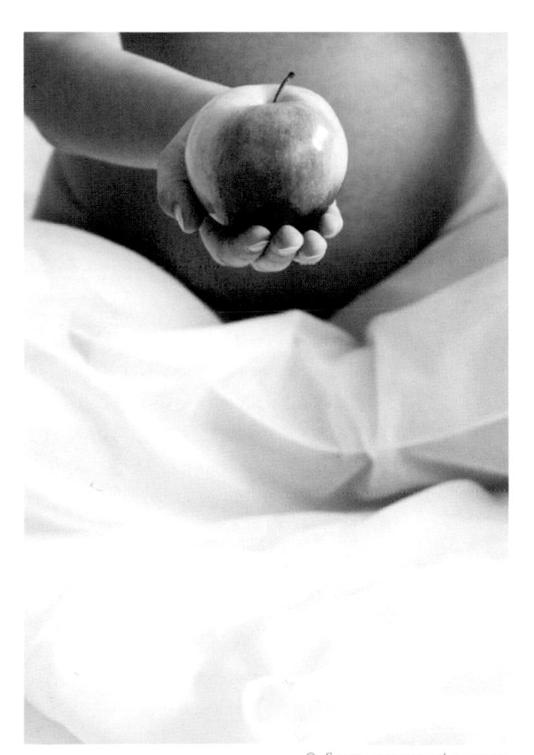

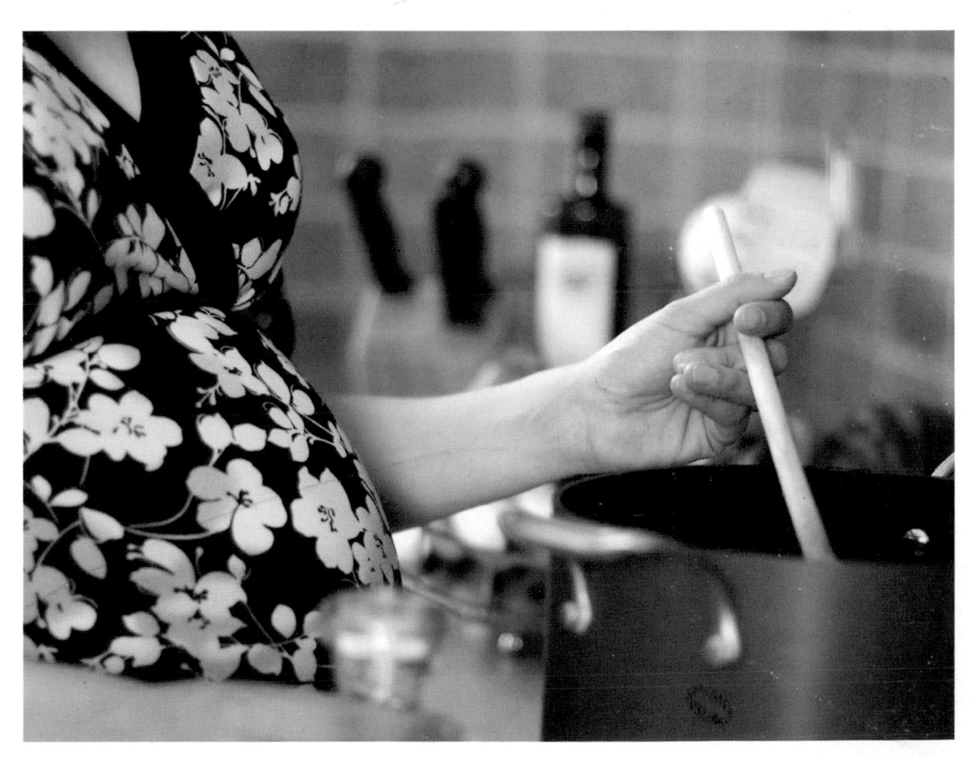

Library and Archives Canada Cataloguing in Publication

Douglas, Leah, 1975–
Gourmet pregnancy / Leah Douglas.

Includes index.
ISBN 978-0-470-73643-2

1. Pregnancy—Nutritional aspects. 2. Cookery. 3. Mothers—Nutrition. I. Title.

RG559.D685 2010 641.5'6319 C2009-905807-3

Production Credits
Cover Design and Interior Design: Michael Douglas
Typesetter: Adrian So
Printer: PrintPlus Ltd.

Editorial Credits
Editor: Leah Fairbank
Project Coordinator: Pauline Ricablanca

Photo Credits
All photography by Michael Douglas unless otherwise credited.
Front cover: © iStockphoto.com/pascalgenest
Back cover: © iStockphoto.com/oscargalway

John Wiley & Sons Canada, Ltd.
6045 Freemont Blvd.
Mississauga, Ontario
L5R 4J3

Printed in China

1 2 3 4 5 PP 14 13 12 11 10

acknowledgements

FOR MY HUSBAND Mike, without whom this book would have been only a passing fancy. You provided remarkable inspiration and countless hours of photography and design work, and made the late nights and hard work both meaningful and enjoyable. Many thanks as well to Avery for love, many hugs and her home-cooked pretend meals.

Special gratitude to my sister, Angie Brennand, and sister-in-law Andrea Douglas, who both contributed fantastic recipes. Michelle Nelson provided tremendous recipe support and assistance, and created five fabulous recipes sent from her very happy kitchen to mine. Our families have been incredibly kind and caring throughout, and I offer many thanks to the Douglas, Trela, Malowaniec and Nelson clans. Pat Nelson, Betty Lou Douglas and Irene Trela are true culinary inspirations and certainly shaped my cooking approach.

Thanks as well to all of my friends who ate the food, critiqued the food, but always returned for more of it! So many of you wonderful women told me about pregnancy cravings, wrote stories, cheered me on and provided much-needed encouragement and support. Alyson Brucker and Tova Wolinsky were gorgeous pregnant models and true friends. Kristina, Denise, Amrin and Sarah are fantastic women who listened, shared and inspired.

Finally, my sincere and heartfelt thanks to my incredible agent Carolyn Swayze, a mover and shaker who makes wonderful things happen. Leah Fairbank got the ball rolling at Wiley, Judy Phillips provided exceptional copyediting and Pauline Ricablanca managed the project in a very organized fashion.

Cheers!

"A grand adventure is about to begin."

~Winnie the Pooh

contents

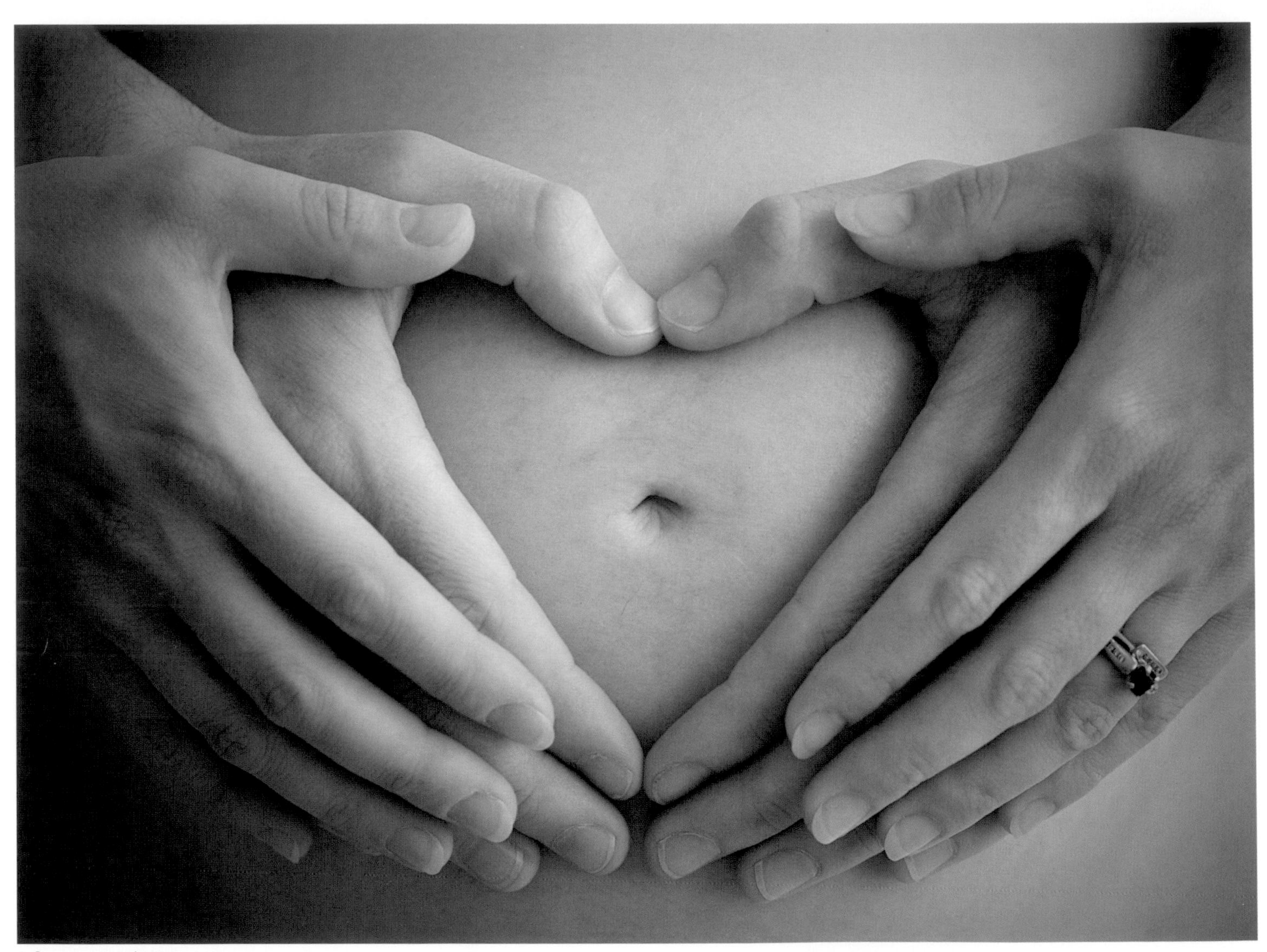

© iStockphoto.com/shmuel

Acknowledgements ... iii
Foreword ... 1
Introduction ... 3
On the Guest List ... 5
Not Invited to the Party ... 7
What Are You Craving? ... 8

if morning sickness has passed you by:
breakfasts and brunch

Herbed Cream Cheese Eggs Benedict ... 14
Ham and Grilled Pineapple Bagel with Honey Mustard Cream Cheese ... 16
Salmon, Zucchini and Sweet Corn Latkes with Dill Sour Cream ... 18
Italian Omelet with Artisan Bread ... 20
Black Bean Scramble with Fresh Tomato Salsa ... 22
Garden Vegetable Frittata ... 24
Roasted Sweet Potato and Pepper Eggs ... 25
Bacon, Apple, Lettuce, Tomato, Cheddar and Avocado Sandwich ... 26
Chorizo Chive Buttermilk Biscuits ... 28
Ultimate Peanut Butter Sandwich ... 30
Sweet and Savoury Crêpes ... 32
Sourdough French Toast with Blueberry Crème ... 34
Orchard Fruit Muffins ... 36
Exotic Fruit Salad with Sweet Citrus Guacamole ... 37

yummy nibbles to soothe those cravings:
snacks and sidekicks

Tempura Dill Pickles with Sambal Oelek Dip ... 40
Asparagus with Truffle Oil and Toasted Pine Nuts ... 42
Green Olives with Roasted Chickpeas and Mixed Nuts ... 44
Cumin Pita Chips with Peanut Sweet Chili Dip ... 46
Sweet Potato Fries with Truffle Aioli ... 48
Corn on the Cob with Spiced Maple Butter ... 50
Grilled Peaches with Pink Grapefruit and Mint ... 52
Mango Cilantro Salsa ... 54
Granny Smith Honey Cornbread ... 56
Tangerine Dream Muffins ... 58
M&M Granola Bars ... 60
Slightly Naughty Biscotti ... 62
Chocolate Chip Blueberry Almond Cookies ... 64
Maple Walnut Caramel Corn ... 66
Banana, Yogurt and Juice Layered Popsicles ... 67

mini-bites for you and your mini-me:
appetizers

Sushi Vegetables with Asian and Wasabi Yogurt Dipping Sauces ... 70
Roasted Butternut Squash Wedges with Honey Green Curry Drizzle ... 72
Bacon-Wrapped Dried Plums Stuffed with Maple Toasted Pecans ... 74
Baked Grape Leaves with Sumac Chicken, Apricots and Rice ... 76
Sun-Dried Olive and Tomato Tuna Zucchini Rounds ... 78
Caramelized Onion and Balsamic Cherry Jam ... 80
Gourmet Seven Layer Dip ... 82
Roasted Garlic, Sirloin Meatball and Toasted Pita Skewers ... 84
Rustic Sesame Vegetable Tart ... 86
Hazelnut, Avocado and Garlic Whole-Wheat Crostinis ... 88
Apple Slices, Belgian Endive, Flatbreads and Portobello Mushroom Pâté ... 90
Meyer Lemon and Blueberry Salad in Parmesan Baskets ... 92
Fresh Tomato, Basil and Bocconcini Skewers with Lemon Olive Oil ... 94
White Cheddar with Pear Compote and Walnuts ... 96

since your tummy might already feel full:

lighter fare

French Fusion Onion Soup ... 100
Butternut Squash and Carrot Ginger Soup with Crème Fraîche ... 102
Salmon, White Asparagus and Dill Pea Salad ... 104
Lemongrass Tiger Prawn and Chickpea Salad ... 106
Sesame Cashew Red Cabbage Noodle Salad ... 108
Spiced Caramelized Cauliflower and Candied Curry Pecan Salad ... 110
Roasted Balsamic Vegetable Panini with Roasted Garlic Aioli ... 112
Grilled Pear and Thai Basil Sandwich ... 114
Toasted Three-Cheese Sandwich on Homemade Dill Onion Bread ... 115
Chicken Rosemary Horseradish Cream Wrap ... 116
Ginger Wasabi Sliders ... 118
Mild Curry Chicken Pizza on Naan ... 120
Succulent Crab Cakes with Tarragon Sour Cream ... 122
Panko-Crusted Stuffed Grilled Portobello ... 124

delicious food to nourish your body and soul:

entrées

Sautéed Sablefish with Eggplant Caviar ... 128
Chocolate Sesame Salmon with Steamed Broccoli ... 130
Tilapia Fillets with Coconut Curry Cream Sauce ... 132
Seared Scallops with Cilantro Honey Pesto and Baby Arugula Salad ... 134
Garlic Shrimp and Feta Linguine ... 136
Butternut Squash Ravioli with Fig Brown Butter Sauce ... 138
Eggplant and Spinach Lasagna with Béchamel Sauce ... 140
Gnocchi with Truffle Butter Sauce ... 142
Bacon, Leek and Toasted Almond Risotto ... 144
Rosemary Garlic Roast Beef ... 146
Tempura Beets, Mushrooms and Onions ... 148
Apple and Anjou Pear Beef with Smashed Yams ... 149
Grilled New York Striploin Steak Salad ... 150
Moroccan Spiced Chicken Quesadilla with Dried Fruits ... 152
Ancho Chili Chicken and Zucchini with Garlic Roasted Potatoes ... 154

a bite for you, a bite for baby, a bite for you:

desserts

Chocolate Truffle Soufflés ... 158
Chocolate Mousse Cake with Chocolate Cookie Toffee Crust ... 160
Dulce de Leche Sex in a Pan ... 162
Orange Ginger Pumpkin Cheesecake ... 164
Cherry and Fresh Mint Tart with Rustic Vanilla Shortbread Crust ... 166
White Peach Crumble Pie with Caramel Drizzle ... 168
Berry Kiwi Citrus Cream Meringues ... 170
Layered Banana Butterscotch Pudding ... 172
Duet of Dried Cranberry Shortbread and Candy Cane Ice Creams ... 174
Decadent Chocolate Anise Sauce with Vanilla Ice Cream and Fresh Raspberries ... 176
Cashew Brittle Frost ... 177
Toffee Coffee Chocolate Chip Cookies ... 178
Chocolate Raspberry Fudge ... 180
Almond Mocha Nanaimo Bars ... 182
London Fog Cupcakes ... 184

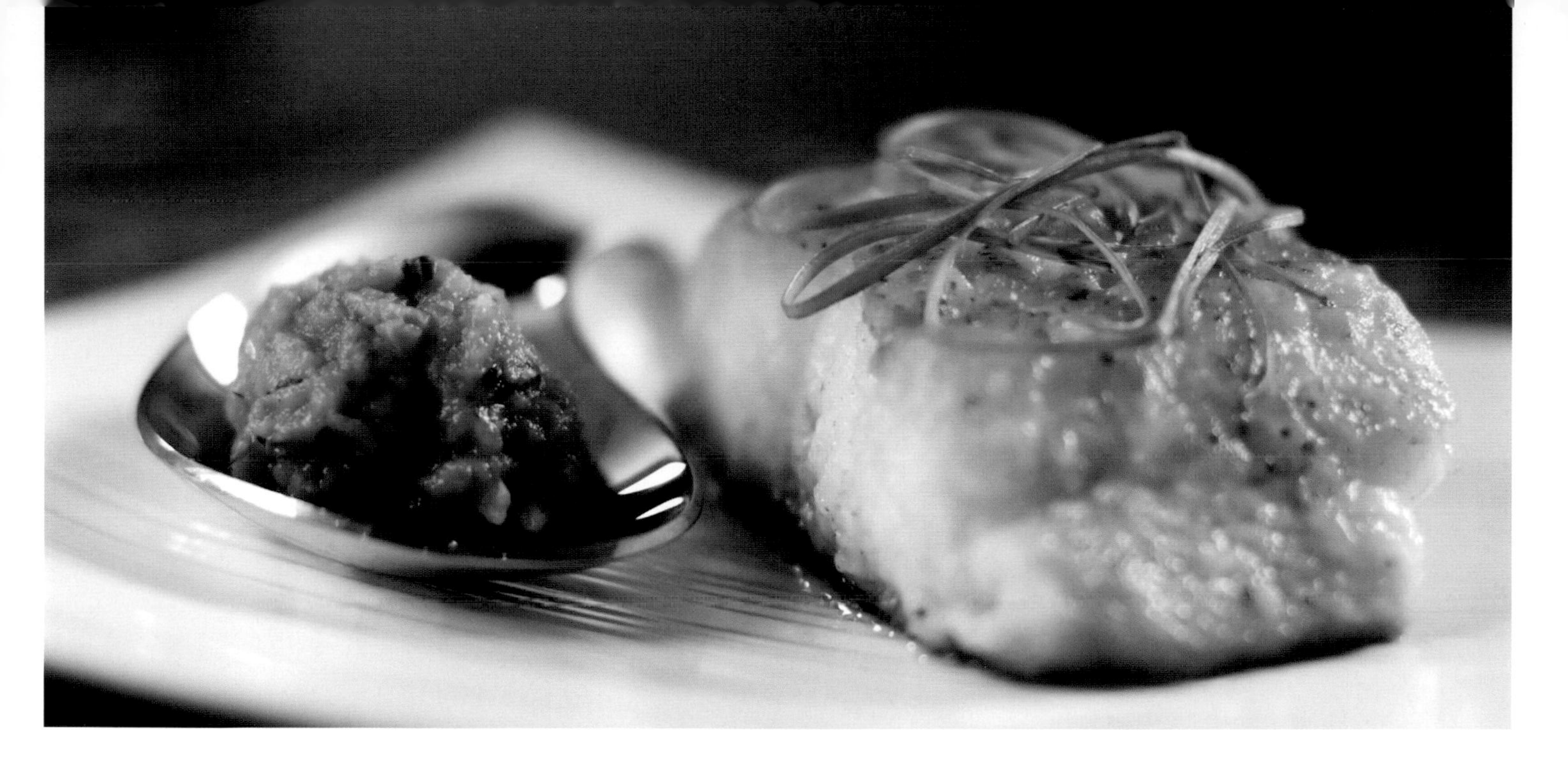

all the flavour, none of the booze:

drinks

Fresh Mango Strawberry Lemonade 188
Blueberry Lychee Kiss 190
Ginger Beer No-jito 190
White Peach Bellini 192
Lemon Drop Cosmopolitan 192
Pickled Mary 194
Sparkling Raspberry Float 195
Vanilla Rooisbos and Passion Fruit Teaser 196
Iced Mint Tea with Cucumber 196
Watermelon Refresher 198
Good Morning, Sunshine! 198
Blueberry Coconut Smoothie 200
Chocolate Chai White Tea 200
Vanilla Cinnamon Latte 201
Rich Hazelnut Hot Cocoa 202

menus

Romantic Picnic 205
Fine Dining 205
Baby Shower 205
Girlfriends' Brunch 205

Imperial/Metric Conversions 206
Index 208

foreword

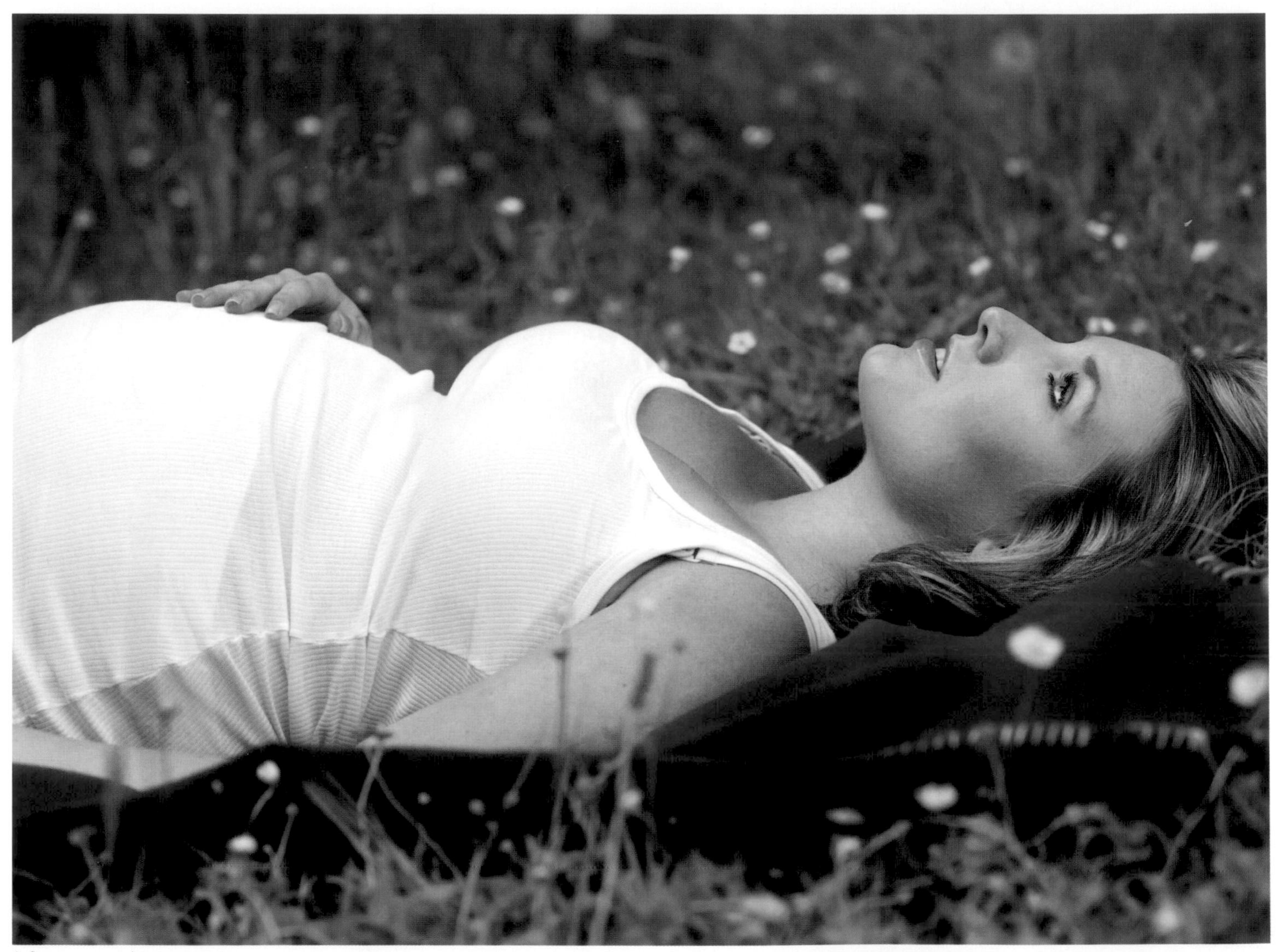

I'M SO PLEASED to introduce you to this wonderful book. *The Gourmet Pregnancy* is a book that finally helps pregnant women not only to eat well while they are pregnant, but to enjoy eating (and their beautifully changing bodies) throughout this distinct period of life.

Health really is a lifelong project. In fact, it starts before we are born. Your baby's health is determined by factors that begin prior to you becoming pregnant and continue throughout your pregnancy, nutrition being one of the most important. "You are what you eat" applies even more to the developing fetus than it does later in life.

However, healthy eating is more complicated when pregnant; our immune systems are less robust, an adaptation that lets the pregnant body accept a growing visitor. Yet this same adaptation means that we are more susceptible to some infections such as salmonella and listeriosis. As well, pregnancy is a time when tiny changes in cell metabolism can have huge consequences, and hence toxins and substances such as alcohol can have effects far beyond what they normally would.

Every year, there is more available research to help us face these issues. In fact there is so much information that it can be really difficult for anyone who doesn't do this full time to stay up to date! That's why having access to a cookbook such as this is essential — it helps you to eat within safe guidelines while still celebrating your food. The brilliance of this innovative, fun cookbook is that it gives you so much information and so many great ideas in one place. The recipes are consistent with the guidelines presently endorsed by professional organizations around the world, and many of the recipes introduce exciting variations on our favourite meals in order to make them safe during pregnancy.

Of course, every pregnancy is different. Your nutritional needs will vary with each pregnancy and even within your pregnancy, depending on the stage and many other factors. In early pregnancy, organs and other structures are just forming. In later stages muscles, organs and bones are growing, increasing the need for many nutrients. Because of this, it is always a good idea to talk to your health care provider about what foods are best for you, and whether or not you should consider taking supplements such as folic acid, iron or calcium.

Part of eating well is enjoying what you eat: I hope you enjoy this cookbook and enjoy your pregnancy, knowing that the effort you put into your deliciously healthy diet helps to get your baby off to the best start possible!

Dr. Jan E. Christilaw, MD, FRCSC, MHSc

Obstetrician-Gynecologist
President, BC Women's Hospital & Health Centre
Vancouver, British Columbia

introduction

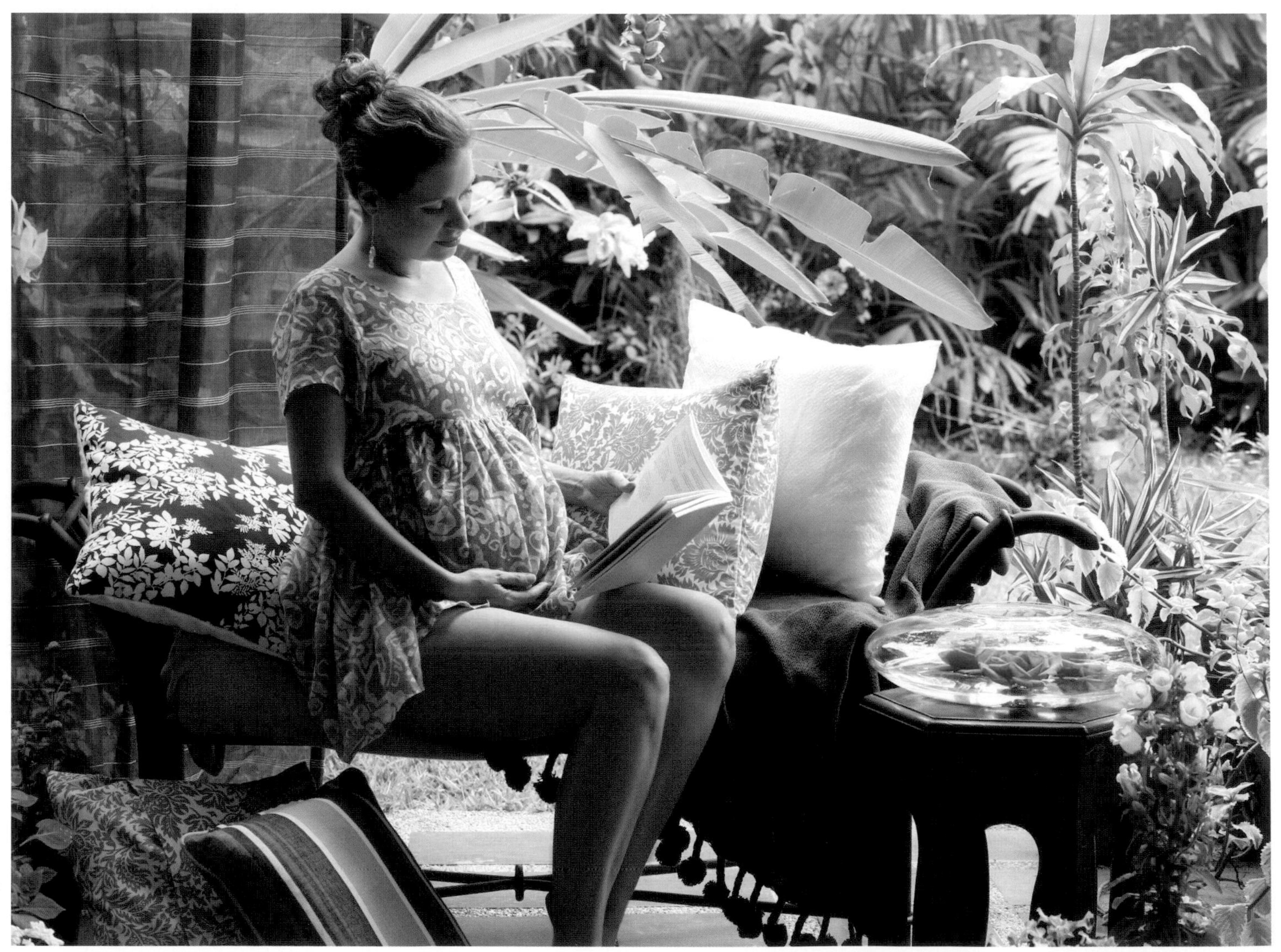

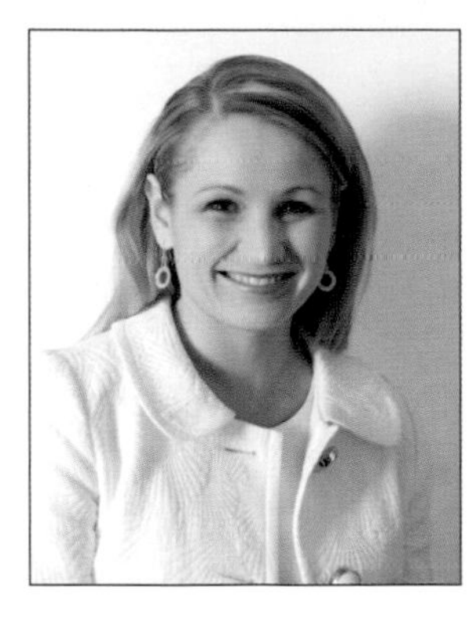

WHAT WOULD LIFE BE without great food? I love food and am always happy to prepare, share and enjoy meals with family and friends. Eating local, flavourful and healthy meals became even more of a priority when I found out I was expecting a baby. Like many women, I wanted to eat what would be best for my baby and steer clear of any foods or drinks that could cause harm or increase risk. But I couldn't always keep track of what foods were to be avoided and was often confused by advice or the most recent recommendations for nutrition during pregnancy. I also worried that I would inadvertently eat something I wasn't supposed to have, especially at restaurants. I felt much happier and comfortable making meals at home and having a fun dinner party instead of an expensive meal out. And some days I could barely manage to eat at all, as the "morning" sickness lasted all day. I've heard from many other women who felt the same way.

I put together this collection of fun, relatively simple but gourmet recipes for all the other pregnant gals out there who also want to keep eating well without confusion. I am incredibly thankful to Dr. Jan Christilaw, who has reviewed the recipes and given them all a stamp of approval for expectant women. I hope this book will save you time, energy and stress in deciding what to eat, as I know you've got other important things to do. You don't need any special training to make these gourmet meals, just high-quality ingredients and the time to prepare the dishes. You can certainly continue eating these meals after your baby is born — you'll want to make the recipes for your children and family for years to come. There are lots of good food movies to watch if you need extra inspiration — a few of my favourites are *Like Water for Chocolate*, *Eat Drink Man Woman*, *Chocolat*, *Babette's Feast*, *Ratatouille* and *Julie & Julia*. You'll be in the mood to whip up a feast after watching any one of them. I hope you also get your partner and friends in the kitchen to cook with (or for!) you. Put on some music, shift into a creative and playful frame of mind, and have fun in the kitchen. Cooking can be such great entertainment — and the eating part that follows is pretty good, too. Enjoy!

> "Happy and successful cooking doesn't rely only on know-how; it comes from the heart, makes great demands on the palate and needs enthusiasm and a deep love of food to bring it to life."
>
> *~Georges Blanc, Ma Cuisine des Saisons*

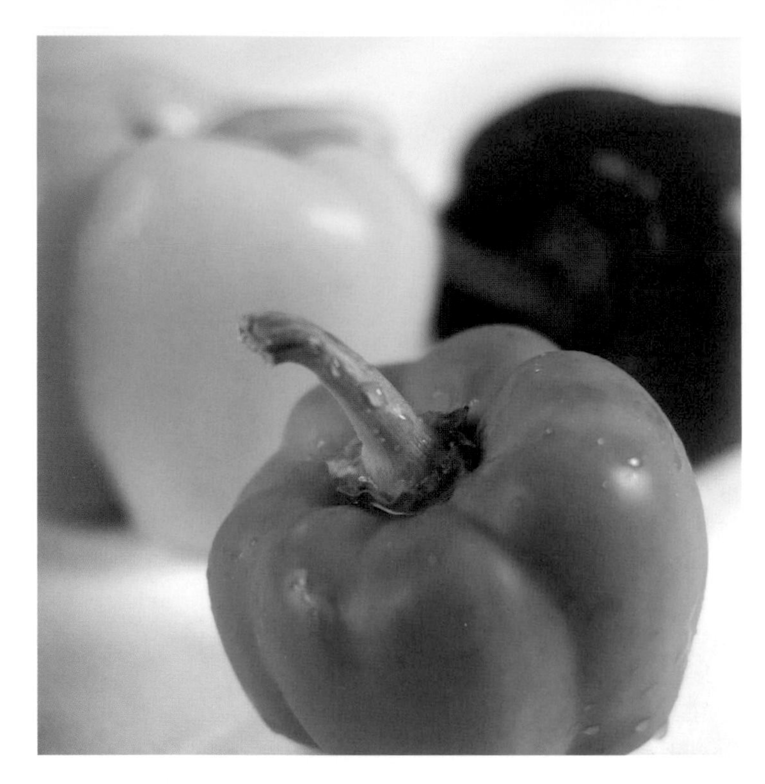
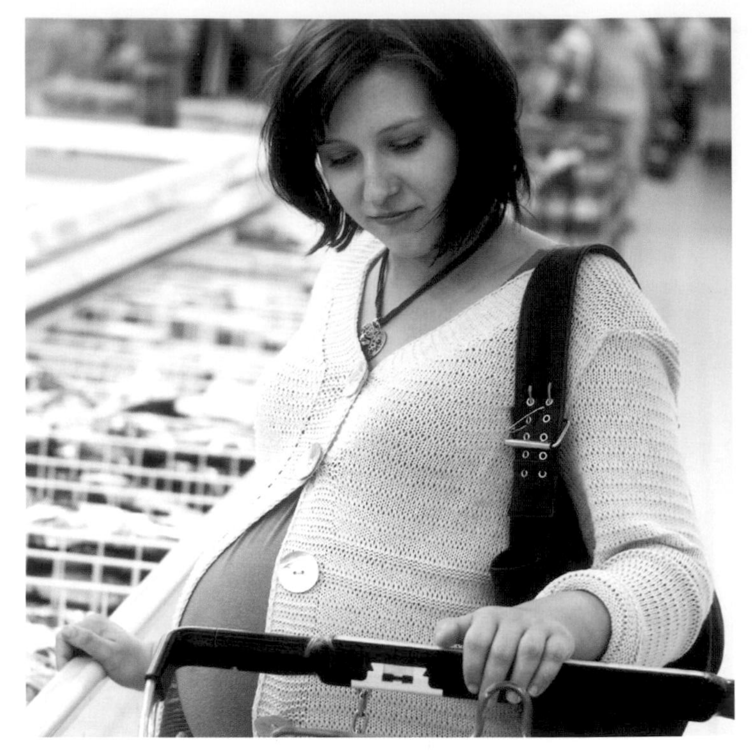
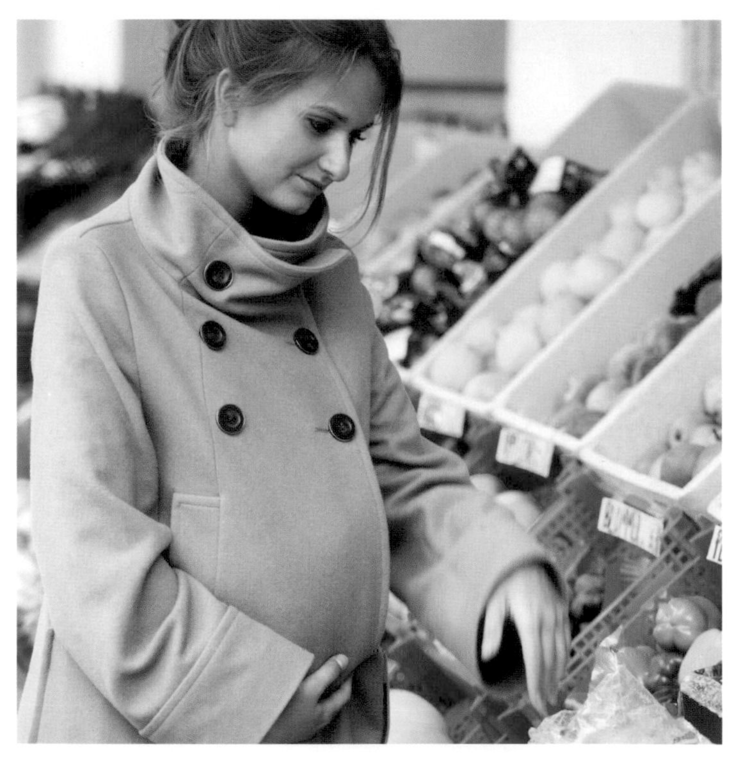
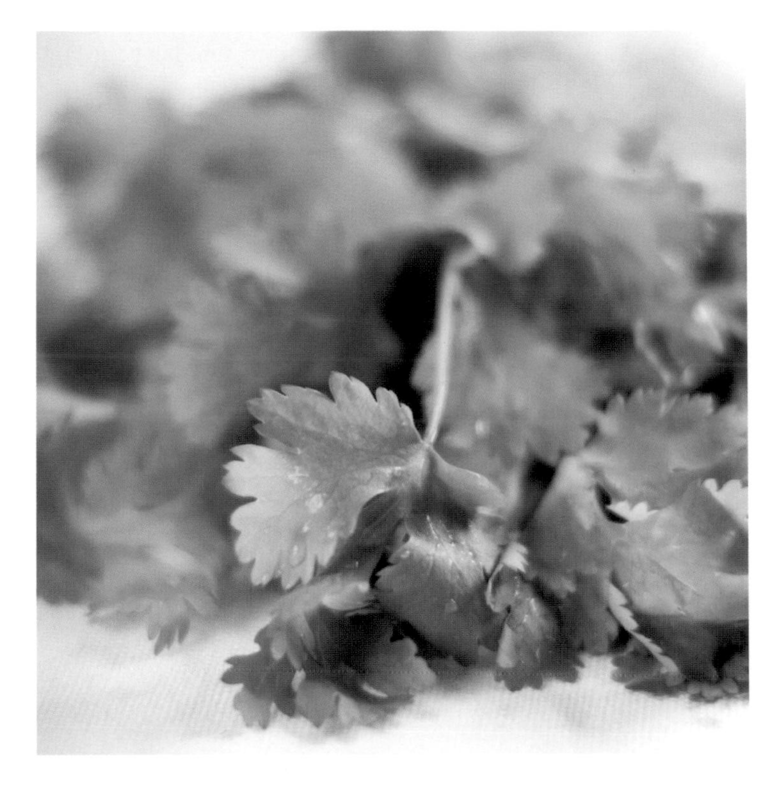

on the guest list

CONGRATULATIONS! YOU'RE PREGNANT. Isn't it wonderful? In less than nine months you'll have a tiny baby bundle of joy to hold, love and care for. Until then, you'll be blessed with a growing belly, an altered lifestyle, morning sickness, and food cravings and aversions. Your relationship with food and your body may change significantly — luckily, there are many opportunities to make changes in a fun and healthy way.

Maintaining a healthy diet during your pregnancy is important, and you should eat a wide variety of nutritious foods. Between cravings, food aversions and morning sickness, try to focus on a balanced diet of protein, fruits and vegetables, calcium-rich dairy products, whole grains and good fats (such as those found in fish, olive oil, avocado and nuts). Make sure you are getting enough iron in your diet, drink lots of water and take your prenatal vitamin. Remember to be good to your body. Visit your doctor, dietician or public health unit for detailed information about nutrition during pregnancy. But I bet you knew that already.

So maybe it's time to lose the guilt, stop stressing about every bite that goes into your mouth and start enjoying what you eat. The next few months are a unique and special time, and your pregnancy won't last forever — even though it may feel that way sometimes. You only need a few hundred extra calories a day, so skip the giant portions and delight in small servings of delicious, fabulous food that will truly, genuinely satisfy you. Take pleasure in preparing and eating fantastic and healthy meals, and in spending time with friends and family. Early on, I searched high and low for a cookbook for pregnant women. The only ones I found were aimed specifically at those who enjoy eating lots of brown rice and granola — and that's just not me. The recipes in this book will help you avoid the stress of eating the "right" foods by focusing on the sensual tastes of nourishing and sumptuous meals. They've all been screened by an obstetrician/gynecologist to ensure they are safe to eat during pregnancy. You may be giving up a lot been these nine special months, so perhaps it's time to add in some excitement and culinary adventure. I hope the positive and luxurious focus of this book will help you to feel posh, sexy and connected with your body, baby and partner. As a bonus, many people believe that exposing baby to lots of foods and flavours in utero is a surefire way to have a child who is open to eating lots of different foods. So why not have some fun with gourmet cooking? Celebrate your pregnant body, pamper your palate and start loving up your kitchen!

"The most important thing she'd learned over the years was that there was no way to be a perfect mother and a million ways to be a good one."

~Jill Churchill

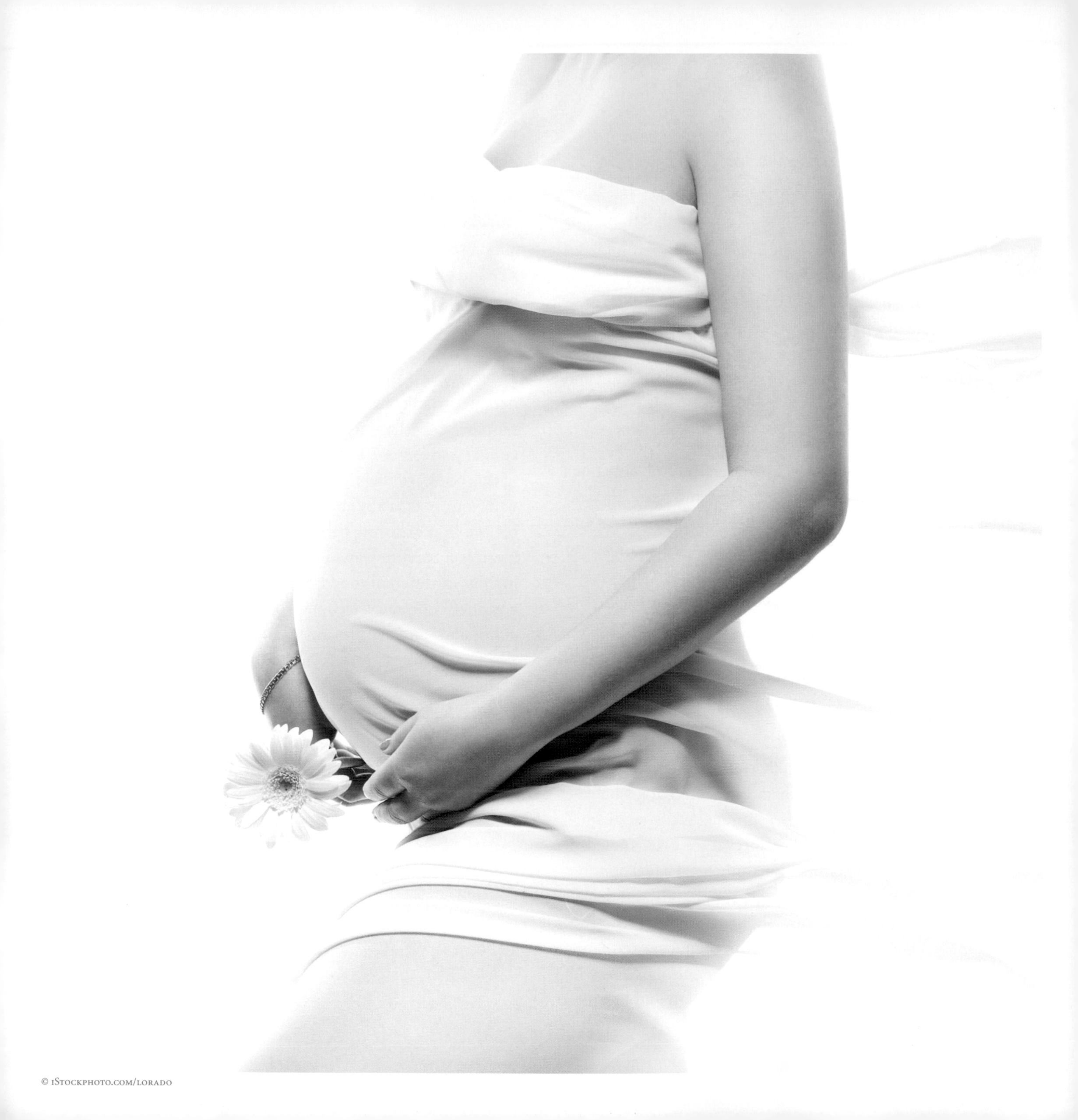

not invited to the party

THERE ARE MANY FOODS you may have enjoyed before you were expecting that are now off-limits — at least until your darling baby is born. Some of these foods (such as raw eggs or undercooked meats) can potentially be contaminated with bacteria that can make you or your baby sick; others (such as alcohol) may disrupt your baby's healthy growth. Foods to definitely avoid when you are pregnant include:

- Alcohol.
- Sushi (cooked rolls are fine; anything containing raw fish/seafood/shellfish is not).
- Raw, rare or undercooked meat.
- Raw eggs (the yolk and egg white should be cooked solid).
- Foods containing raw eggs. Avoid uncooked cookie dough, some mousses, cakes and custards, and homemade ice cream. Store-bought mayonnaise is considered safe but homemade is not. Caesar salad dressing and Hollandaise and Béarnaise sauces also contain raw eggs.
- Cold smoked seafood or other smoked fresh meats. They are safe in cooked dishes or from a tin.
- Any unpasturized juice, milk or milk product.
- Soft cheeses, including blue cheese, stilton, feta, brie and Camembert. They are safe if noted on the label to be pasteurized.
- Fish containing high levels of mercury (shark, swordfish, king mackerel, tilefish) or high levels of the pollutant PCB (bluefish, striped bass and freshwater fish such as salmon, pike, trout and walleye from contaminated lakes and rivers).
- Cold deli meats, including sandwich meats and hot dogs. Deli meats that have been reheated to steaming hot do not pose a threat.
- Liver or liver products, or pâté of any meat type.
- Unwashed fruits and vegetables (Be sure to wear gloves if you are gardening).
- Raw sprouts (alfalfa, clover or radish).
- Prepared (store-bought) salads such as coleslaw and potato salad.

As well as avoiding certain foods altogether, there are a few you should limit your consumption of, including:

- Caffeine, to 300 milligrams/day (found in coffee, tea, cola and chocolate).
- Herbal teas (some may potentially have toxic or pharmacologic effects on mother-to-be or baby-to-be).
- Artificial sweeteners (aspartame, acesulfame potassium, sucralose, isomalt, lactitol, maltitol, mannitol, sorbitol, thaumatin, xylitol). Although these do not pose a health risk to your baby, they should not be used in place of nutrient-dense, natural foods.

what are you craving?

THEORIES ABOUND as to why pregnant women crave certain foods — is it hormones? A vitamin or mineral deficiency? Your baby needing a certain food? Who knows! I asked plenty of women what they were craving during pregnancy, and the most commonly reported food cravings were for chocolate; ice or a Slurpee; ice cream; salty snacks; peanut butter; steaks, burgers or other red meat; ham, bacon or sausage; tangy or tart foods; spicy foods; coffee; vegetables; olives; fruit; seafood; sushi; candy or licorice. I added pickles, just for fun. I've included lots of recipes in this book that focus on those delicious, fantastic and sometimes slightly wacky ingredients. No harm in indulging, as long as it is part of a balanced diet. If you're looking for something that tickles your fancy, just check the recipe list below.

if you're craving chocolate, try:

M&M Granola Bars 60
Chocolate Chip Blueberry Almond Cookies 64
Chocolate Sesame Salmon with Steamed Broccoli 130
Chocolate Truffle Soufflés 158
Chocolate Mousse Cake with Chocolate Cookie Toffee Crust 160
Decadent Chocolate Anise Sauce with Vanilla Ice Cream and Fresh Raspberries 176
Cashew Brittle Frost 177
Toffee Coffee Chocolate Chip Cookies 178
Chocolate Raspberry Fudge 180
Good Morning, Sunshine! 298
Chocolate Chai White Tea 200
Rich Hazelnut Hot Cocoa 202

if you're craving ice or a Slurpee, try:

Banana, Yogurt and Juice Layered Popsicles 67
Fresh Mango Strawberry Lemonade 188
Ginger Beer No-jito 190
White Peach Bellini 192
Sparkling Raspberry Float 195
Watermelon Refresher 198

if you're craving ice cream, try:

Duet of Dried Cranberry Shortbread and Candy Cane Ice Creams 174
Decadent Chocolate Anise Sauce with Vanilla Ice Cream and Fresh Raspberries 176
Cashew Brittle Frost 177
Sparkling Raspberry Float 195

if you're craving salty snacks, try:

Asparagus with Truffle Oil and Toasted Pine Nuts 42
Green Olives with Roasted Chickpeas and Mixed Nuts 44
Cumin Pita Chips with Peanut Sweet Chili Dip 46
Sweet Potato Fries with Truffle Aioli 48
Mango Cilantro Salsa 54
Gourmet Seven Layer Dip 84

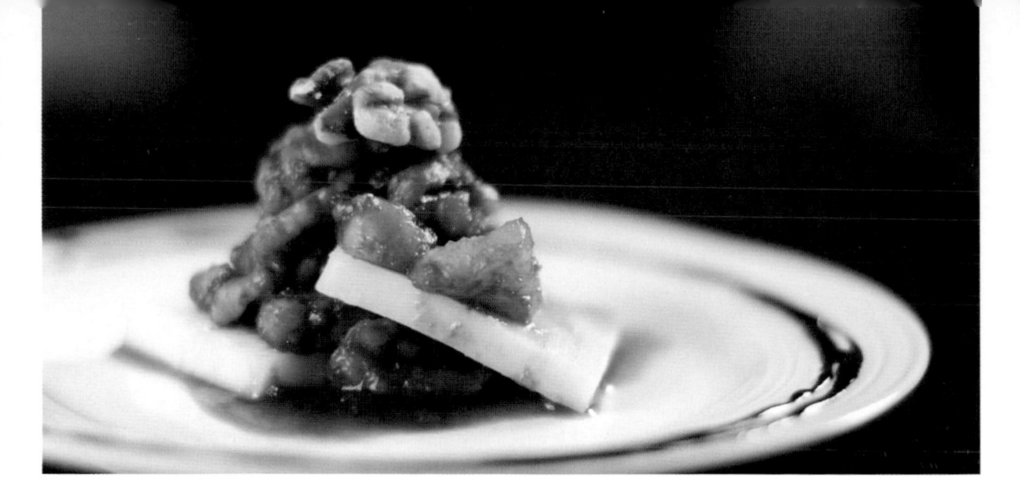

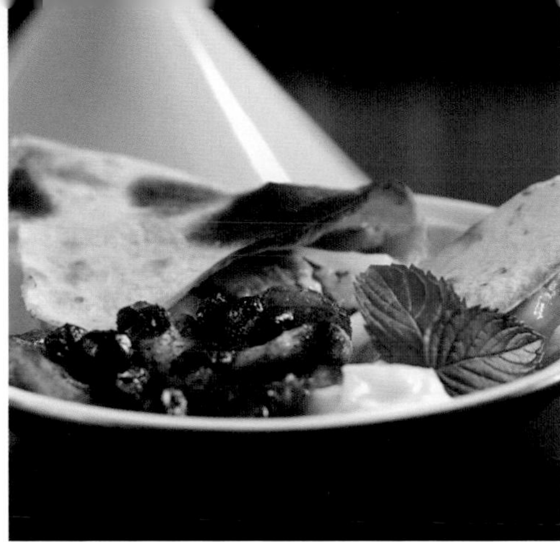

if you're craving peanut butter, try:

Ultimate Peanut Butter Sandwich 30
Cumin Pita Chips with Peanut Sweet Chili Dip 46

if you're craving steaks, burgers or other red meat, try:

Roasted Garlic, Sirloin Meatball and Toasted Pita Skewers 82
Ginger Wasabi Sliders 118
Rosemary Garlic Roast Beef 146
Apple and Anjou Pear Beef with Smashed Yams 149
Grilled New York Striploin Steak Salad 150

if you're craving ham, bacon or sausage, try:

Ham and Grilled Pineapple Bagel with Honey Mustard Cream Cheese 16
Italian Omelet with Artisan Bread 20
Bacon, Apple, Lettuce, Tomato, Cheddar and Avocado Sandwich 36
Chorizo Chive Buttermilk Biscuits 28
Bacon-Wrapped Dried Plums Stuffed with Maple Toasted Pecans 74
Bacon, Leek and Toasted Almond Risotto 144

if you're craving tangy or tart foods, try:

Grilled Peaches with Pink Grapefruit and Mint 52
Granny Smith Honey Cornbread 56
Tangerine Dream Muffins 58
Apple Slices, Belgian Endive, Flatbreads and Portobello Mushroom Pâté 90
Meyer Lemon and Blueberry Salad in Parmesan Baskets 92
Fresh Tomato, Basil and Bocconcini Skewers with Lemon Olive Oil 94
Berry Kiwi Citrus Cream Meringues 170
Fresh Mango Strawberry Lemonade 188
Lemon Drop Cosmopolitan 192
Good Morning, Sunshine! 198

if you're craving spicy foods, try:

Tempura Dill Pickles with Sambal Oelek Dip 40
Cumin Pita Chips with Peanut Sweet Chili Dip 46
Roasted Butternut Squash Wedges with Honey Green Curry Drizzle 72
Mild Curry Chicken Pizza on Naan 120
Ancho Chili Chicken and Zucchini with Garlic Roasted Potatoes 154

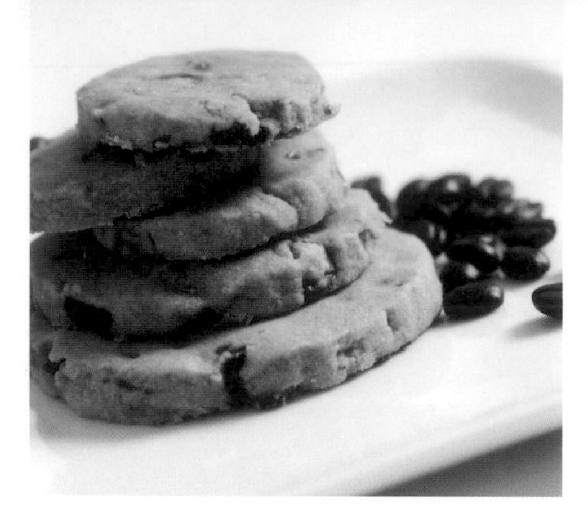

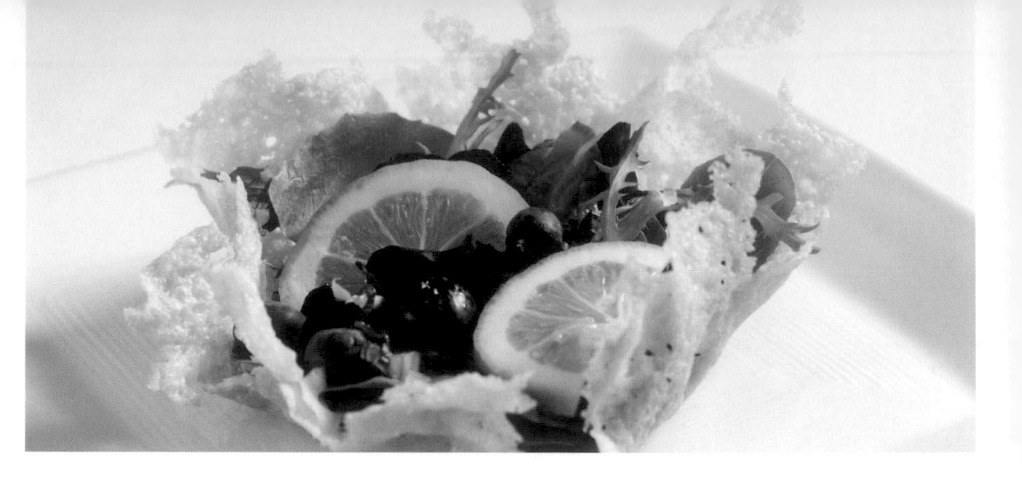

if you're craving coffee, try:

Toffee Coffee Chocolate Chip Cookies ... 178
Vanilla Cinnamon Latte ... 201

if you're craving vegetables, try:

Salmon, Zucchini and Sweet Corn Latkes with Dill Sour Cream ... 18
Italian Omelet with Artisan Bread ... 20
Black Bean Scramble with Fresh Tomato Salsa ... 22
Garden Vegetable Frittata ... 24
Roasted Sweet Potato and Pepper Eggs ... 25
Tempura Dill Pickles with Sambal Oelek Dip ... 40
Asparagus with Truffle Oil and Toasted Pine Nuts ... 42
Green Olives with Roasted Chickpeas and Mixed Nuts ... 44
Sweet Potato Fries with Truffle Aioli ... 48
Corn on the Cob with Spiced Maple Butter ... 50
Sushi Vegetables with Asian and Wasabi Yogurt Dipping Sauces ... 70
Roasted Butternut Squash Wedges with Honey Green Curry Drizzle ... 72
Bacon-wrapped Dried Plums Stuffed with Maple Toasted Pecans ... 74
Baked Grape Leaves with Sumac Chicken, Apricots and Rice ... 76
Sun-dried Olive and Tomato Tuna Zucchini Rounds ... 78
Caramelized Onion and Balsamic Cherry Jam ... 80
Gourmet Seven Layer Dip ... 84
Rustic Sesame Vegetable Tart ... 86
Apple Slices, Belgian Endive, Flatbreads and Portobello Mushroom Pâté ... 90
Meyer Lemon and Blueberry Salad in Parmesan Baskets ... 92
Fresh Tomato, Basil and Bocconcini Skewers with Lemon Olive Oil ... 94
Butternut Squash and Carrot Ginger Soup with Crème Fraîche ... 102
Salmon, White Asparagus and Dill Pea Salad ... 104
Lemongrass Tiger Prawn and Chickpea Salad ... 106
Sesame Cashew Red Cabbage Noodle Salad ... 108
Spiced Caramelized Cauliflower and Candied Curry Pecan Salad ... 110
Roasted Balsamic Vegetable Panini with Roasted Garlic Aioli ... 112
Panko-crusted Stuffed Grilled Portobello ... 124
Eggplant and Spinach Lasagna with Béchamel Sauce ... 140
Tempura Beets, Mushrooms and Onions ... 148
Iced Mint Tea with Cucumber ... 196

if you're craving olives, try:

Italian Omelet with Artisan Bread 20

Green Olives with Roasted Chickpeas and Mixed Nuts 44

Sun-dried Olive and Tomato Tuna Zucchini Rounds 78

if you're craving fruit, try:

Orchard Fruit Muffins 36

Exotic Fruit Salad with Sweet Citrus Guacamole 37

Grilled Peaches with Pink Grapefruit and Mint 52

Mango Cilantro Salsa 54

Granny Smith Honey Cornbread 56

Tangerine Dream Muffins 58

White Cheddar with Pear Compote and Walnuts 96

Grilled Pear and Thai Basil Sandwich 114

Moroccan Spiced Chicken Quesadilla with Dried Fruits 152

Cherry and Fresh Mint Tart with Rustic Vanilla Shortbread Crust 166

White Peach Crumble Pie with Caramel Drizzle 168

Berry Kiwi Citrus Cream Meringues 170

Layered Banana Butterscotch Pudding 172

Fresh Mango Strawberry Lemonade 188

Blueberry Lychee Kiss 190

White Peach Bellini 192

Sparkling Raspberry Float 195

Watermelon Refresher 198

Blueberry Coconut Smoothie 200

if you're craving seafood, try:

Salmon, Zucchini and Sweet Corn Latkes with Dill Sour Cream 18

Salmon, White Asparagus and Dill Pea Salad 104

Lemongrass Tiger Prawn and Chickpea Salad 106

Succulent Crab Cakes with Tarragon Sour Cream 122

Sautéed Sablefish with Eggplant Caviar 128

Chocolate Sesame Salmon with Steamed Broccoli 130

Tilapia Fillets with Coconut Curry Cream Sauce 132

Seared Scallops with Cilantro Honey Pesto and Baby Arugula Salad 134

Garlic Shrimp and Feta Linguine 136

if you're craving sushi, try:

Sushi Vegetables with Asian and Wasabi Yogurt Dipping Sauces 70

if you're craving candy or licorice, try:

M&M Granola Bars 60

Maple Walnut Caramel Corn 66

Dulce de Leche Sex in a Pan 162

Duet of Dried Cranberry Shortbread and Candy Cane Ice Creams 174

Decadent Chocolate Anise Sauce with Vanilla Ice Cream and Fresh Raspberries 176

Cashew Brittle Frost 177

if you're craving pickles, try:

Tempura Dill Pickles with Sambal Oelek Dip 40

Pickled Mary 194

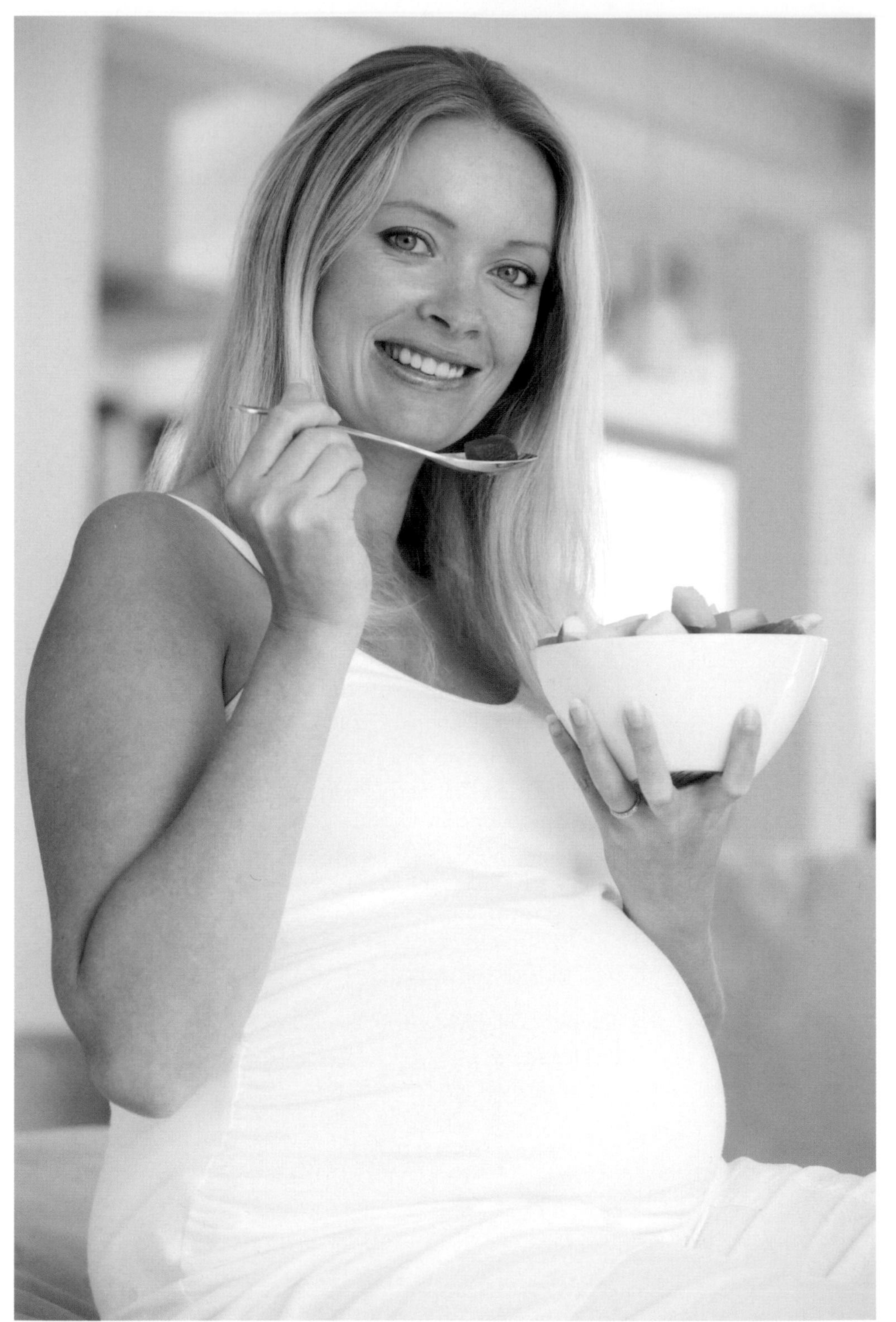

if morning sickness
has passed you by:

breakfasts & brunch

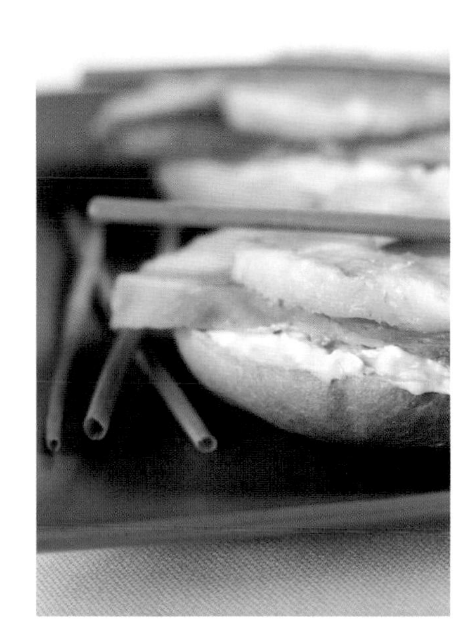

"Life is always a rich and steady time when you are waiting for something to happen or to hatch."

~ E.B. White, Charlotte's Web

herbed cream cheese eggs benedict

SERVES 2 | TOTAL TIME 15 MINUTES | ACTIVE TIME 15 MINUTES

No hollandaise sauce for us pregnant ladies! I lovingly refer to these eggs as "Eggs Benny Baby." This version is safe to eat when expecting and equally as delicious — the fresh herbed cream cheese adds a ton of flavour. Enjoy your leisurely weekend mornings with this scrumptious dish, great music and your favourite book or newspaper — you won't have as much time to relax once your new baby arrives!

INGREDIENTS

4 tablespoons cream cheese, softened

1 teaspoon chopped fresh dill (or combination of dill, basil and rosemary)

1 teaspoon butter

4 eggs

2 English muffins, halved

Salt and freshly ground black pepper

Sliced watermelon, honeydew and/or cantaloupe melons, for garnish (optional)

METHOD

In a small bowl, combine cream cheese and herbs. Set aside.

Add a dab of butter to each cup of a 4-egg poacher. Poach eggs over boiling water until cooked through, about 5 minutes (until the yolks are firm).

Meanwhile, toast English muffins halves. Spread each half with a generous amount of the herbed cream cheese. Top each with a poached egg. Season with salt and ground pepper.

TO SERVE

Serve 2 Eggs Benny per plate. Fan slices of melon (if using) beside eggs on plate.

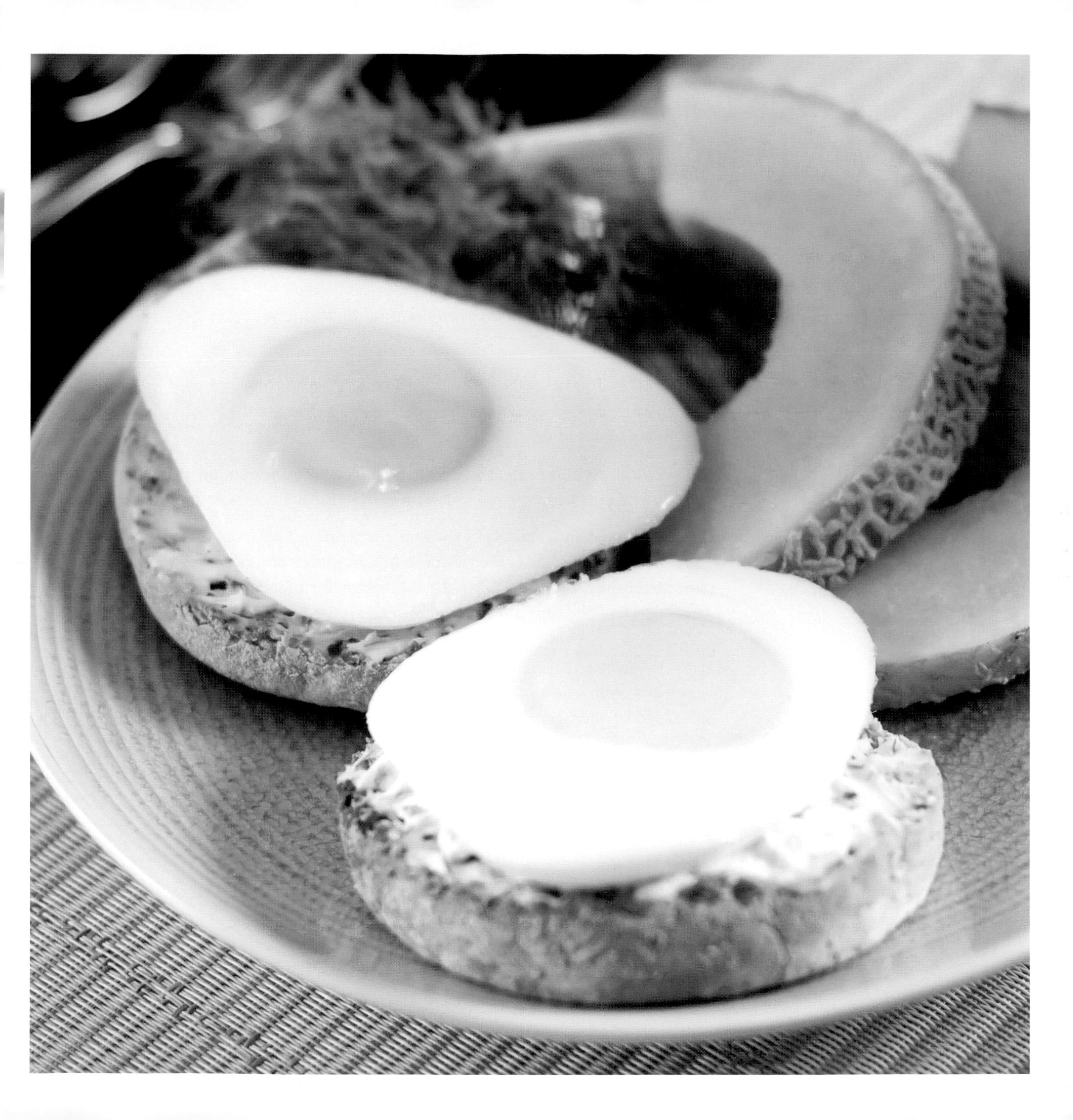

ham and grilled pineapple bagel with honey mustard cream cheese

SERVES 2 TO 4 | TOTAL TIME 40 MINUTES | ACTIVE TIME 15 MINUTES

The grilled pineapple takes this bagel sandwich to an amazing new level. It's fairly simple to make but will certainly impress your guests (or your sweetie). Make sure the ham has been cooked to steaming for all of us pregnant gals. This is a delicious and modern way to use up leftover ham from any family celebration.

INGREDIENTS

3 tablespoons cream cheese, softened

2 teaspoons honey

½ teaspoon Dijon mustard

4 thick slices cooked ham

4 pineapple rings

2 bagels

Fresh chives, for garnish

METHOD

In a small bowl, combine cream cheese, 1 teaspoon of the honey and the Dijon mustard. Set aside.

Preheat oven to 325°F. Place cooked ham in an ovenproof dish; pour in ½ cup water. Cover ham with foil and warm in oven for 30 minutes or until steaming hot.

Brush pineapple rings lightly with the remaining 1 teaspoon of honey. Cook on an indoor grill or barbecue for 2 to 4 minutes per side over medium heat. Meanwhile, slice bagels in half and toast lightly. Spread cream cheese on each bagel half and top with a slice of ham and grilled pineapple.

TO SERVE

Those with smaller appetites will likely eat only a half bagel, but others may enjoy a whole one. Serve on a breakfast plate and garnish each with a long chive.

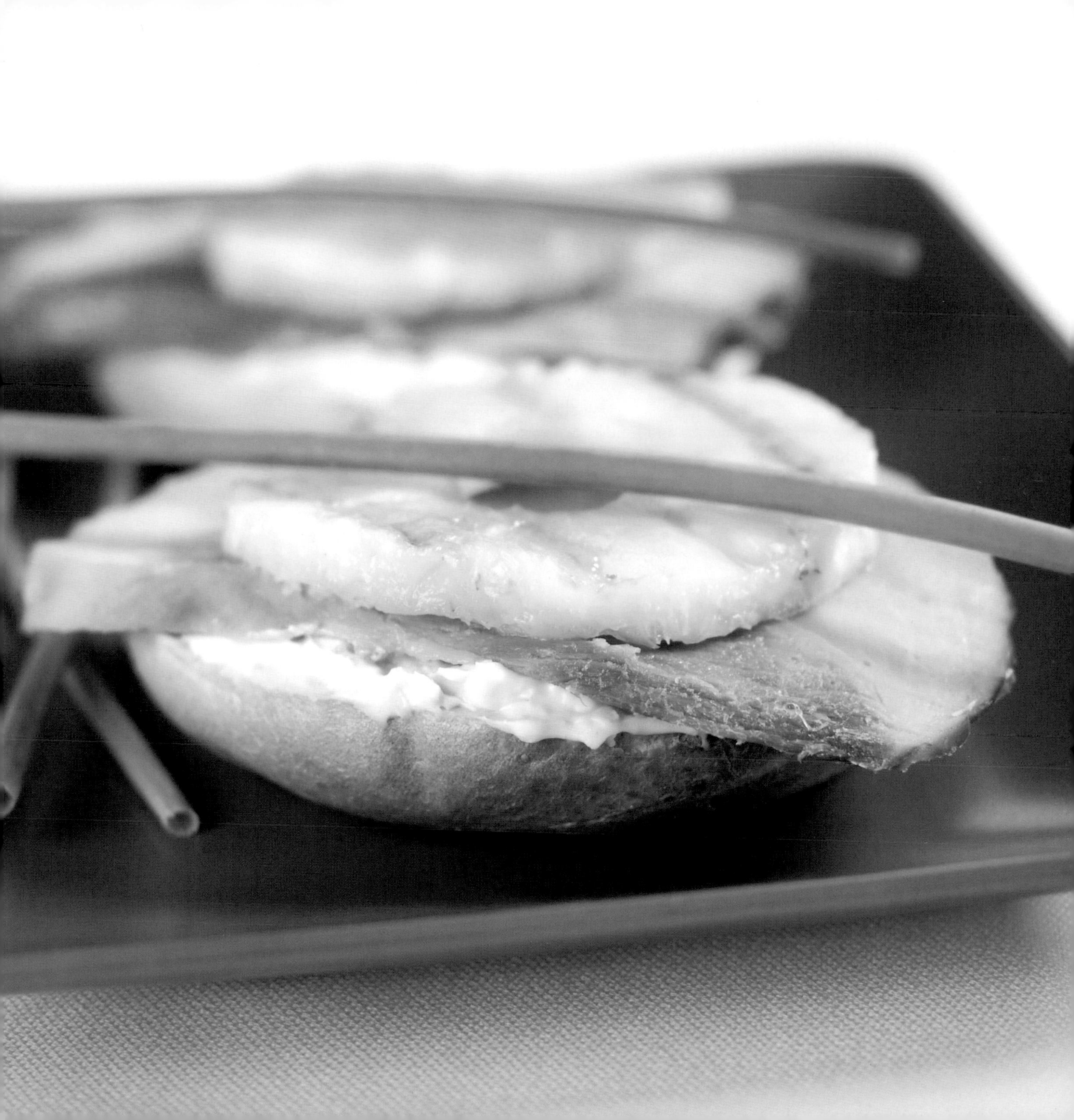

salmon, zucchini and sweet corn latkes with dill sour cream

SERVES 4 | TOTAL TIME 40 MINUTES | ACTIVE TIME 40 MINUTES

Mmm … You can't go wrong with comfort food that has a gourmet twist. These delicious latkes will make you feel like your sweet and kind grandmother is giving you a warm hug. The succulent flavour comes from fresh salmon and dill, and the latkes are sautéed until crisp.

DILL SOUR CREAM

1 cup sour cream

½ shallot, minced

2 teaspoons finely chopped fresh baby dill

½ teaspoon fresh lime juice

Freshly ground black pepper

LATKES

5 ounces fresh wild salmon

1 large zucchini, grated

½ cup sweet corn niblets

1 egg, lightly beaten

⅓ cup all-purpose flour

2 tablespoons olive oil

METHOD

To make the dill sour cream, in a small bowl, combine sour cream, shallot, dill and lime juice. Season with ground pepper. Keep in the refrigerator until ready to use.

To make the latkes, remove skin from salmon and discard. Finely chop the salmon and transfer to a bowl. Add the zucchini, corn niblets, egg and flour, stirring well to combine.

Heat olive oil in a large frying pan over medium heat. Using a wooden spoon, scoop 4 large spoonfuls (about half of the mixture) into the pan and gently flatten with a spatula or back of the spoon. Cook for 5 to 6 minutes per side or until browned and crisp, flipping carefully. Repeat with remaining mixture.

TO SERVE

Serve 2 latkes per plate, with a dollop of dill sour cream.

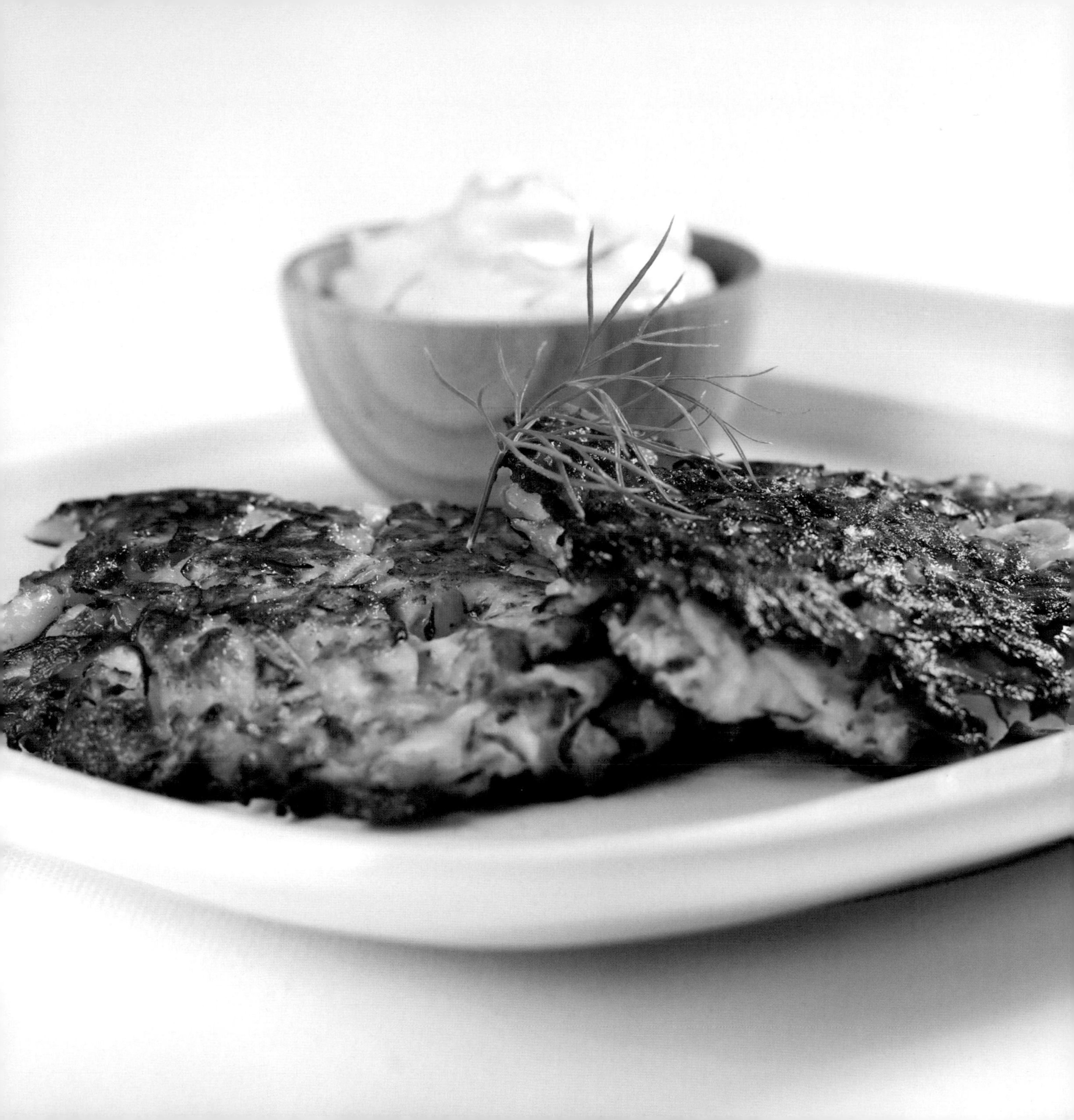

italian omelet with artisan bread

SERVES 2 | TOTAL TIME 15 MINUTES | ACTIVE TIME 15 MINUTES

This hearty and flavourful omelet will make you feel like you are brunching in the patio of a small Tuscan café, under the warm sun. The olives and Italian sausage are a wonderful combination, and buttery toasted artisan breads complete the meal. This also makes a nice light dinner.

INGREDIENTS

1 tablespoon olive oil

1 Italian sausage

1 clove garlic, crushed

¼ onion, chopped

¼ yellow pepper, diced

3 eggs

Dash of salt and freshly ground black pepper

1 tablespoon water

2 ounces Asiago cheese

1 handful chopped oil-packed black olives

4 slices artisan bread

METHOD

Heat olive oil in a large frying pan over medium heat. Cook sausage for 3 to 4 minutes. Remove from pan and slice into 10 to 12 pieces. Cook for another 2 to 3 minutes, turning once. Add garlic, onion and yellow pepper; cook for 3 to 4 minutes.

Meanwhile, crack the eggs into a mixing bowl; season with salt and pepper. Whisk in the water. Pour the egg mixture over the sausage and vegetables.

Shred Asiago cheese over half of the omelet. Top with olives. When egg is becoming firm, fold omelet in half. Continue to cook until egg is cooked through. Meanwhile, toast the bread slices.

TO SERVE

Cut omelet in half and carefully transfer to individual plates. Serve with buttered toasted bread.

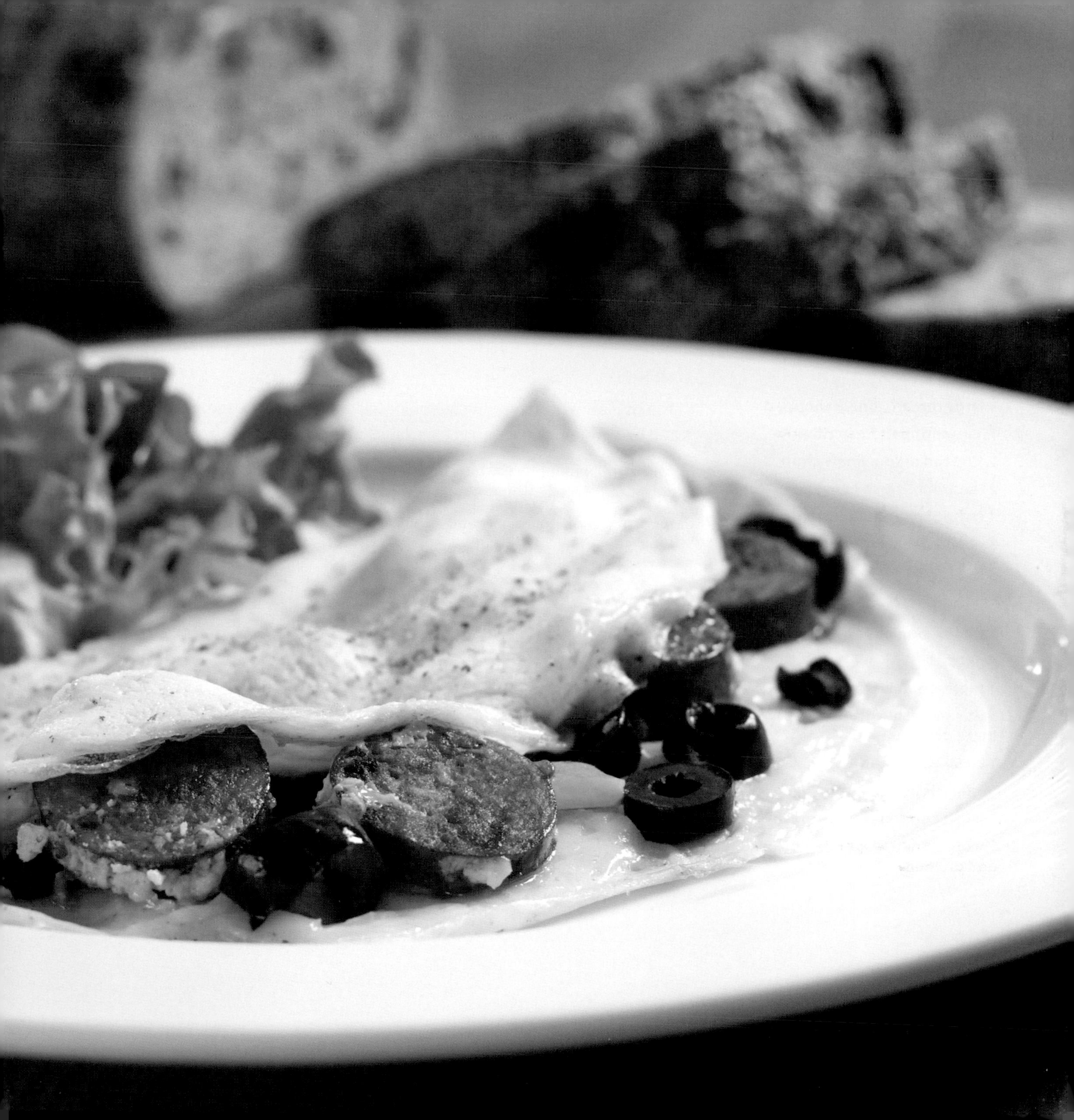

black bean scramble with fresh tomato salsa

SERVES 2 | TOTAL TIME 15 MINUTES | ACTIVE TIME 15 MINUTES

Healthy, fresh and delicious, this yummy scramble will energize you on busy days and keep you well fuelled. The simple tomato salsa is outstanding and can be added to other dishes or served with pita or chips. Add a bit of jalapeño pepper if you're in the mood for some spice.

SALSA

1 large tomato, finely chopped

½ cup chopped fresh cilantro

¼ cup red onion, finely chopped

2 teaspoons fresh lime juice

1 teaspoon granulated sugar

Salt and freshly ground black pepper

SCRAMBLE

1 tablespoon olive oil

4 eggs

1 tablespoon water

Salt and freshly ground black pepper

1 clove garlic, minced

½ cup chopped baby spinach

¼ cup chopped cremini mushrooms

½ cup canned black beans, rinsed and drained

METHOD

In a small bowl, combine tomato, onion, cilantro, lime juice and sugar. Season with salt and ground pepper. Heat olive oil in a large frying pan over medium heat.

Meanwhile, in a bowl, whisk together eggs, water, and salt and ground pepper. In the pan, sauté garlic, spinach and mushrooms for 3 to 4 minutes. Add egg mixture; cook for 1 minute. Add black beans and cook for another 1 to 2 minutes, stirring often to break up mixture.

TO SERVE

Serve black bean scramble on breakfast plates, with the salsa on the side.

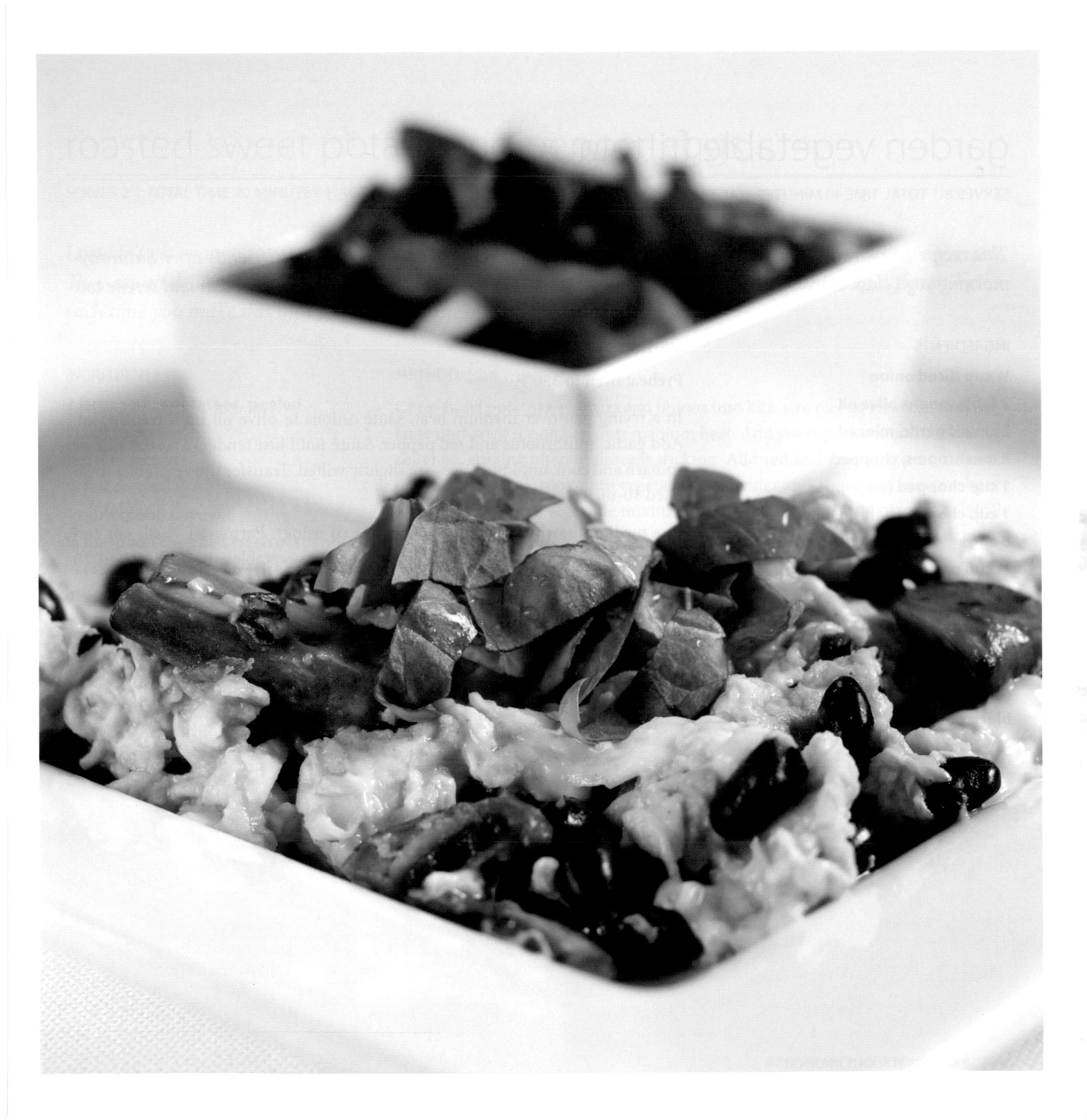

bacon, apple, lettuce, tomato, cheddar and avocado sandwich

SERVES 2 | TOTAL TIME 15 MINUTES | ACTIVE TIME 15 MINUTES

How to improve on the classic BLT? Just ask a pregnant woman! Add avocado and sautéed apples for a sandwich that is very close to perfection. This will be sure to satisfy a number of your cravings.

INGREDIENTS

6 slices bacon, cut in half

1 Red Delicious apple, peeled, cored and thinly sliced

4 slices calabrese bread

1 tablespoon mayonnaise

2 lettuce leaves

½ tomato, sliced

6 thick slices extra-old white cheddar

½ ripe avocado, pitted, peeled and sliced

METHOD

In a large frying pan over medium heat, fry bacon to desired doneness. Remove from pan and blot on paper towel to remove excess grease. Reduce heat to low, drain off excess drippings and add apple slices to pan. Cook for 2 minutes, flip apples and cook for another 2 minutes. Transfer to a paper towel. Toast bread; spread each slice with mayonnaise. For each sandwich, layer half of the lettuce, tomato, cheese, bacon, avocado and apple slices. Top with another slice of bread.

TO SERVE

Use 2 cocktail toothpicks per sandwich to hold the sandwich together. Slice in half and serve.

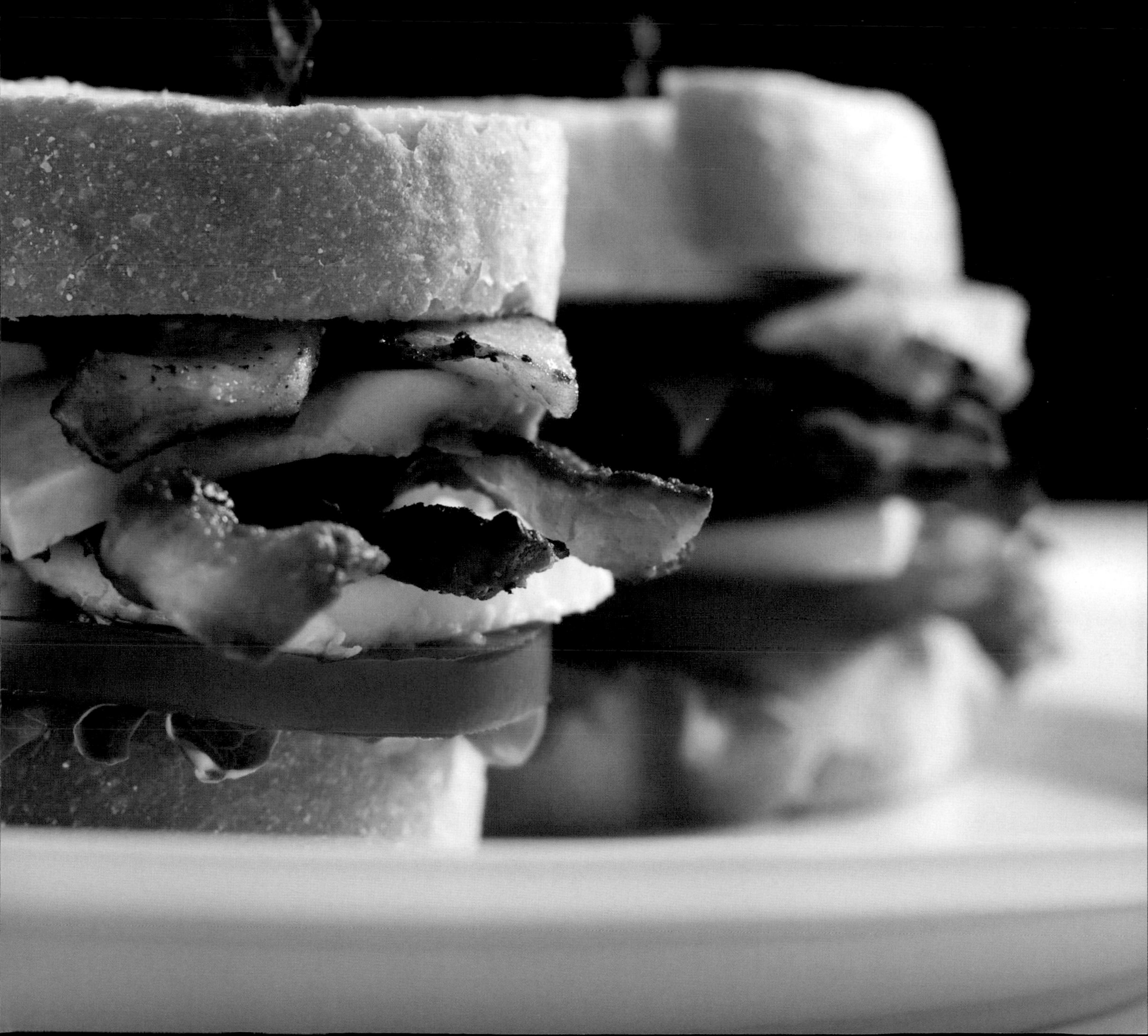

chorizo chive buttermilk biscuits

MAKES 12 TO 15 | TOTAL TIME 45 MINUTES | ACTIVE TIME 30 MINUTES

This comforting country classic has moved to swanky new digs in the big city! The chorizo and aged cheddar up the ante for this rich and flaky biscuit. These are a great breakfast or side dish for soup or salad.

INGREDIENTS

½ teaspoon vegetable oil

1 chorizo sausage

2 cups all-purpose flour

3 teaspoons baking powder

½ teaspoon baking soda

½ teaspoon salt

6 tablespoons butter

1 cup buttermilk

¼ cup shredded aged cheddar cheese

2 tablespoons chopped chives

METHOD

Preheat oven to 450°F.

Heat vegetable oil in a frying pan over medium heat. Cook sausage, turning often, until casing is browned. Slice sausage and cook for another 1 to 3 minutes, until cooked through. Remove from heat and let cool before cutting into small pieces.

In a mixing bowl, combine flour, baking powder, baking soda and salt. Using a pastry cutter, cut in butter, until just worked into the flour mixture. Add buttermilk, stirring with a fork until just combined. Add cheese, chives and the chopped sausage, mixing just until combined. Transfer dough to a floured surface and pat out to ½-inch thickness; cut into rounds (12 to 15 in total) with a biscuit cutter. Place on a parchment-lined baking sheet and bake for 12 to 15 minutes, until light golden brown.

TO SERVE

Serve biscuits warm, with butter for spreading.

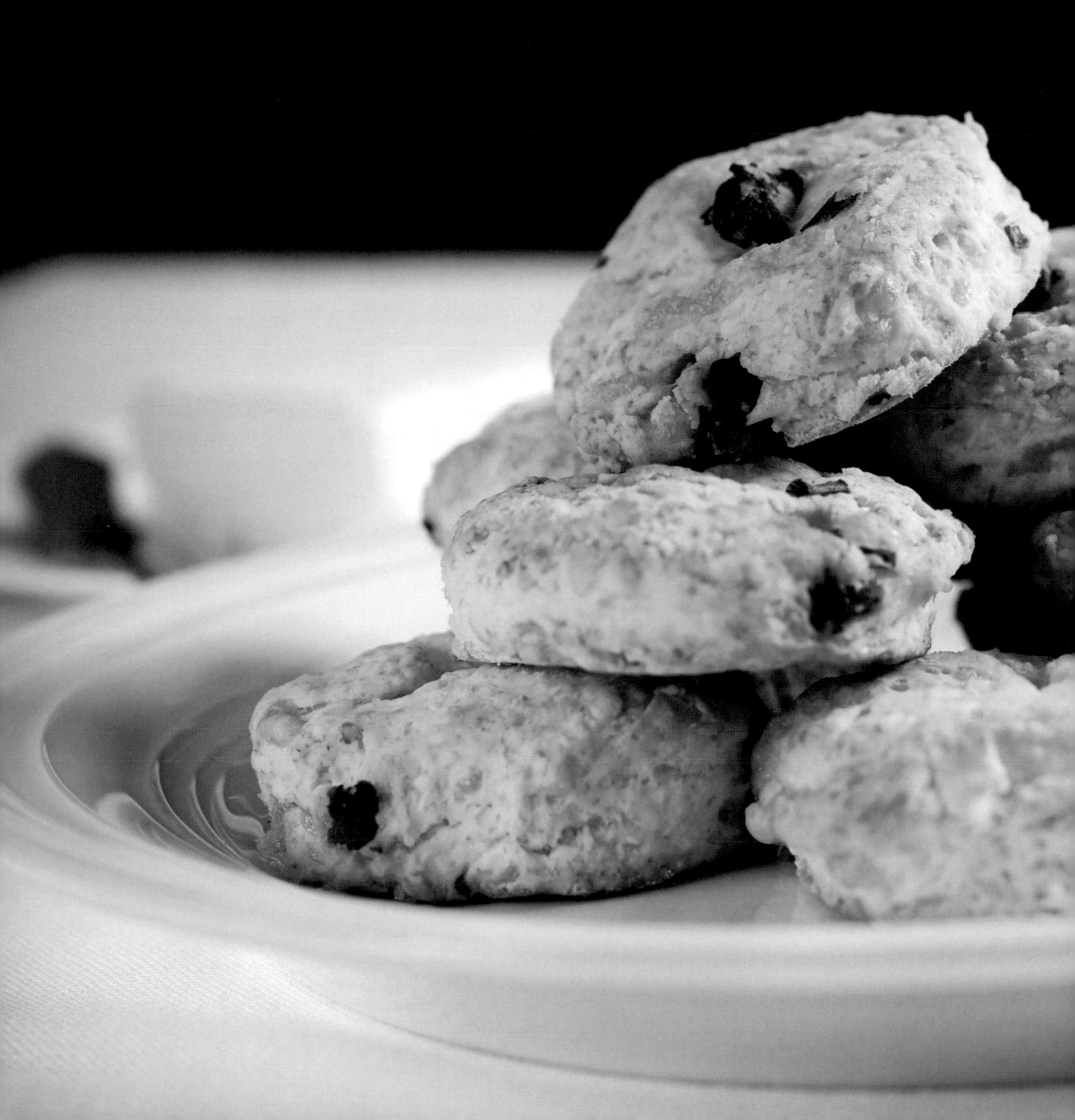

ultimate peanut butter sandwich

SERVES 2 | TOTAL TIME 25 MINUTES | ACTIVE TIME 15 MINUTES

Lots of women crave peanut butter when they are pregnant — it is so nutty and flavourful. This version is the absolute pinnacle of perfection for a peanut butter sandwich. Start with the basics and add toasted hazelnuts and cinnamon honey for a taste you'll surely love. Try it on toasted challah bread for extra enjoyment.

INGREDIENTS

¼ cup hazelnuts

2 tablespoons pasteurized honey

¼ teaspoon cinnamon

4 thick slices bread

2 tablespoons natural peanut butter

METHOD

Preheat oven to 350°F. Toast hazelnuts on a baking sheet for 15 minutes. Remove from oven and, once cool to the touch, rub off the skins using a towel or your fingers. Using a mortar and pestle, crush the nuts into small pieces.

In a small bowl, combine honey and cinnamon. Lightly toast bread. Spread peanut butter on 2 slices and top with crushed hazelnuts. Spread honey onto the remaining 2 slices and place face down on the first two slices, to make sandwiches.

TO SERVE

Cut sandwiches in half and serve individually.

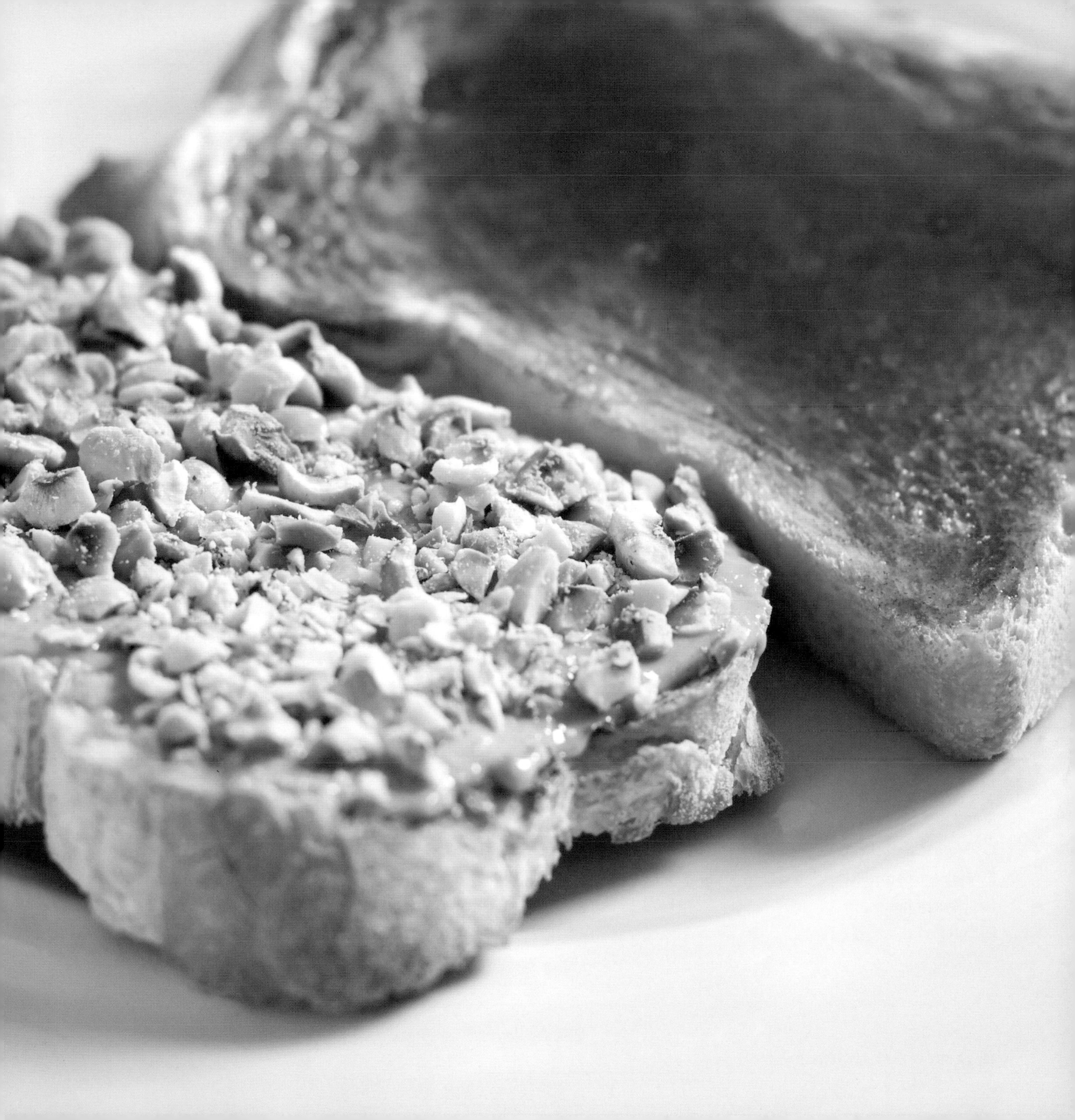

sweet and savoury crêpes

SERVES 4 | TOTAL TIME 20 MINUTES | ACTIVE TIME 20 MINUTES

Can't decide if you fancy something sweet or savoury? Have both! These easy-to-make delicacies are so versatile they can be filled with anything you are craving. Have fun deciding what to use!

SAVOURY CRÊPES

1 cup all-purpose flour

2 eggs

1 cup milk

¼ teaspoon salt

2 tablespoons butter, melted

FOR SWEET OR DESSERT CRÊPES, ADD TO SAVOURY CRÊPE RECIPE:

1 egg

3 tablespoons granulated sugar

½ teaspoon pure vanilla extract

SUGGESTED SAVOURY FILLINGS

Bacon and cheddar cheese

Grilled vegetables and Swiss cheese

Baked beans and cheddar cheese

Chorizo sausage and grilled onions

SUGGESTED SWEET FILLINGS

Chocolate and sliced bananas

Strawberries and whipped cream

Raspberry jam

Nutella

METHOD

In a large bowl, whisk together all ingredients until smooth and well combined. Prepare your choice of fillings and set aside. In a crêpe pan or non-stick frying pan, melt about 1 additional teaspoon of the butter; brush in pan to evenly coat. Pour about ¼ cup crêpe batter in the pan, tilting the pan to evenly distribute the batter. Cook for 2 to 3 minutes, until golden brown; flip crêpe with a spatula and cook on other side until golden brown, about 1 to 2 minutes. Transfer to a plate and keep warm in a 250°F oven until ready to assemble. Repeat with remaining batter, adding more butter to the pan as necessary to prevent sticking.

TO SERVE

Spoon a small amount of filling in a line down one side of the crêpe. Fold edge of crêpe over, then continue rolling up.

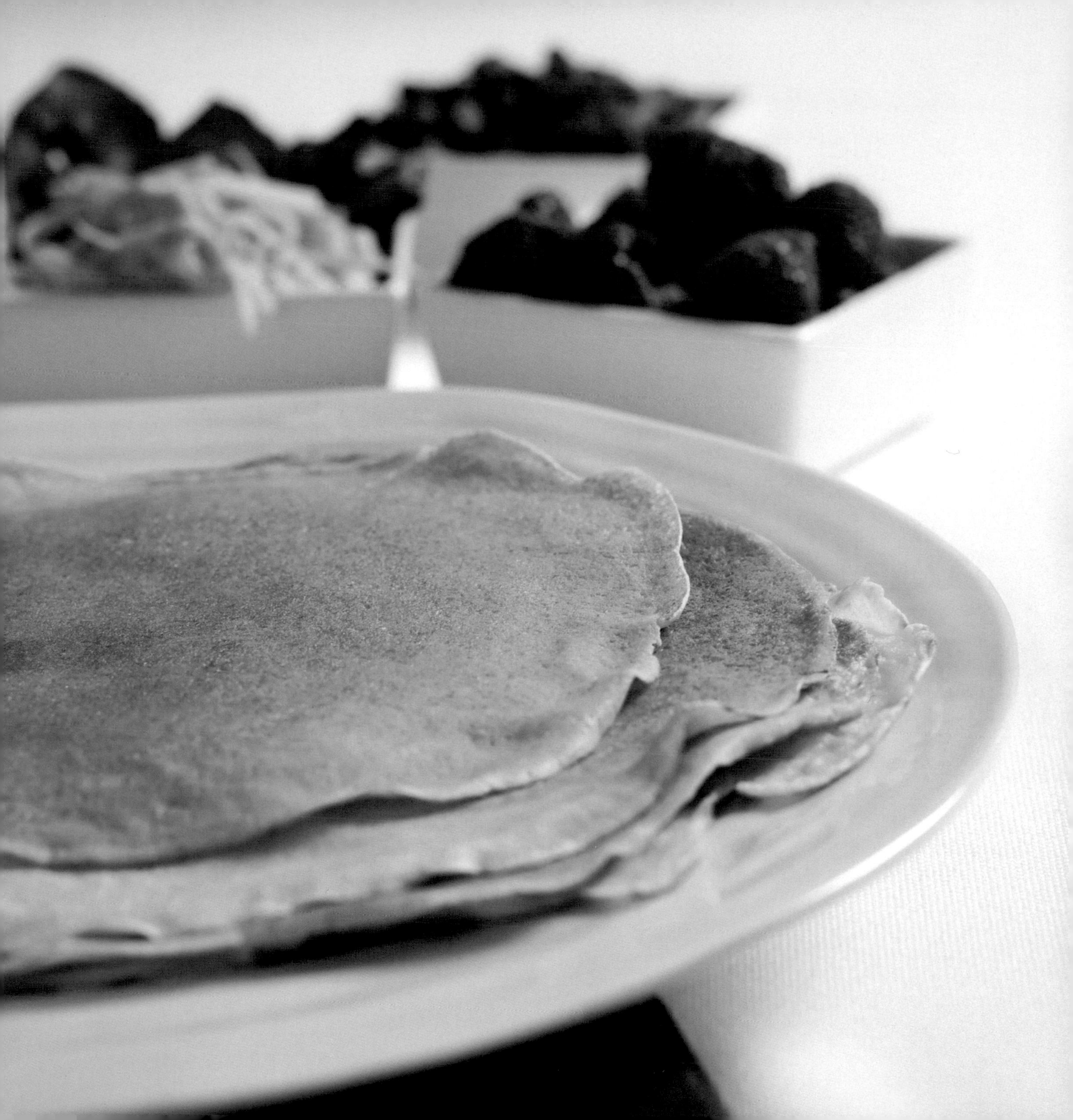

sourdough french toast with blueberry crème

SERVES 2 | TOTAL TIME 20 MINUTES | ACTIVE TIME 20 MINUTES

This is one of my husband's specialties, and he offers this suggestion: Make sure your refrigerator is well stocked with the necessary ingredients, leave the book open to this page, and stay warm and cozy in bed while your sweetie prepares this heavenly breakfast for you.

BLUEBERRY CRÈME

1 cup whipping cream
½ cup blueberries
3 tablespoons icing sugar
½ teaspoon pure vanilla extract

FRENCH TOAST

3 eggs
3 tablespoons milk
½ teaspoon pure vanilla extract
1 teaspoon vegetable oil or butter
4 slices sourdough bread
1 teaspoon cinnamon
½ cup blueberries for garnish

METHOD

To make the blueberry crème, in a deep bowl, beat whipping cream with a hand mixer until stiff peaks form, about 5 minutes. If you're using frozen blueberries, thaw them and discard any liquid. Beat in blueberries. Beat in icing sugar and vanilla; refrigerate until ready to use.

To make the French toast, in a flat-bottomed bowl, whisk together eggs, milk and vanilla. Melt vegetable oil or butter in a large non-stick frying pan over medium heat. Dip each slice of bread in egg mixture, coating both sides; transfer to the pan. Sprinkle with cinnamon and cook 1 to 2 minutes on each side, until golden brown.

TO SERVE

Arrange slices of French toast on individual plates. Top each with blueberries and a dollop of the blueberry crème. Eat with as much maple syrup as you like.

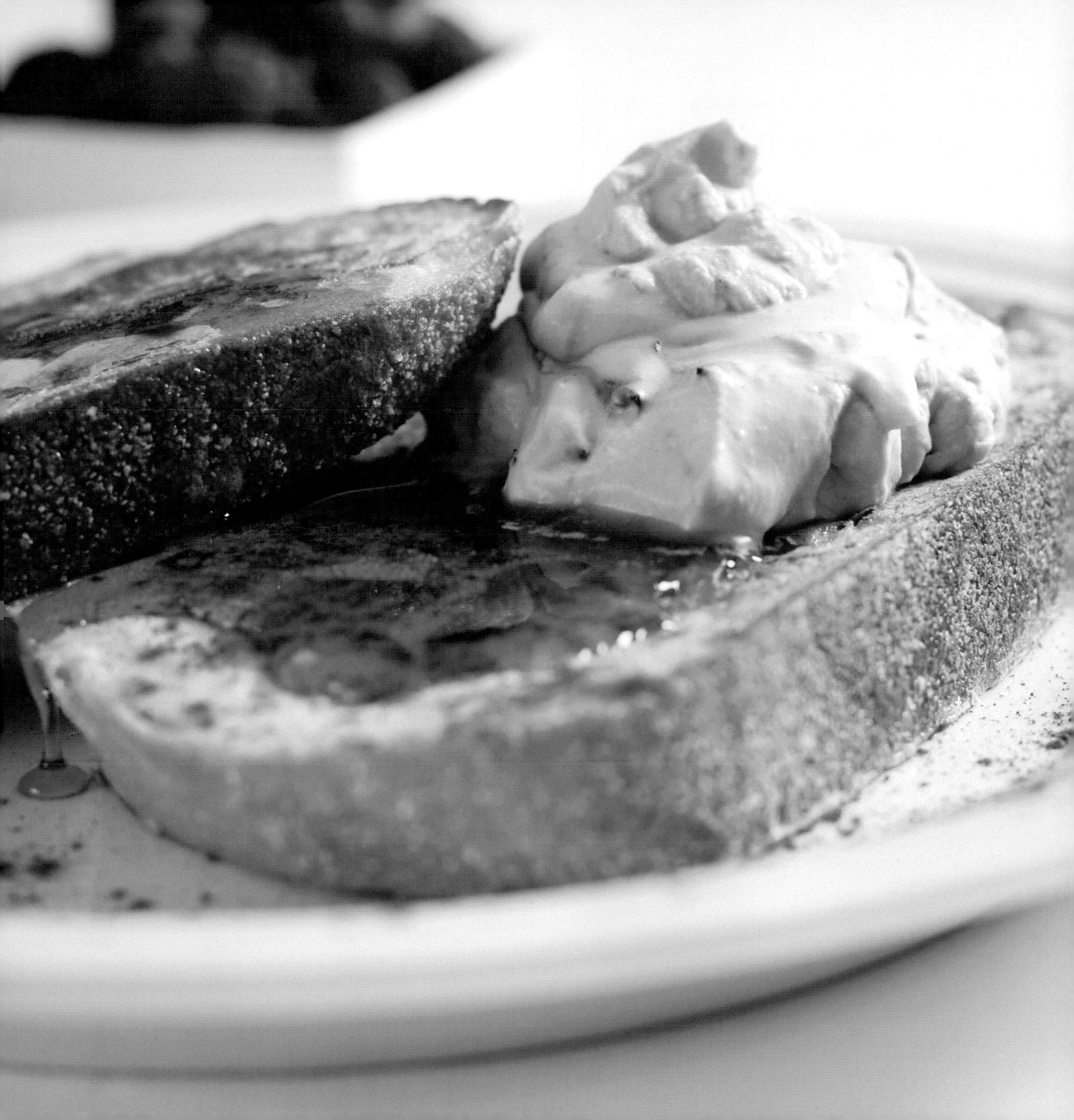

orchard fruit muffins

MAKES 12 MUFFINS | TOTAL TIME 35 MINUTES | ACTIVE TIME 15 MINUTES

You'll love the aroma that fills your kitchen after baking these deliciously spiced muffins. Your fragranced candles can get moved to the bedroom to heat up things there! My good friend Michelle Nelson shared this original recipe — she's a wonderful chef.

INGREDIENTS

2 large eggs

¼ cup peach-flavoured yogurt

½ cup milk

½ cup butter, melted and cooled

¾ cup granulated sugar

1 teaspoon pure vanilla extract

1 Granny Smith apple, peeled, cored and grated

¼ cup dried sour cherries, quartered

¼ cup dried apricots, chopped

¼ cup walnuts, chopped

1½ cups all-purpose flour

¼ cup wheat bran

¼ cup oatmeal

2 teaspoons flax seeds

2 teaspoons baking powder

¼ teaspoon salt

Dash of freshly ground black pepper

1½ teaspoon cinnamon

1 teaspoon ginger

½ teaspoon nutmeg

METHOD

Preheat oven to 375°F. In a large bowl, whisk together eggs, yogurt, milk, butter, sugar and vanilla. Stir in apple until well distributed. Add cherries, apricots and walnuts.

In a medium bowl, combine flour, wheat bran, oatmeal, flax seeds, baking powder, salt, pepper, cinnamon, ginger and nutmeg. Add dry ingredients to wet ingredients, folding from the bottom until dry ingredients are just moistened — the batter will be lumpy. Grease a 12-cup muffin tin; distribute batter evenly. Bake for 20 minutes or until tops are golden and feel springy when touched.

TO SERVE

Serve muffins warm with butter.

exotic fruit salad with sweet citrus guacamole

SERVES 4 TO 6 | TOTAL TIME 25 MINUTES | ACTIVE TIME 25 MINUTES

If you're too far along to fly to a tropical country, bring the sunny flavours to your home with this exotic fruit salad. No long airport lineups, cramped seats or stiff necks required! Share this salad with friends on a bright warm day for that delightful vacation feeling.

FRUIT SALAD

2 kiwis, peeled and sliced into half-moons

1½ cups fresh pineapple, cored and cubed

2 large navel oranges, segmented

1 ripe mango, chopped into bite-size chunks

1 papaya, chopped into bite-size chunks

1 cup chopped lychees (use canned and drained if fresh are unavailable)

8 to 12 strawberries, for garnish

4 to 6 fresh mint sprigs, for garnish

GUACAMOLE

1 large, very ripe avocado

Juice of 1 large navel orange

Juice of ½ lemon

Zest of 1 lemon

2 teaspoons pure vanilla extract

1 teaspoon honey (optional)

METHOD

Mix all fruits in a bowl; set aside. To make the guacamole, cut avocado in half, remove pit and scoop flesh into a small bowl; mash with a fork until smooth. Add orange juice and lemon juice, stirring to blend. Add lemon zest and vanilla, and the honey (if using), stirring to incorporate well.

TO SERVE

Spoon fruit salad into breakfast bowls. Top each with a large dollop of guacamole (use a piping bag if you have one) and garnish with a sprig of mint and 2 strawberries.

Note: *If preparing the fruit salad and guacamole in advance, store fruit in small separate bags or containers (strawberries will stain the other fruit if mixed). Place plastic wrap directly on the surface of the guacamole in its container to keep it from browning.*

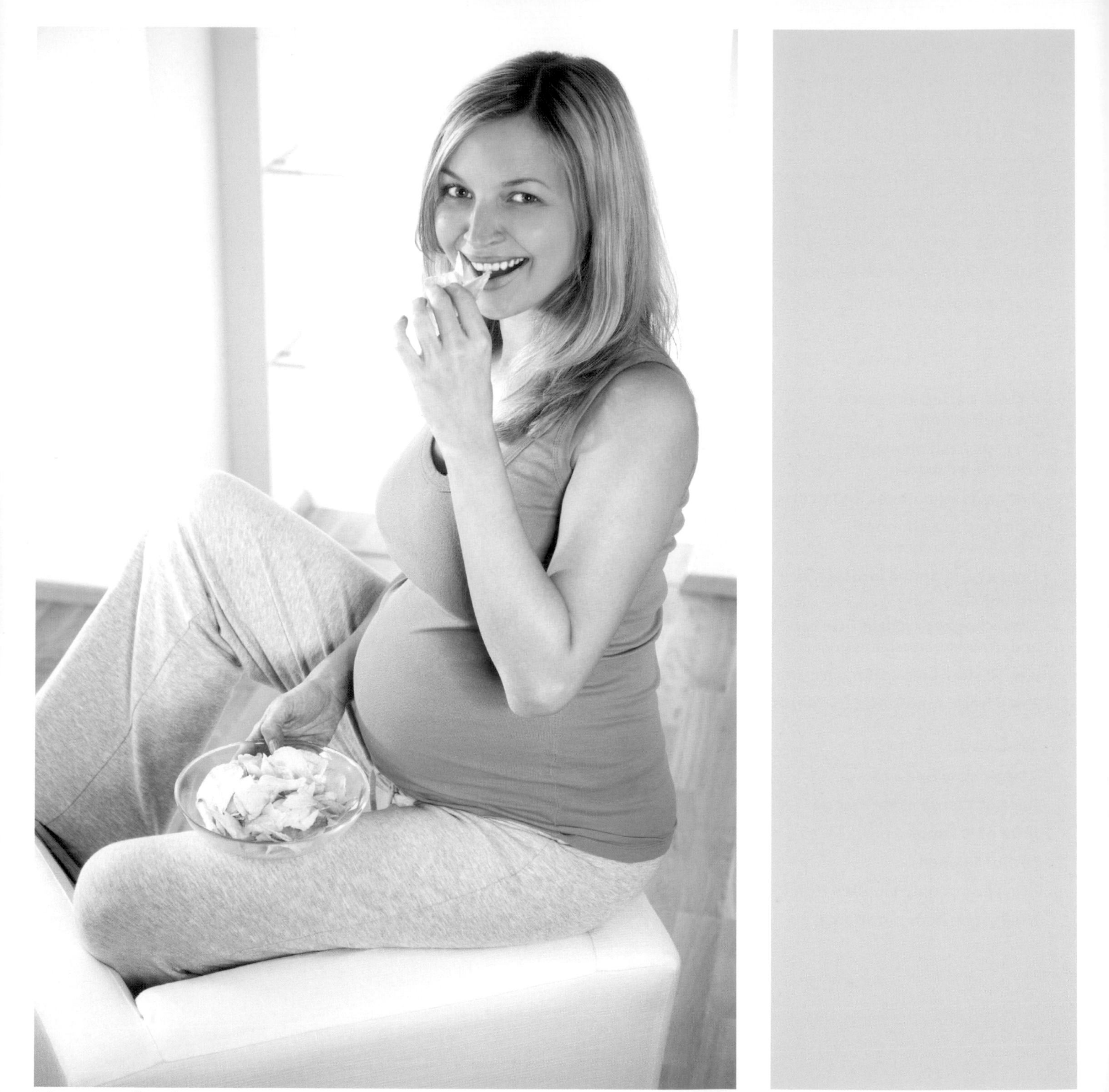

© iStockphoto.com/HannesEichinger

yummy nibbles to
soothe those cravings:

snacks & sidekicks

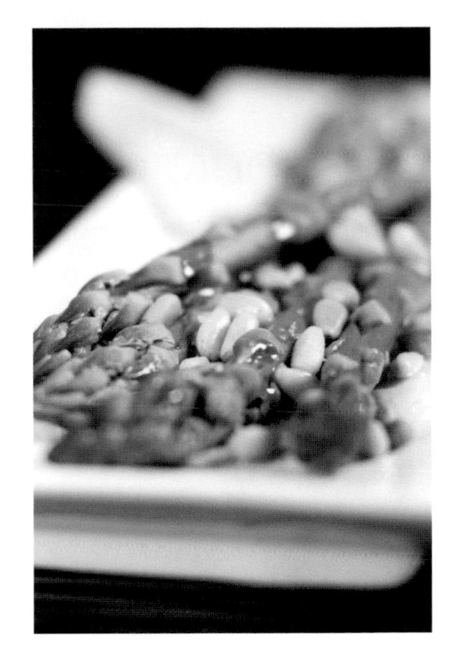

"Feeling fat lasts nine months but the joy of becoming a mom lasts forever."

~ Nikki Dalton

tempura dill pickles with sambal oelek dip

MAKES 32 PIECES | TOTAL TIME 20 MINUTES | ACTIVE TIME 20 MINUTES

I don't know anyone who actually craved pickles while they were pregnant, despite the cliché, but you will probably start to crave them after tasting these modern tempura-style nibbles with spicy dip. Serve these to your friends for a delicious appetizer and a good laugh. Sambal oelek is a mixture of chilies, brown sugar and salt, available at Asian food markets.

PICKLES

Vegetable oil

8 large dill pickles

1 (5-ounce) pkg tempura batter mix

DIP

¼ cup mayonnaise

1 tablespoon sambal oelek

METHOD

Pour vegetable oil into a medium saucepan to 1 inch deep; warm over medium heat. Meanwhile, slice each pickle lengthwise into 4 pieces; pat dry with a paper towel. Follow instructions on tempura batter mix package to achieve a thick batter. Test oil temperature by dropping in a small amount of batter — it should start to fry and brown if oil is hot enough.

Dip pickles in batter, coating completely. Fry for 1 minute, turning if needed to cook all sides. Remove and blot on paper towel to remove excess oil. Do not allow oil to overheat, as the pickles will brown too quickly.

To make the dip, in a small bowl, combine mayonnaise and sambal oelek.

TO SERVE

Serve tempura pickles immediately. On a small plate, pile tempura pickles with sliced plain pickles and the sambal oelek dip.

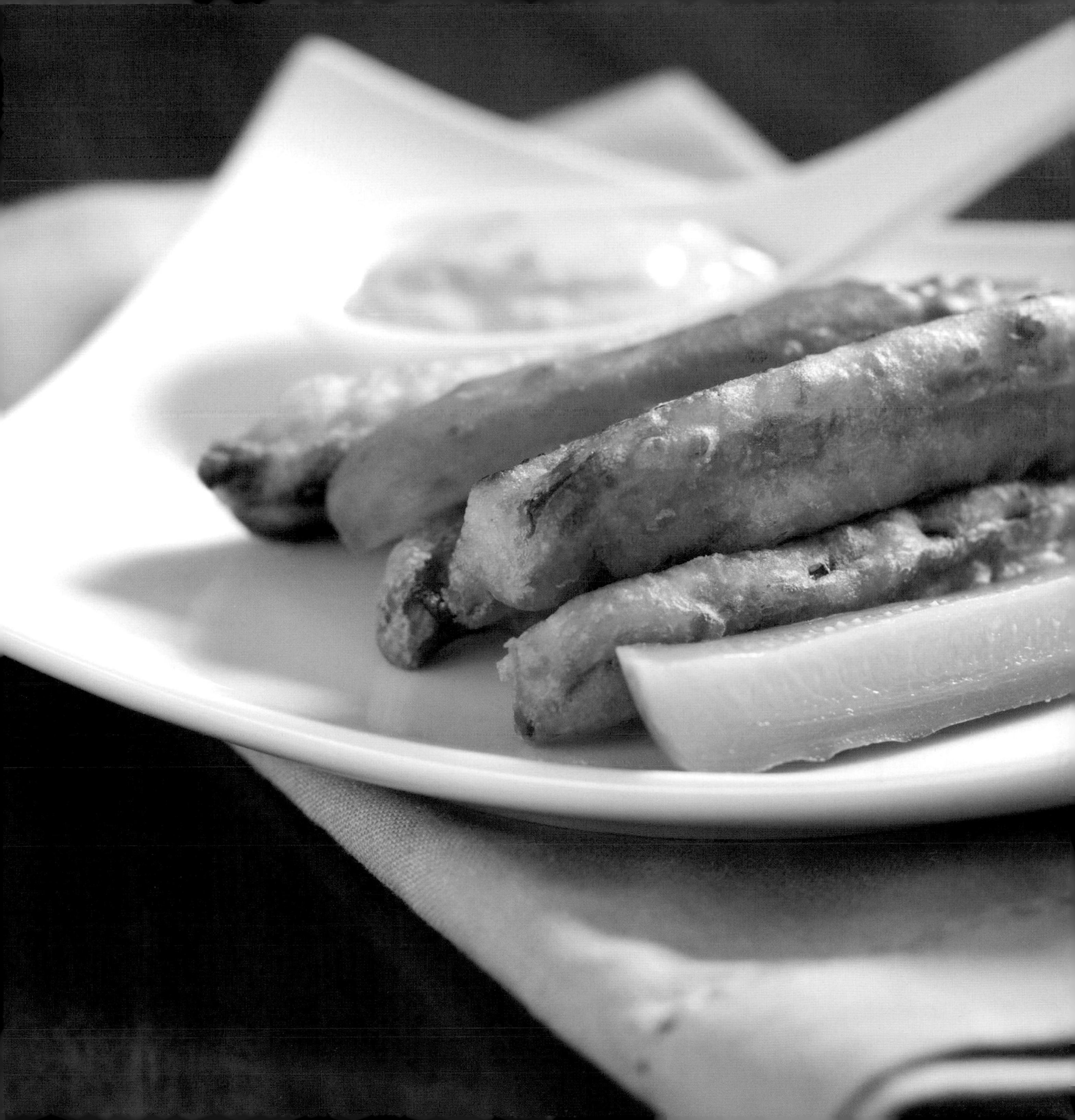

asparagus with truffle oil and toasted pine nuts

SERVES 4 | TOTAL TIME 10 MINUTES | ACTIVE TIME 10 MINUTES

Traditionally, asparagus is eaten with your fingers, although you'll probably want to use a knife and fork with this glammed-up version. The truffle oil adds tremendous depth of flavour and is wonderful with the pine nuts and asparagus. It's a tantalizing way to eat your vegetables! This is a great snack or side dish.

INGREDIENTS

1 small bunch asparagus
⅓ cup pine nuts
Sea salt
2 tablespoons truffle oil

METHOD

Cut or snap the ends off asparagus. To a large frying pan, add water to about 1 inch deep; bring to a boil over high heat. Boil asparagus for about 2 minutes. Remove and dry gently on a paper towel. Meanwhile, spread pine nuts on a baking sheet and sprinkle with sea salt. Broil pine nuts in the oven or toaster oven for about 3 to 5 minutes, until golden.

TO SERVE

Artfully arrange asparagus on a platter and top with the toasted pine nuts. Drizzle truffle oil over top and sprinkle with sea salt.

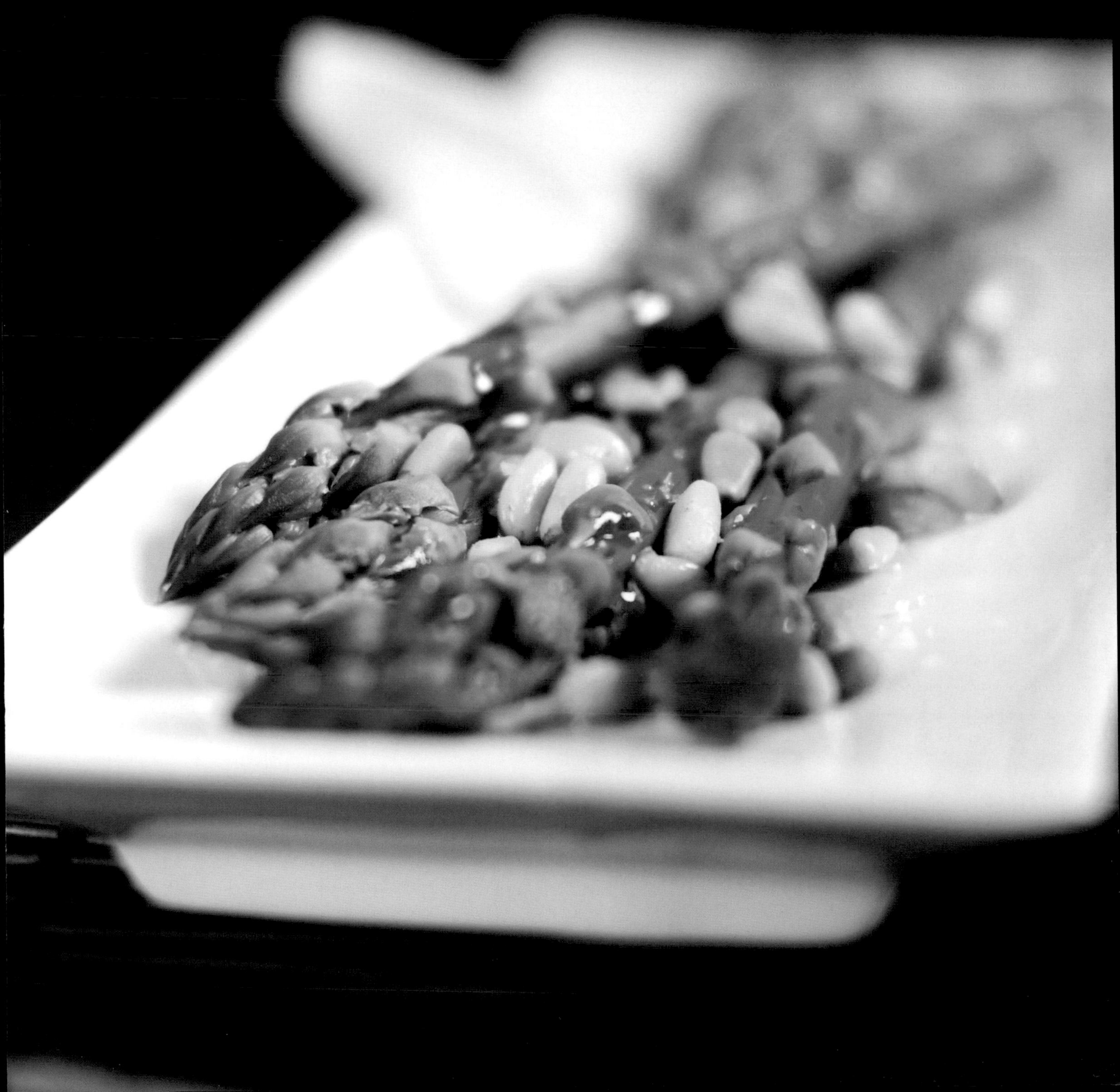

green olives with roasted chickpeas and mixed nuts

SERVES 6 TO 8 | TOTAL TIME 45 MINUTES | ACTIVE TIME 35 MINUTES

What a perfect snack platter for pregnant gals! Salty, delectable olives, spicy toasted nuts and savoury crunchy and crispy chickpeas will appeal to all of your senses and gastronomic needs. It's like a Superbowl buffet for us ladies.

CHICKPEAS

1 (19-ounce) can chickpeas, drained and rinsed

1 tablespoon olive oil

Salt and freshly ground black pepper

1 teaspoon chopped fresh savory

½ teaspoon fresh lemon juice

NUTS

⅓ cup pine nuts

¼ teaspoon chopped fresh savory

⅓ cup walnuts

⅓ cup pecans

¼ teaspoon ancho chili powder

Salt and freshly ground black pepper

1 cup oil-packed pitted green olives

METHOD

Preheat oven to 400°F. In a large bowl, combine chickpeas and olive oil. Season with salt and ground pepper. Spread on a baking sheet and bake for 30 minutes or until crisp.

Meanwhile, toast the nuts. Preheat toaster oven to 375°F and spread pine nuts on tray with savory. Toast for about 3 to 5 minutes, until golden. Transfer to a bowl. Spread walnuts and pecans on baking sheet and toast for 10 to 12 minutes, until fragrant. Add to pine nuts. Season with chili powder, and salt and ground pepper.

Remove chickpeas from the oven and stir well. Add savory and drizzle with lemon juice. Bake for another 5 minutes. Remove from oven and stir well.

TO SERVE

Arrange chickpeas, nuts and olives separately on a serving platter.

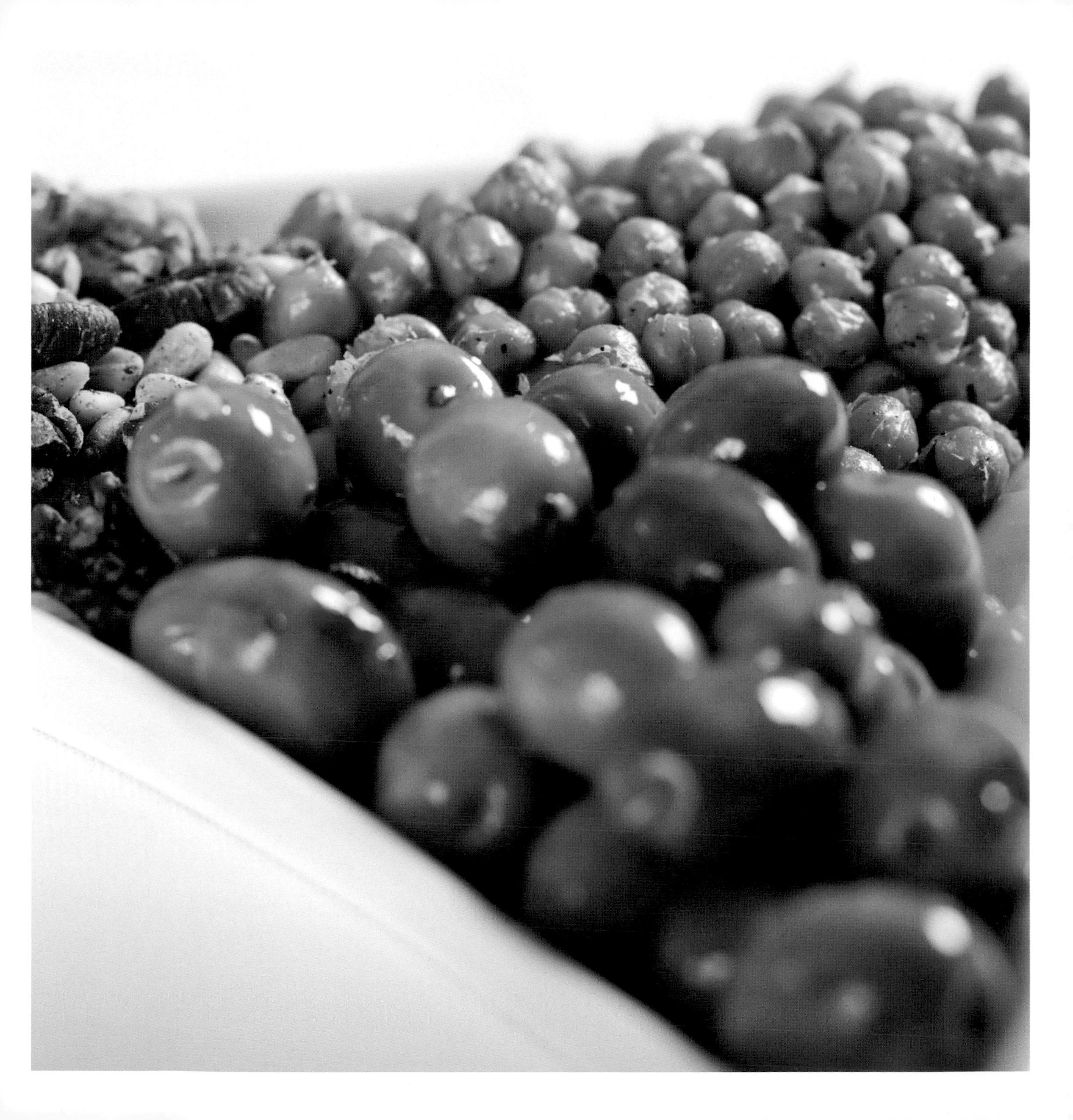

cumin pita chips with peanut sweet chili dip

SERVES 4 | TOTAL TIME 45 MINUTES | ACTIVE TIME 45 MINUTES

This spicy and smooth dip is heavenly — it's made with peanut butter — yum. The homemade pita chips get a fierce kick from cumin. These chips and dip won't last long if you make them for a party (or even for just you and your sweetie). You can mix things up by using both white and whole-wheat pitas.

PITA CHIPS

4 pita pockets

¼ cup extra-virgin olive oil

Sea salt or kosher salt

Ground cumin

DIP

4½ ounces spreadable cream cheese

3 tablespoons natural peanut butter

3 tablespoons Thai sweet red chili sauce

½ teaspoon ground cumin

METHOD

Preheat oven to 400°F. Cut each pita pocket into 8 triangles and separate each triangle into 2 pieces. Place triangles on a baking sheet with the inside of pitas facing up, making sure they don't overlap (you may need to do this in batches). Brush lightly with olive oil; sprinkle with salt and cumin to taste. Bake on middle rack in oven for 4 to 6 minutes, checking often to ensure they don't burn. Transfer to a cooling rack, repeating until all triangles are baked.

To make the dip, in a small bowl, combine cream cheese, peanut butter, chili sauce and cumin.

TO SERVE

Transfer dip to a serving dish. Arrange pita chips around the edges of a large plate and place dip in the centre.

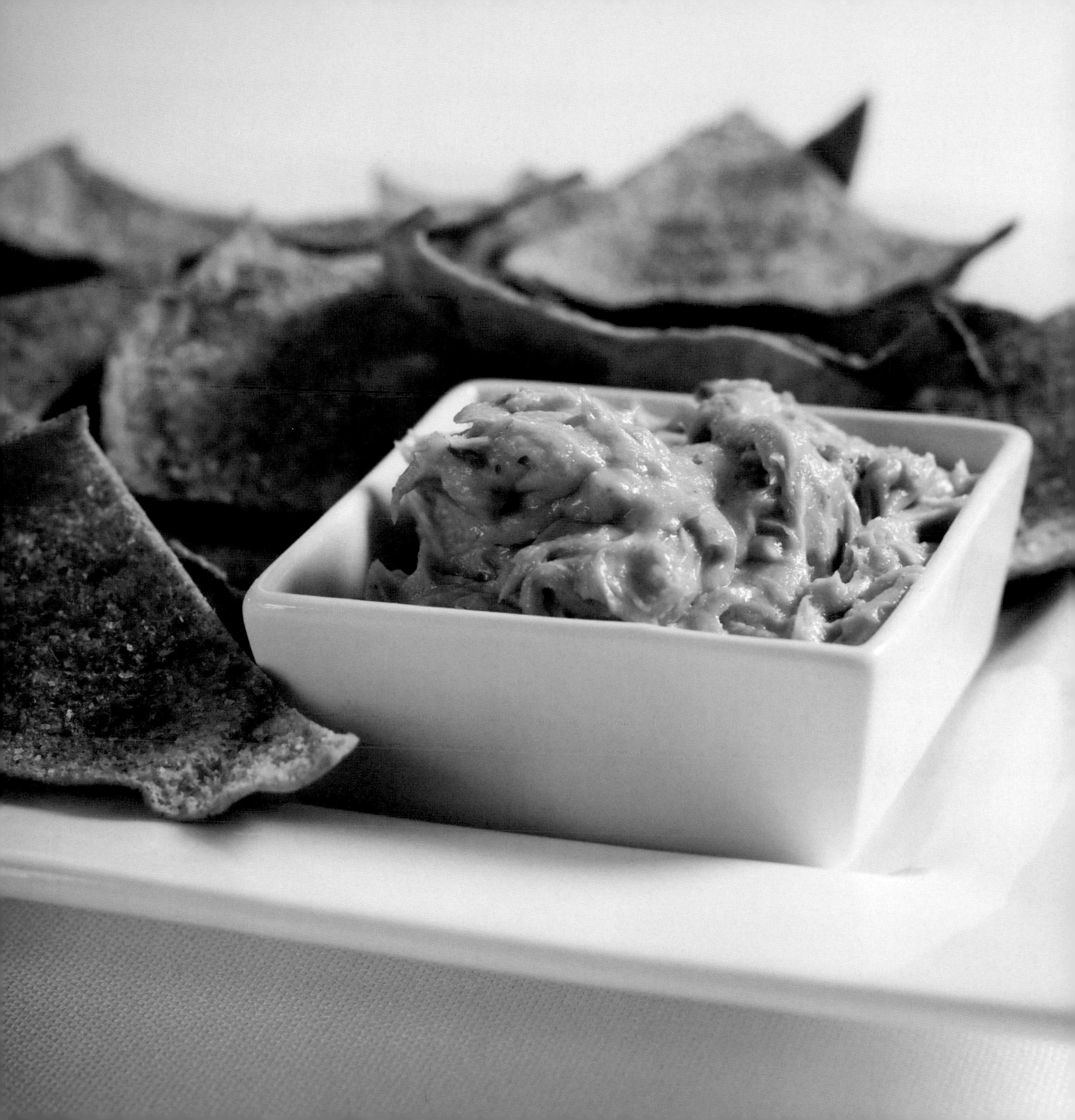

sweet potato fries with truffle aioli

SERVES 4 | TOTAL TIME 25 MINUTES | ACTIVE TIME 10 MINUTES

Far more satisfying than regular fries, these warm sweet potato nibbles are baked with a delicate hint of sesame oil. They are a great standalone snack, or serve them with a burger or sandwich. We pregnant gals must avoid traditional aioli, as it's made with raw eggs. This recipe for earthy and complex truffle aioli uses store-bought mayonnaise — still delicious and completely safe to eat!

FRIES

2 large sweet potatoes (large, thick-skinned variety with orange flesh)

2 tablespoons sesame oil

Dash of salt and freshly ground black pepper

AIOLI

2 tablespoons low-fat mayonnaise

1 teaspoon truffle oil

Salt and freshly ground black pepper

METHOD

Turn broiler to high. Peel sweet potatoes and cut into even chip-size wedges. In a large mixing bowl, toss with sesame oil, salt and pepper to coat.

Spread fries in a single layer on a lightly oiled baking sheet. Bake for 10 to 15 minutes, to desired doneness — tender or crisp — turning halfway through (the thinner they are, the faster they will cook). They tend to burn quickly, so keep an eye on them.

Meanwhile, prepare the truffle aioli. In a small bowl, gently combine mayonnaise and truffle oil. Season with salt and ground pepper.

TO SERVE

Spoon aioli into a condiment cup and serve alongside the sweet potato fries.

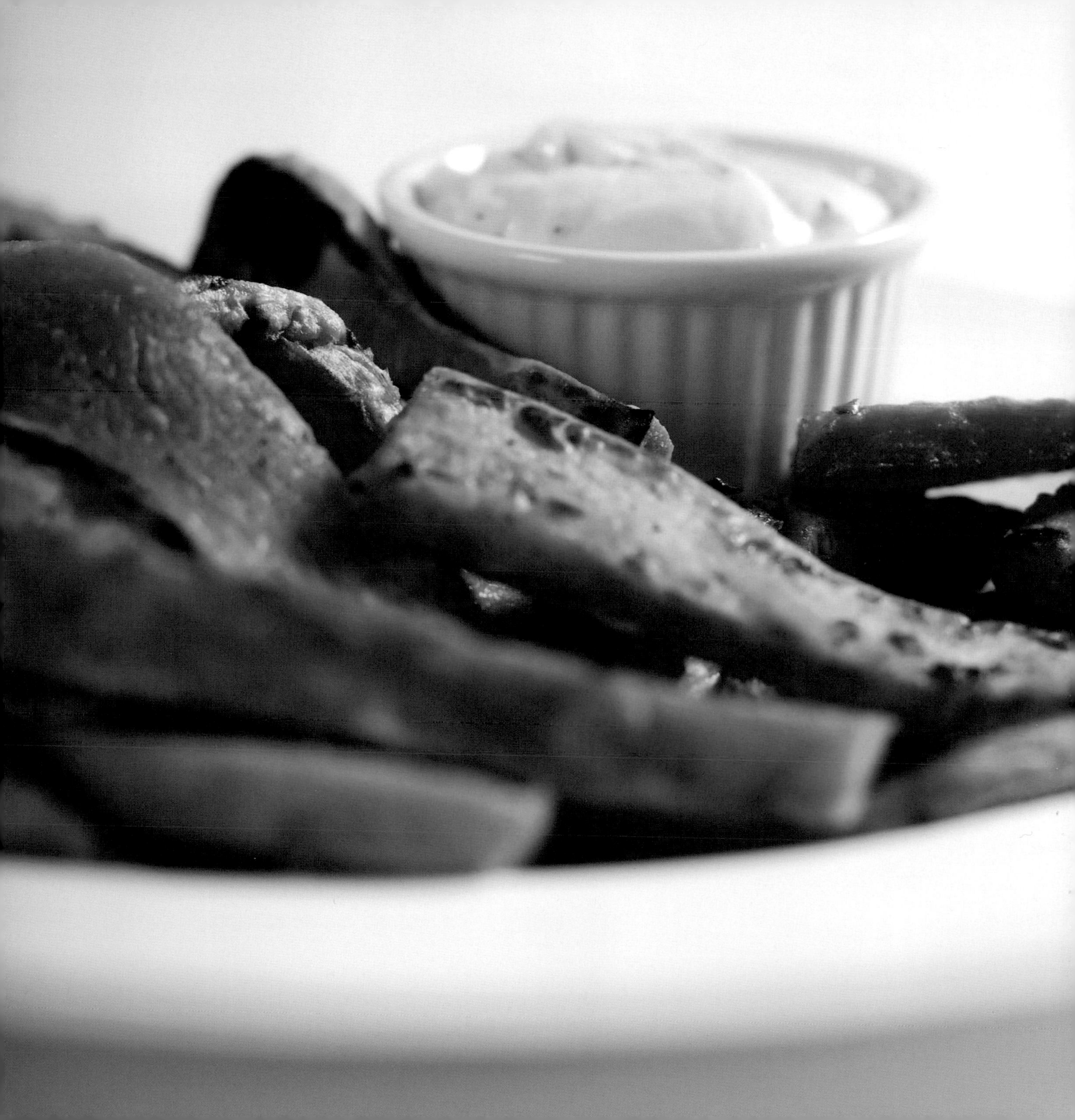

corn on the cob with spiced maple butter

MAKES 4 COBS | TOTAL TIME 1 HOUR 30 MINUTES | ACTIVE TIME 30 MINUTES

Evoking so many memories of summer barbecues, picnics and long lazy evenings with family and friends, corn on the cob is always a delight. It is so much more delicious with this sweet and fragrant maple spice butter. Try roasting the corn on the barbecue with the husks on — the taste is fantastic. You can skip the barbecue and boil the corn if you're short on time.

INGREDIENTS

4 fresh corn cobs, husks on
½ teaspoon cinnamon
¼ teaspoon allspice
⅛ teaspoon ground cloves
½ cup butter, softened
2 tablespoons maple syrup

METHOD

Pull off any excess silk hanging from the corn husks. In a large pot or cooler, soak corn in cold water for 1 hour, placing a heavy object on top of cobs to keep them submerged. Heat barbecue to medium-high. Barbecue corn for 15 minutes, turning every 5 minutes. Husks may char or burn, but this won't affect the corn.

Meanwhile, prepare spice mixture. In a small bowl, combine cinnamon, allspice and cloves. Divide spice mixture in half.

In a small bowl using a fork, cream the butter, maple syrup and half of the spice mixture. Keep the spiced butter in the refrigerator until ready to use.

When corn is cooked, strip off husks and sprinkle corn cobs with remaining spice mixture. Serve immediately, or return to the barbecue to add grill marks, rotating every 2 to 3 minutes.

TO SERVE

Arrange corn on a serving platter. Allow guests to slather maple spiced butter on corn and be sure to have extra napkins on hand.

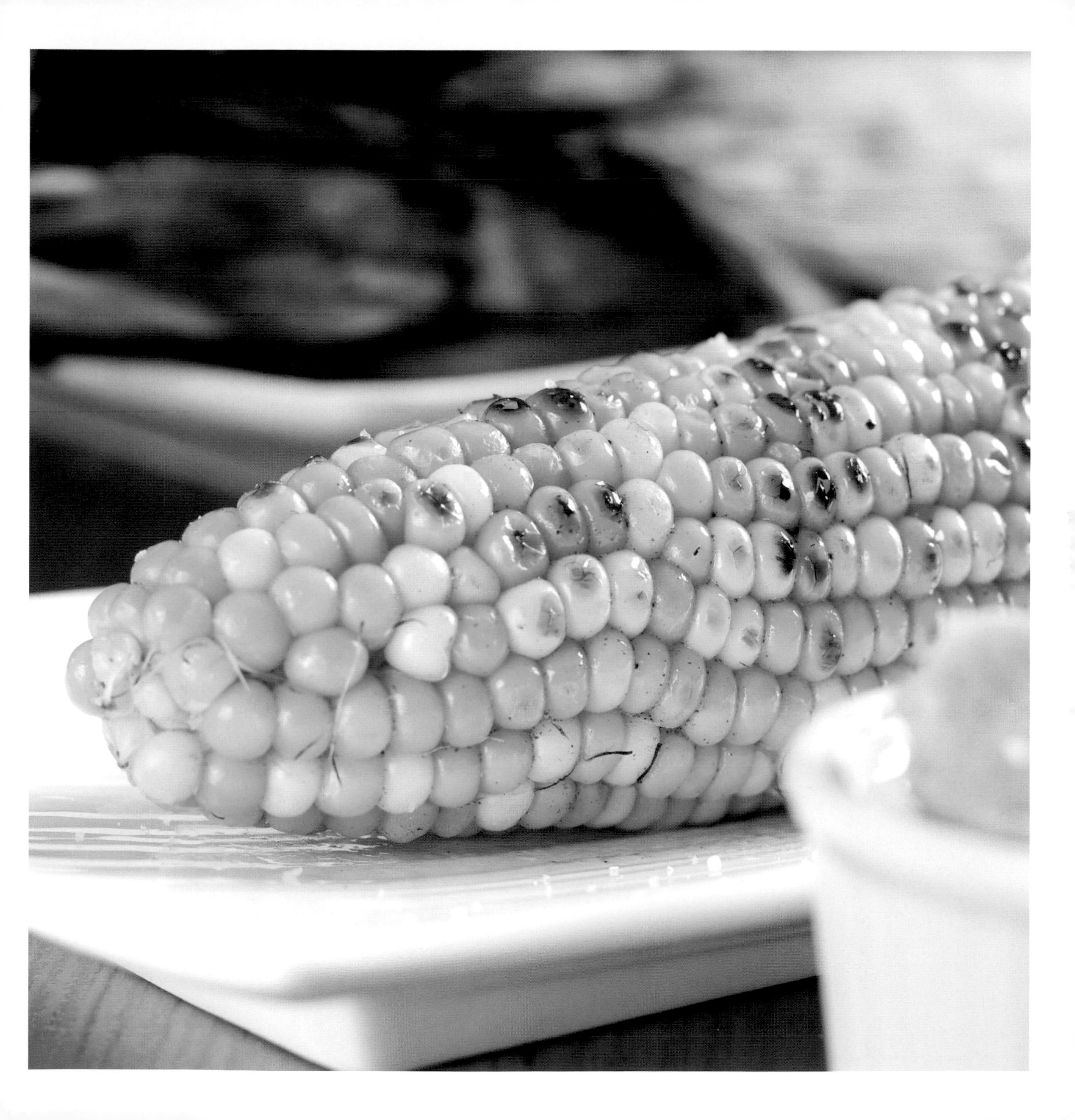

grilled peaches with pink grapefruit and mint

SERVE 4 | TOTAL TIME 15 MINUTES | ACTIVE TIME 15 MINUTES

These luscious, juicy peaches are incredible, and the pink grapefruit and mint are a perfect contrast. This elegant and flavourful dish can be served alone or with chicken or fish. Grilled fruits taste so fabulous, so if you're feeling adventurous, throw whatever other fruits you have on the barbecue as well.

INGREDIENTS

2 ripe peaches

1 tablespoon olive oil

2 tablespoons champagne vinegar

2 tablespoons brown sugar

1 pink grapefruit, peeled and sectioned

2 tablespoons diced red onion

8 fresh mint leaves

METHOD

Peel peaches. Cut in half and discard pits. Brush peach halves lightly with olive oil and place on barbecue or indoor grill over medium-high heat. Barbecue for 3 minutes; flip and grill on the other side for another 3 minutes.

Meanwhile, in a saucepan over high heat, bring champagne vinegar and sugar to a boil, stirring constantly. Remove from heat.

Cut each grapefruit section into 3 or 4 pieces. In a bowl, mix grapefruit chunks and onion. Chop 4 of the mint leaves and add to grapefruit mixture. Pour vinegar mixture into the bowl, stirring to mix lightly.

TO SERVE

Serve each peach half individually, topped with a spoonful of the grapefruit mixture and garnished with a mint leaf.

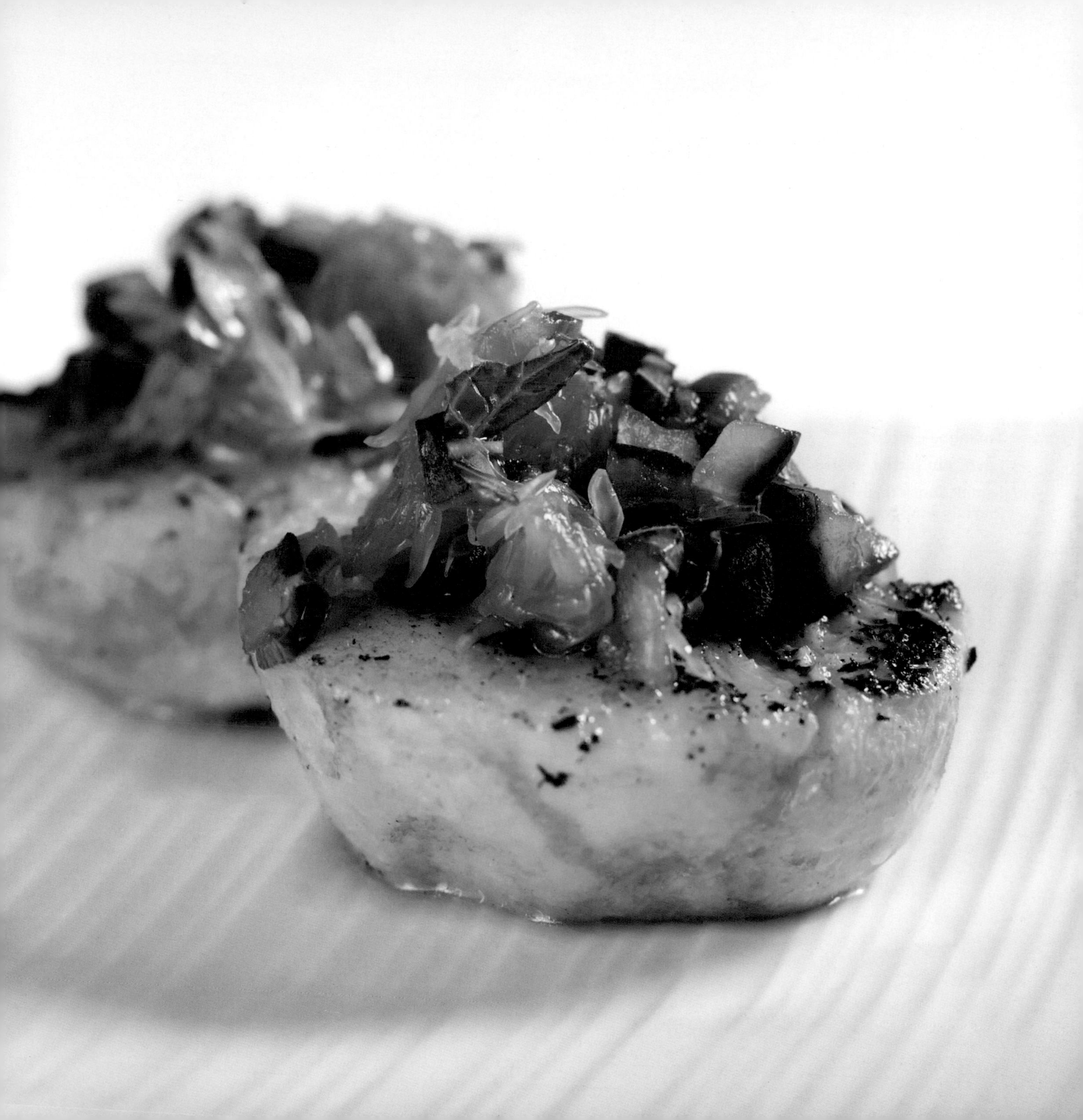

mango cilantro salsa

SERVES 4 | TOTAL TIME 5 MINUTES | ACTIVE TIME 5 MINUTES

Gentle and glorious in both taste and texture, this fresh and simple salsa is addictively delicious. Unlike some spicy salsas, which can upset the gentle tummies of pregnant ladies, this version is mild yet still perfect with corn chips (add diced vine-ripened tomato for a more savoury salsa, if you like). Close your eyes and imagine you are on a warm tropical island, with no worries or stress — and a sexy scuba instructor, of course!

INGREDIENTS

2 mangoes, diced

1 avocado, pitted, peeled and diced

1 small bunch fresh cilantro, coarsely chopped

METHOD

In a bowl, combine mangoes, avocado and cilantro.

TO SERVE

Serve immediately with chips, as an accompaniment to white fish, as a starter salad, or in crêpes.

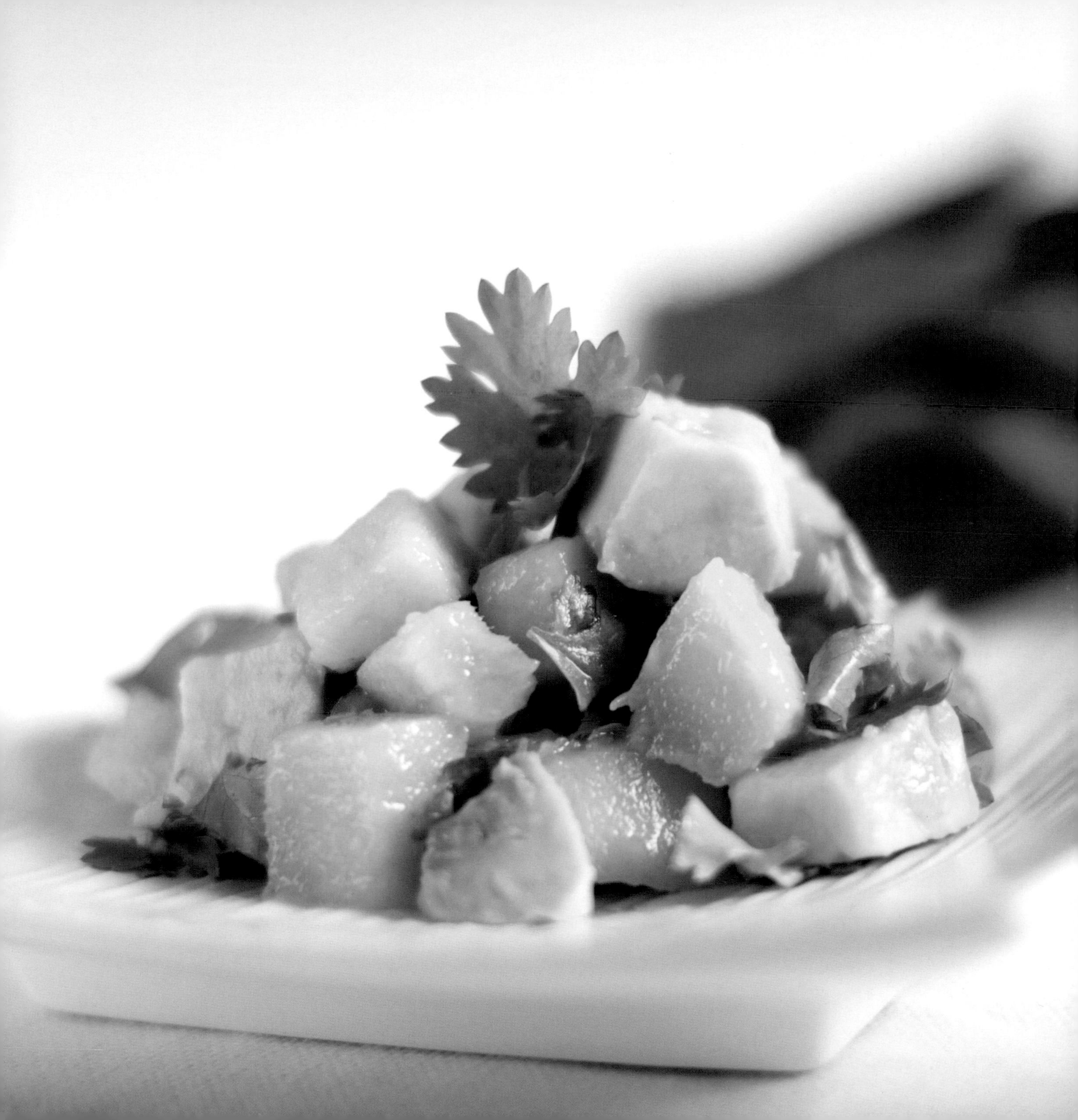

granny smith honey cornbread

MAKES 16 PIECES | TOTAL TIME 45 MINUTES | ACTIVE TIME 15 MINUTES

Ultimately comforting, this cornbread is sweetened with honey and tart Granny Smith apples. A great side or snack, try it warm and topped with melted butter or cheddar cheese. Then show your sweetie some real Southern charm!

INGREDIENTS

2 cups cornmeal

1 cup all-purpose flour

1 tablespoon baking powder

½ teaspoon salt

2 eggs

1 cup whipping cream

¼ cup butter, melted

⅓ cup pasteurized honey

½ cup corn niblets

1 Granny Smith apple, peeled, cored and diced

METHOD

Preheat oven to 400°F. Grease a 9-inch square baking dish.

In a large bowl, combine the cornmeal, flour, baking powder and salt. In a separate bowl, beat the eggs. Stir in the whipping cream, butter and honey.

Stir the corn and apple into flour mixture. Add the whipping cream mixture and stir until just combined. Do not overmix — the batter should be lumpy. Pour into the baking dish and bake for 25 to 30 minutes or until a toothpick inserted into the centre comes out clean.

TO SERVE

Cut into squares and serve warm, with butter.

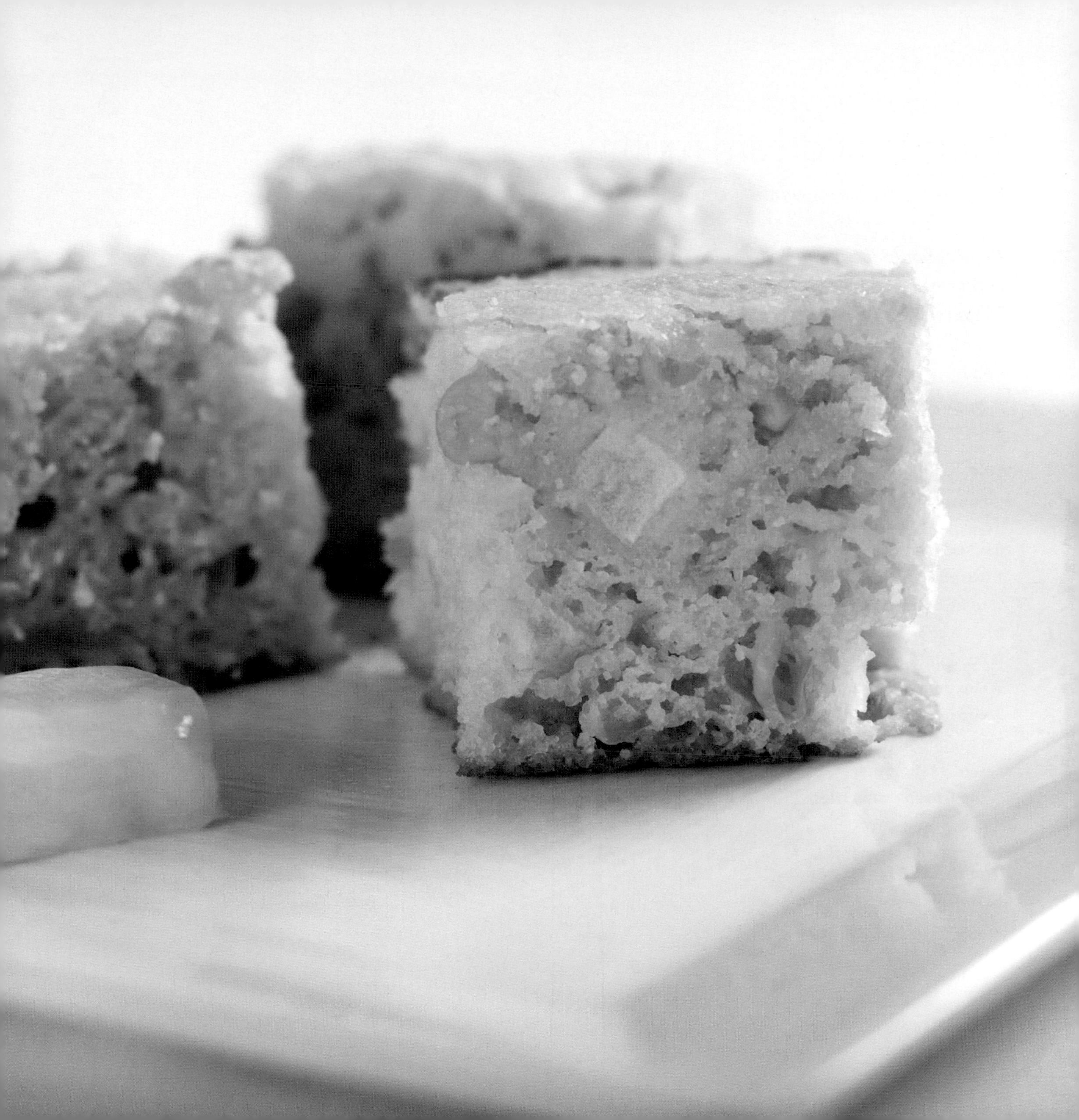

tangerine dream muffins

MAKES 12 | TOTAL TIME 45 MINUTES | ACTIVE TIME 20 MINUTES

In addition to looking gorgeous, these delicious muffins are stuffed with so many yummy, healthy ingredients. Some people believe that eating lots of different foods and flavours while you are pregnant will ensure your child is not too picky an eater. If that's true, then these muffins are a good start!

INGREDIENTS

¼ cup each golden raisins, shredded unsweetened coconut, sunflower seeds and chopped walnuts

1½ cups all-purpose flour

½ cup wheat bran

2 teaspoons each baking powder, flax seeds and ginger powder

1 teaspoon poppy seeds

¼ teaspoon salt

2 large eggs

¾ cup milk

¾ cup granulated sugar

½ cup butter, melted and cooled

1 teaspoon pure vanilla extract

Zest of 1 tangerine

¾ cup frozen cranberries

½ cup grated carrot

12 tangerine segments (approx 1 to 2 tangerines)

12 frozen cranberries

METHOD

Preheat oven to 375°F. In small bowl, combine raisins, coconut, sunflower seeds and walnuts. In another small bowl, use a whisk to combine flour, bran, baking powder, flax seeds, ginger powder, poppy seeds and salt.

In a medium bowl, whisk eggs. Add milk, sugar, butter and vanilla, mixing well. Add tangerine zest, cranberries and carrot; mix until incorporated. Stir in raisin mixture. Add the dry ingredients. Mix quickly until just blended, folding the wet mixture over from the bottom. Don't overmix — the batter should be lumpy. Grease or line a 12-cup muffin tin; distribute batter evenly. On top of each muffin, place 1 tangerine segment and 1 cranberry. Bake for 25 minutes.

TO SERVE

Serve warm with butter.

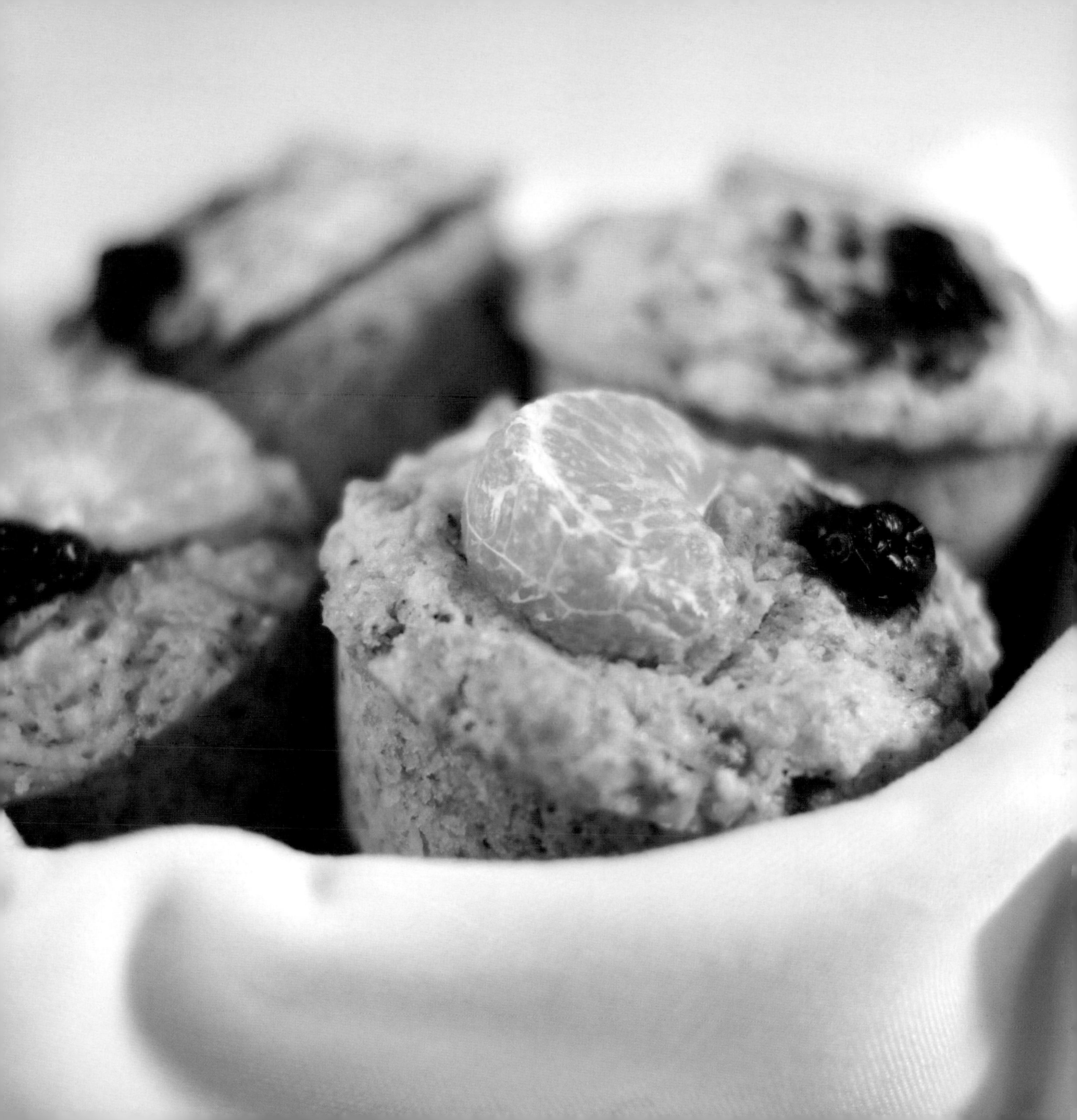

M&M granola bars

MAKES 16 SQUARES | TOTAL TIME 45 MINUTES | ACTIVE TIME 25 MINUTES

This one's for the sisterhood — almost every woman I knew craved M&M's at some point in her pregnancy. Sweet and salty and using both plain and peanut M&M's, these granola bars are way better than store-bought ones. Get some granola with that chocolate fix!

INGREDIENTS

2 cups old-fashioned rolled oats
¾ cup wheat germ
½ cup slivered almonds
½ cup pasteurized honey
½ cup loosely packed brown sugar
4 tablespoons butter
2 teaspoons pure vanilla extract
½ teaspoon salt
½ teaspoon cinnamon
½ cup each plain and peanut M&M's

METHOD

Preheat oven to 350°F. Grease an 8-inch square baking dish. Combine the oats, wheat germ and almonds; spread on a large baking sheet. Toast for 12 to 15 minutes, stirring every 5 minutes, until golden. Remove from oven and reduce oven temperature to 300°F.

Meanwhile, in a medium saucepan over medium heat, combine the honey, sugar, butter, vanilla, salt and cinnamon, stirring occasionally, until sugar has dissolved.

Add oat mixture and M&M's to the saucepan, stirring to combine well. Pour the mixture into the baking dish and press down firmly to spread out evenly. Bake for 20 minutes. Remove from oven and let cool completely.

TO SERVE

Cut into bars. Serve on a dessert plate — with extra M&M's if you wish!

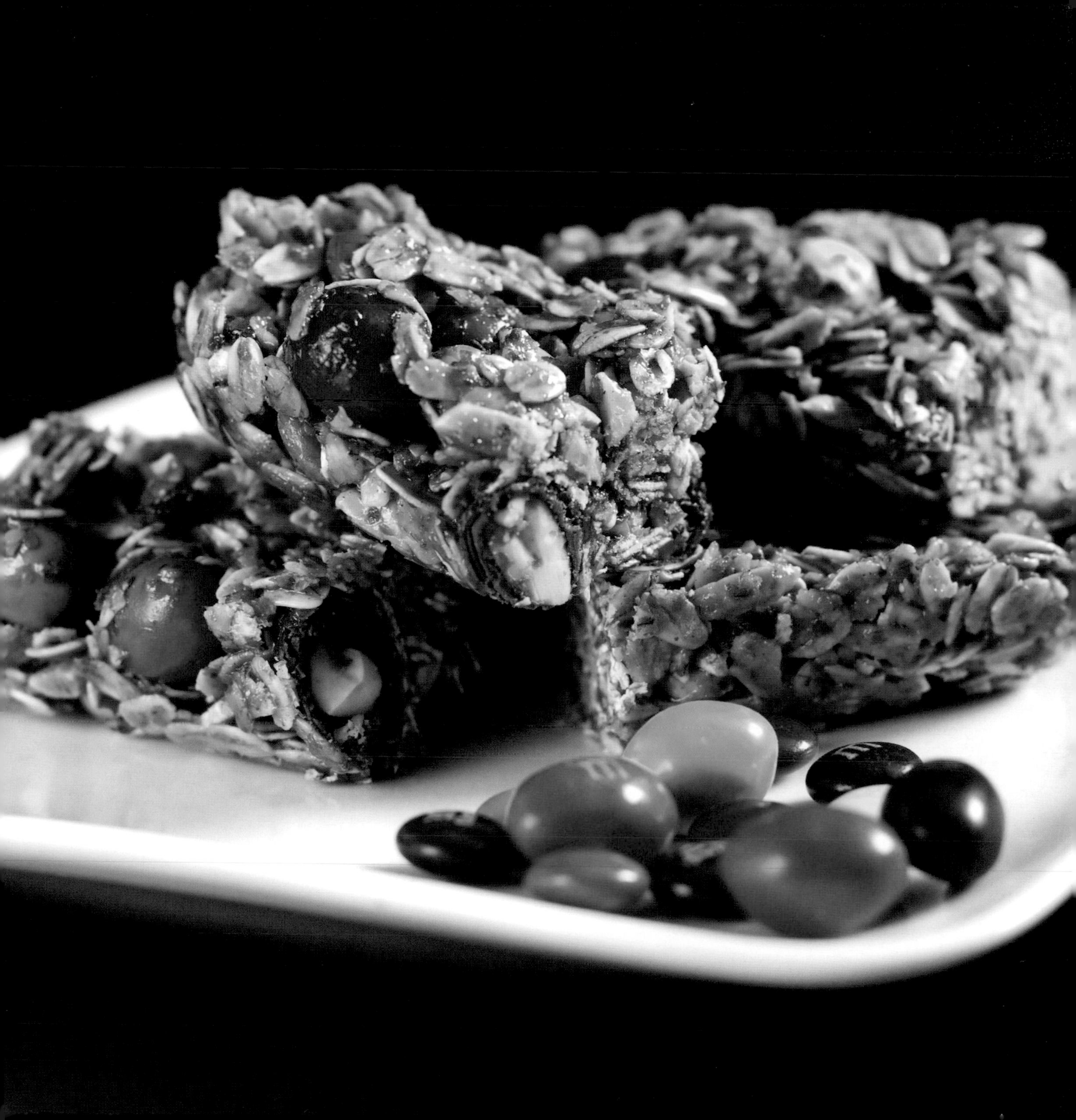

slightly naughty biscotti

MAKES 30 TO 40 | TOTAL TIME 1 HOUR 30 MINUTES | ACTIVE TIME 35 MINUTES

These delightfully crunchy treats are not too sweet, and they go well with both coffee and tea. They are perfect for when you are looking to nibble on something just a little bit naughty! The ginger and orange pair beautifully with the chocolate. Thanks to the ginger, they will help settle your tummy if you are having a bit of morning sickness, and make your tummy feel extra happy if you're already feeling well. This recipe makes enough to serve you plus all your friends and family. As well, the biscotti keep well, so you'll have plenty of time to eat them all!

INGREDIENTS

2 cups all-purpose flour

1 cup granulated sugar

3 tablespoons brown sugar

½ cup unsweetened cocoa powder

1 teaspoon baking soda

½ teaspoon salt

4 eggs

1 tablespoon pure vanilla extract

½ cup candied ginger, chopped into small pieces

1½ cups semisweet chocolate chips

Zest of 1 orange

METHOD

Preheat oven to 350°F. In a large mixing bowl, combine the flour, granulated and brown sugars, cocoa, baking soda and salt. Beat in the eggs and vanilla. Stir in the candied ginger, chocolate chips and orange zest. Do not overmix — the dough should be lumpy.

Form the dough into two flattened logs, each about 12 inches long, 4 inches wide and 2 inches tall. Place on baking sheets lined with parchment paper; bake for 35 minutes or until a toothpick inserted into the centre comes out clean. Remove from oven and set aside to cool for 10 minutes.

Reduce oven temperature to 275°F. Using a serrated knife, cut the cooled logs into ¾-inch-thick slices. Place the slices on their sides on the baking sheet and bake for another 20 to 25 minutes, flipping halfway through baking time. The second baking is to dry out the biscotti to give them their signature crunch.

TO SERVE

Serve biscotti individually on dessert plates or eat directly from the cookie jar! The biscotti will keep in an airtight container for up to 2 weeks, or in the freezer for up to 1 month.

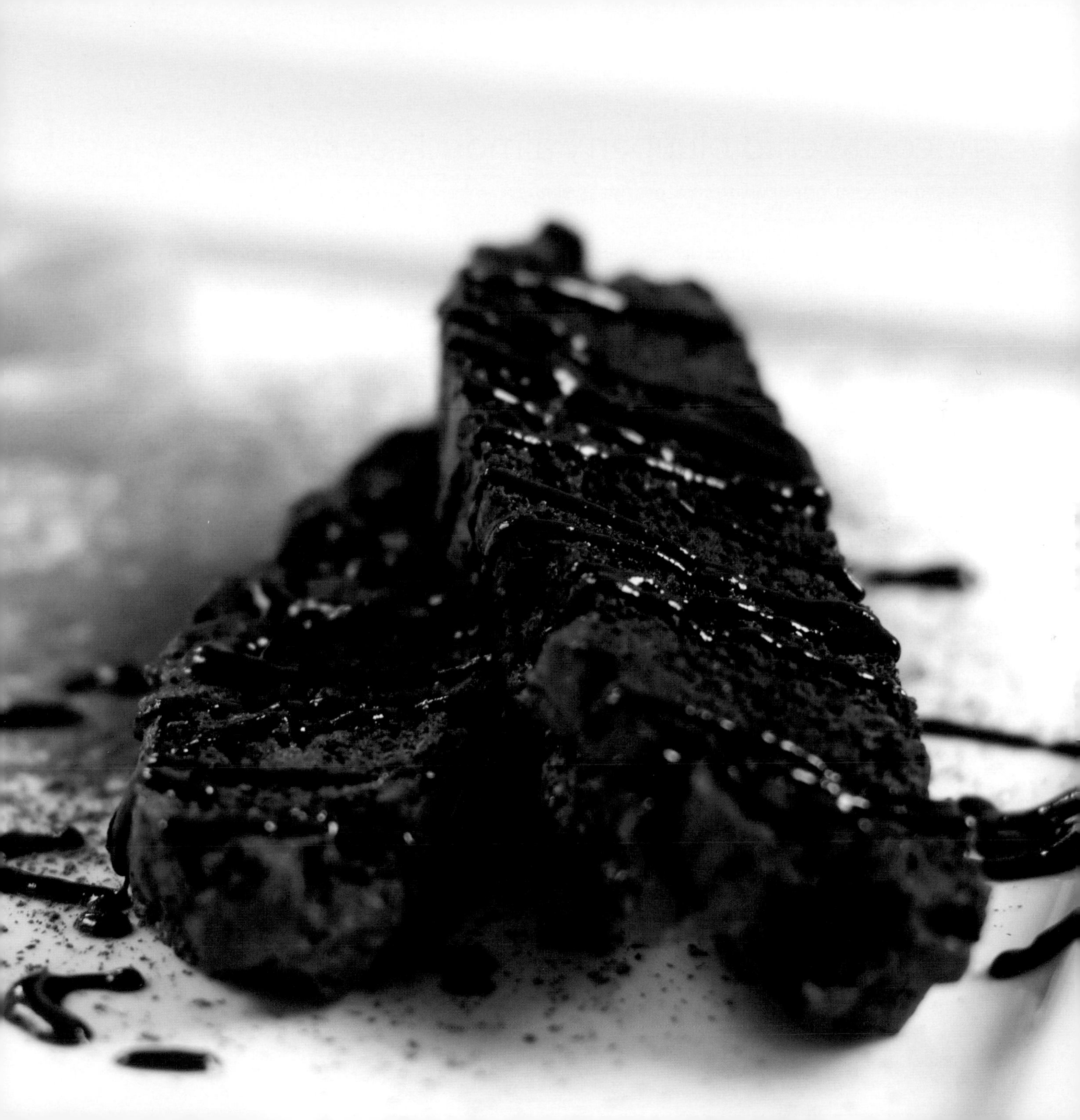

chocolate chip blueberry almond cookies

SERVES 8 TO 10 | TOTAL TIME 40 MINUTES | ACTIVE TIME 15 MINUTES

Adding dried blueberries and toasted almonds gives these familiar and fantastic chocolate chip cookies a whimsical charm. Keep your cookie jar full of them and you'll never be at a loss for what to serve when friends drop in. And in a few years, your little one can help you make them!

INGREDIENTS

⅓ cup slivered almonds
½ cup butter, softened
1 cup loosely packed brown sugar
1 egg
½ teaspoon pure vanilla extract
½ teaspoon almond extract
1 cup all-purpose flour
½ teaspoon salt
½ teaspoon baking soda
¾ cup dark or milk chocolate chunks
½ cup dried blueberries

METHOD

Preheat oven to 375°F. Spread the almonds on a baking sheet and toast for 3 to 5 minutes, turning halfway through baking time. Remove from oven and let cool.

In a large bowl, cream the butter and sugar. Add egg, vanilla and almond extract, beating well.

In a bowl, sift together flour, salt and baking soda; add to butter mixture. Stir in chocolate chunks, blueberries and toasted almonds. Form dough into 2-inch balls and place on a greased baking sheet, flattening each with a fork. Bake for 8 to 10 minutes, until golden.

TO SERVE

Place hand in cookie jar. Remove cookie. Eat!

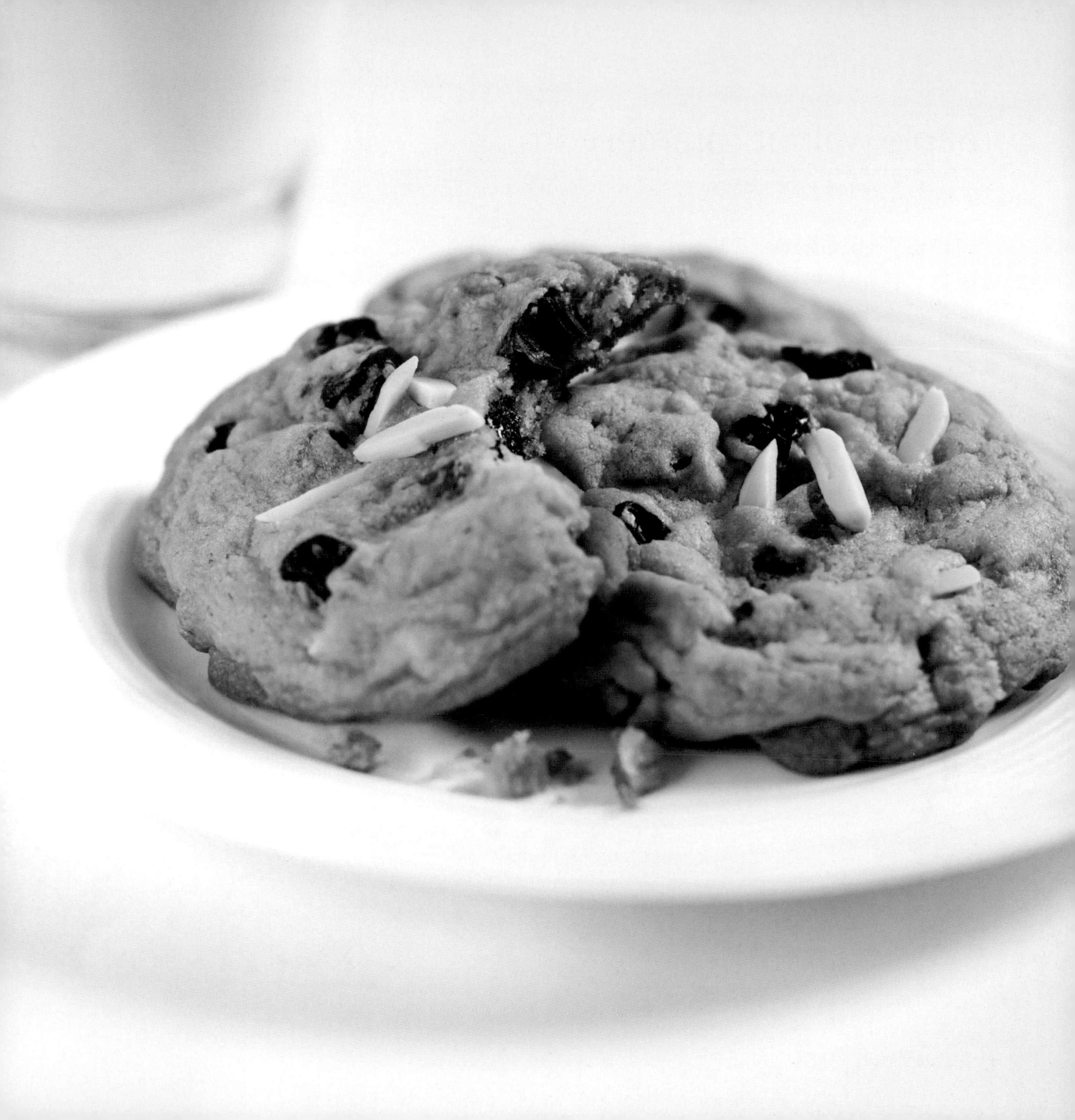

maple walnut caramel corn

SERVES 10 | TOTAL TIME 1 HOUR 20 MINUTES | ACTIVE TIME 20 MINUTES

We just can't stop eating this! It is easy to make and stores well, but you'll be munching on it at every opportunity. Movie night? Friends over? Need a snack before bed? You'll find lots of reasons to indulge.

POPCORN

⅔ cup popping corn

¼ cup vegetable oil

SAUCE

2 cups loosely packed brown sugar

1 cup butter

½ cup maple syrup

½ teaspoon salt

½ teaspoon baking soda

1 teaspoon pure vanilla extract

1 cup whole walnuts

METHOD

Preheat oven to 250°F. In a large, heavy-bottomed pot with a lid, heat the vegetable oil over medium heat. To test the heat, add 3 corn kernels; when they pop, add the remaining popping corn, leaving the lid slightly ajar to vent the steam. When the corn has popped, transfer to baking sheets and keep warm in the oven.

In a medium saucepan over medium-high heat, combine the sugar, butter and maple syrup; bring to a boil. Boil gently for 5 minutes, stirring occasionally. Remove the popcorn from the oven and transfer to a large bowl. Remove the sauce from the heat; stir in the salt, baking soda, vanilla and walnuts. Working quickly before the sauce cools and hardens, pour the sauce over the popcorn, tossing to mix. Transfer the coated popcorn onto oiled baking sheets and bake for 1 hour, stirring every 15 minutes.

TO SERVE

Put popcorn in a large bowl and share with your friends.

banana, yogurt and juice layered popsicles

SERVES 8 | TOTAL TIME 3 TO 4 HOURS | ACTIVE TIME 10 MINUTES

This cheerful childhood treat is a perfect one for pregnant ladies — icy cold, juicy and fruity — just the thing to keep you cool when things start to heat up. The grown-up flavours will appeal to your gourmet palate while also quenching your thirst. Experiment with other juices and frozen fruits to find your favourites.

INGREDIENTS

1 ripe banana

1 cup plain, vanilla or fruit-flavoured yogurt

¼ cup each frozen blueberries and cranberries

¼ cup frozen pineapple chunks

¼ cup each blueberry, orange and cranberry juice

METHOD

Using a fork, mash banana until smooth. Spoon evenly into the bottom of each popsicle mould in a popsicle tray, filling each no more than one-quarter full. Spoon yogurt over the mashed banana, filling each mould to no more than two-thirds full. Chill the popsicles in the freezer for at least 20 minutes to harden. Remove from freezer and distribute frozen fruits among popsicles. Fill each mould with one of the juices, leaving a bit of space at the top. Insert popsicle sticks and return to freezer for 3 to 4 hours or until solid.

TO SERVE

Run warm water over the outside of the popsicle tray to loosen popsicles. Serve individually to guests and have napkins on hand to catch any drips.

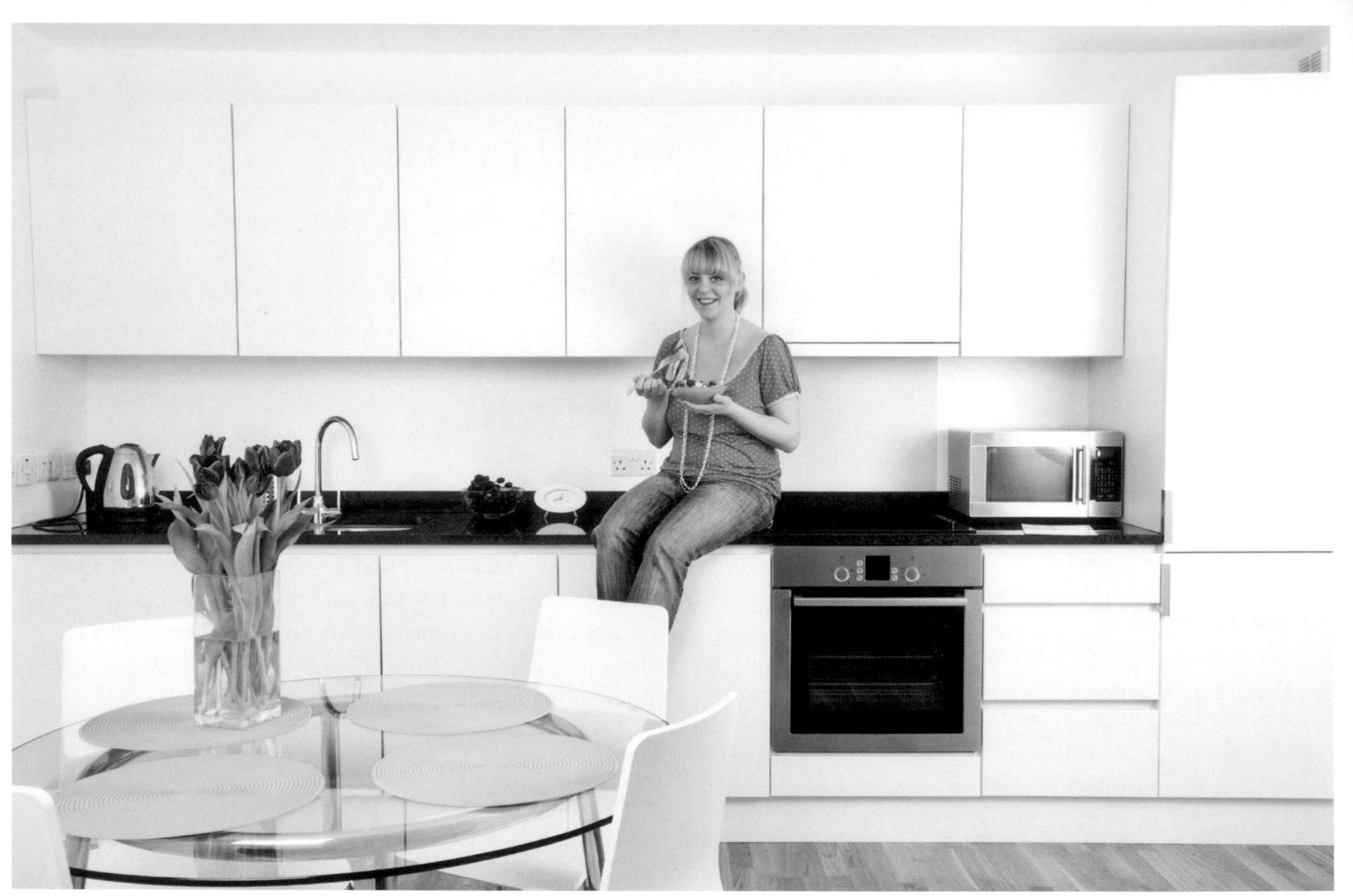

mini-bites for you and your mini-me:

appetizers

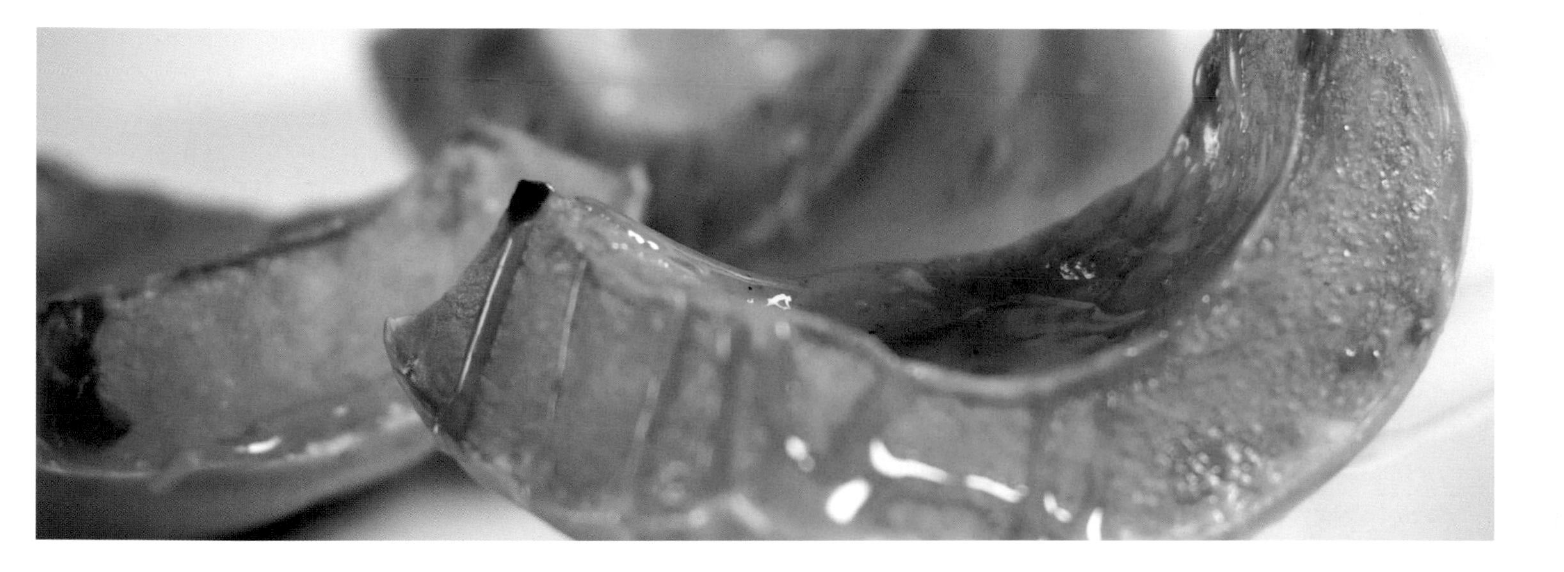

"Men become passionately attached to women who know how to cosset them with delicate tidbits."

~ Honoré de Balzac

sushi vegetables with asian and wasabi yogurt dipping sauces

SERVES 10 TO 12 | TOTAL TIME 25 MINUTES | ACTIVE TIME 25 MINUTES

Yes, I know ... you are dying for sushi! No raw fish allowed, but this is a fun and funky vegetarian appetizer that everyone will love. Chopsticks are optional. It may take you a few tries to get the hang of wrapping the vegetable bundles (unless you have previous training as a sushi chef!), but once you catch on, it'll be easy. Just like parenting, right?

VEGETABLES

1 red pepper

1 yellow pepper

2 celery stalks

2 carrots

1 zucchini

20 sugar peas

3 to 4 sheets toasted nori (Japanese seaweed)

SAUCE

⅓ cup plain yogurt

1 teaspoon pasteurized honey

½ teaspoon freshly grated ginger

¼ teaspoon prepared wasabi

METHOD

Slice peppers lengthwise into ½-inch-thick strips. Cut celery, carrots and zucchini into ½-inch-long strips. Using kitchen shears, cut nori into ½-inch-wide strips. Fill a small bowl with water. Using your fingers, dampen a nori strip and place on a cutting board. Place 3 or 4 vegetable pieces in the centre and gently but firmly wrap nori around them to create a bundle. The nori will seal as it dries.

To make the sauce, in a small bowl, combine the yogurt, honey, ginger and wasabi.

TO SERVE

Arrange bundles on a Japanese-style serving dish accompanied by the dip.

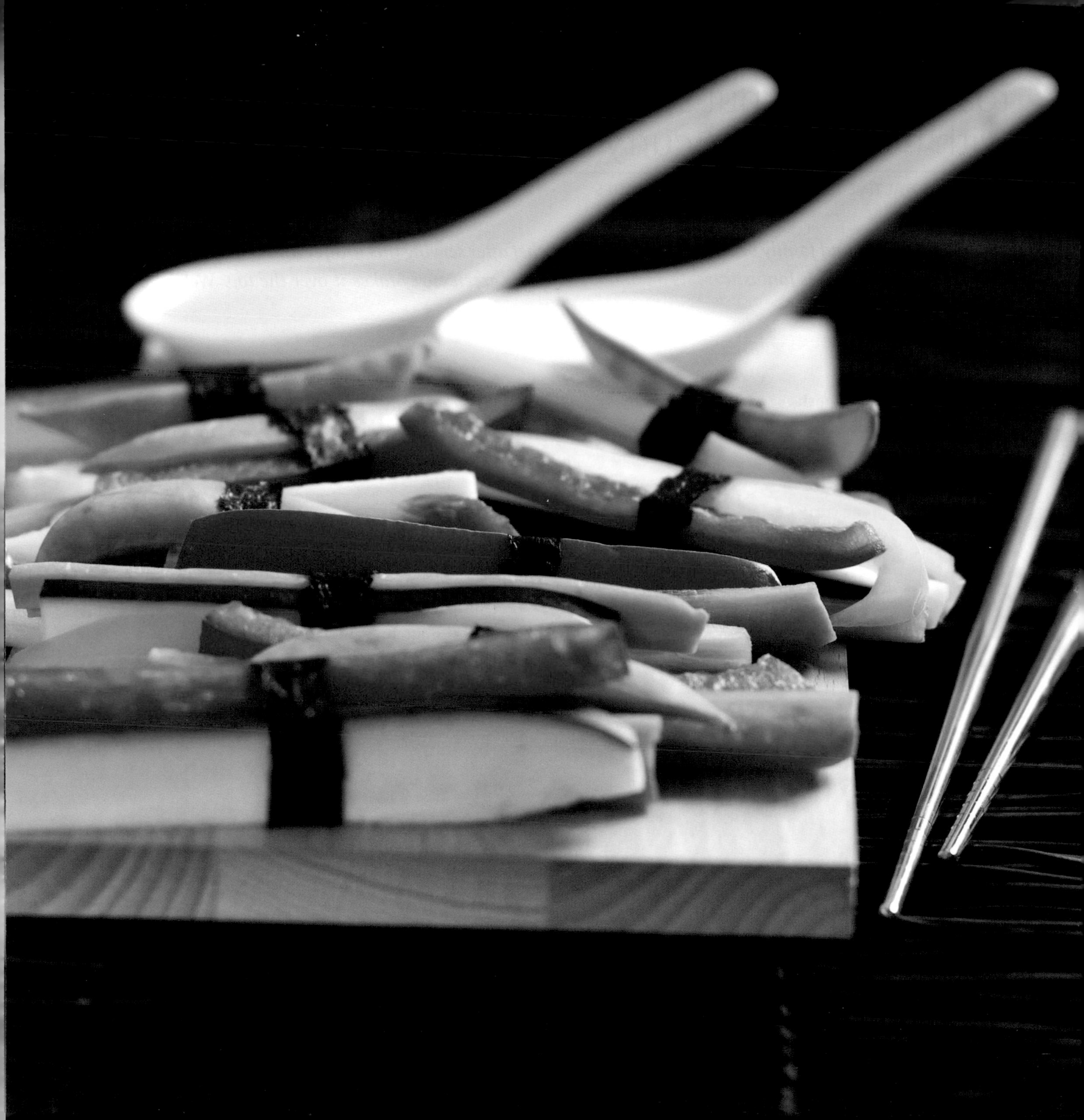

baked grape leaves with sumac chicken, apricots and rice

SERVES 6 TO 8 | TOTAL TIME 1 HOUR 30 MINUTES | ACTIVE TIME 30 MINUTES

We miss you, darling grapes! Since we can't drink your wine, we may as well eat your leaves. These baked grape leaves are fantastic and simpler to prepare than most versions. Sumac is a tart and delicious spice that adds a cool, modern flair.

INGREDIENTS

1 cup white rice (unconverted)
1¼ cups water
1 teaspoon butter
Dash of salt
1 (16-ounce) jar grape leaves
¾ pound ground chicken
½ cup chicken broth
¼ cup chopped dried apricots
2 cloves garlic, minced
½ cup chopped red onion
1 tomato, finely chopped
½ teaspoon ground cinnamon
⅓ teaspoon ground cumin
1½ teaspoon sumac
Dash of salt and freshly ground black pepper

METHOD

In a pot add rice, water, butter and salt; bring to a rapid boil, reduce heat to simmer and cook, covered, until water is absorbed, about 15 minutes. Let stand, covered, for 5 minutes, then fluff with a fork.

Meanwhile, carefully remove grape leaves from jar; separate and soak them in cold water for 20 minutes to reduce saltiness. Pat leaves dry with paper towel.

Preheat oven to 375°F. In a large bowl, combine chicken, cooked rice, broth, apricots, garlic, onion, tomato, cinnamon, cumin and sumac. Season with salt and ground pepper. Form mixture into small logs. Place each at the edge of a grape leaf. Tuck in sides of the leaves, then roll up. Arrange on a baking sheet and bake for 22 to 25 minutes.

TO SERVE

Serve piled on a platter.

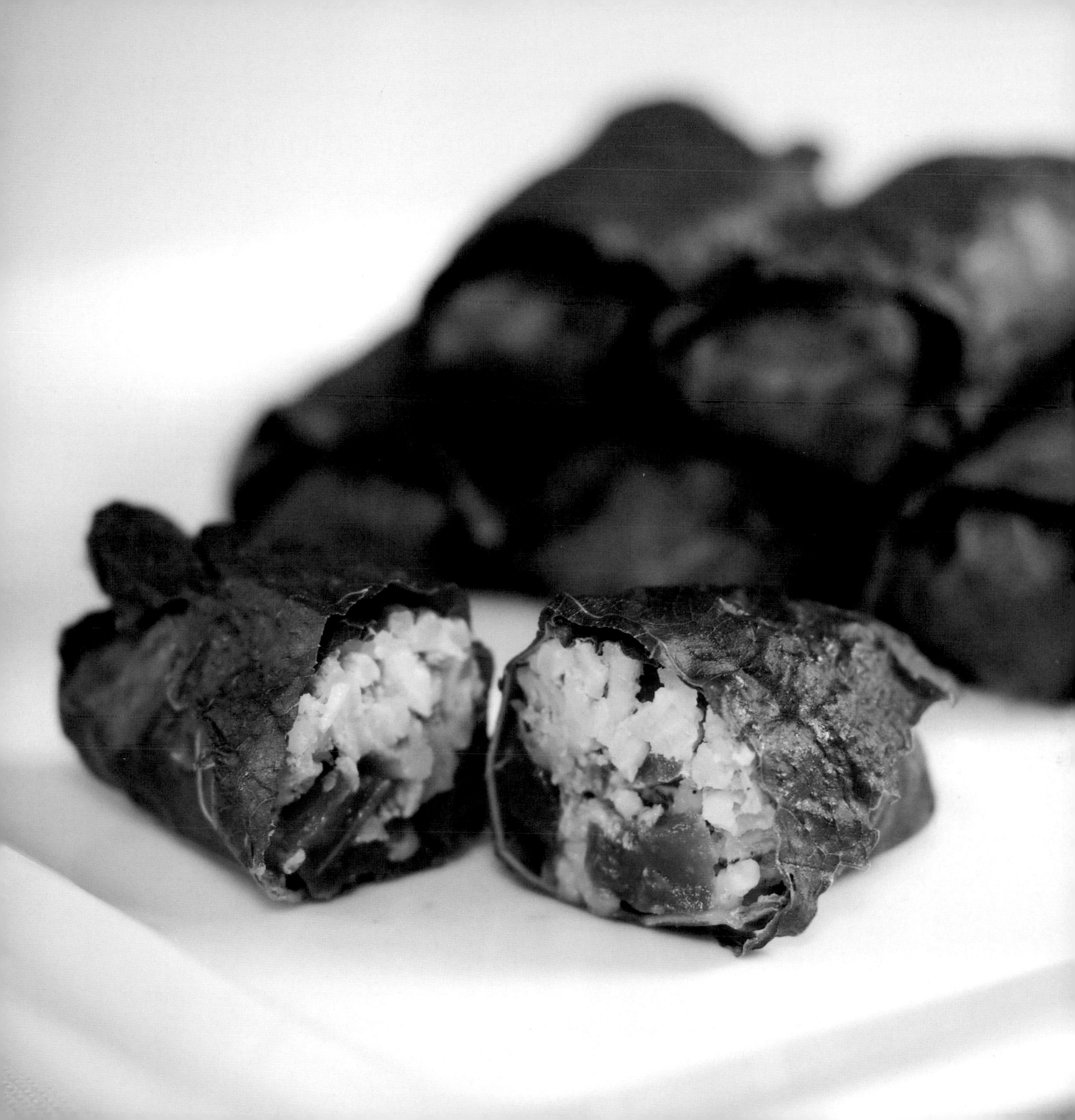

sun-dried olive and tomato tuna zucchini rounds

MAKES 24 ROUNDS | TOTAL TIME 15 MINUTES | ACTIVE TIME 15 MINUTES

Crackers are so passé … using veggie rounds as a base for appetizers is much more fun. These adorable, earthy nibbles are piled with decadent sun-dried olives, tomatoes, herbed tuna and melted cheese. You can use any good black olive if you can't find sun-dried. This Mediterranean-inspired appy is healthy and delicious.

INGREDIENTS

2 large zucchini

2 ounces canned tuna, drained

3 sun-dried black olives, pitted and chopped

1 teaspoon chopped sun-dried tomato

1 teaspoon mayonnaise

3 fresh basil leaves, chopped

½ cup shredded Asiago cheese

Freshly ground black pepper

METHOD

Preheat oven to 400°F. Chop zucchini on an angle into ½-inch-thick rounds; place on a lightly oiled baking sheet. In a small bowl, combine tuna, olives, sun-dried tomato, mayonnaise and basil. Spoon mixture onto zucchini rounds. Top each with 1 teaspoon cheese. Bake for 5 minutes. Remove from oven and season with ground pepper.

TO SERVE

Arrange rounds on a serving platter, and let them cool for 1 to 2 minutes before serving.

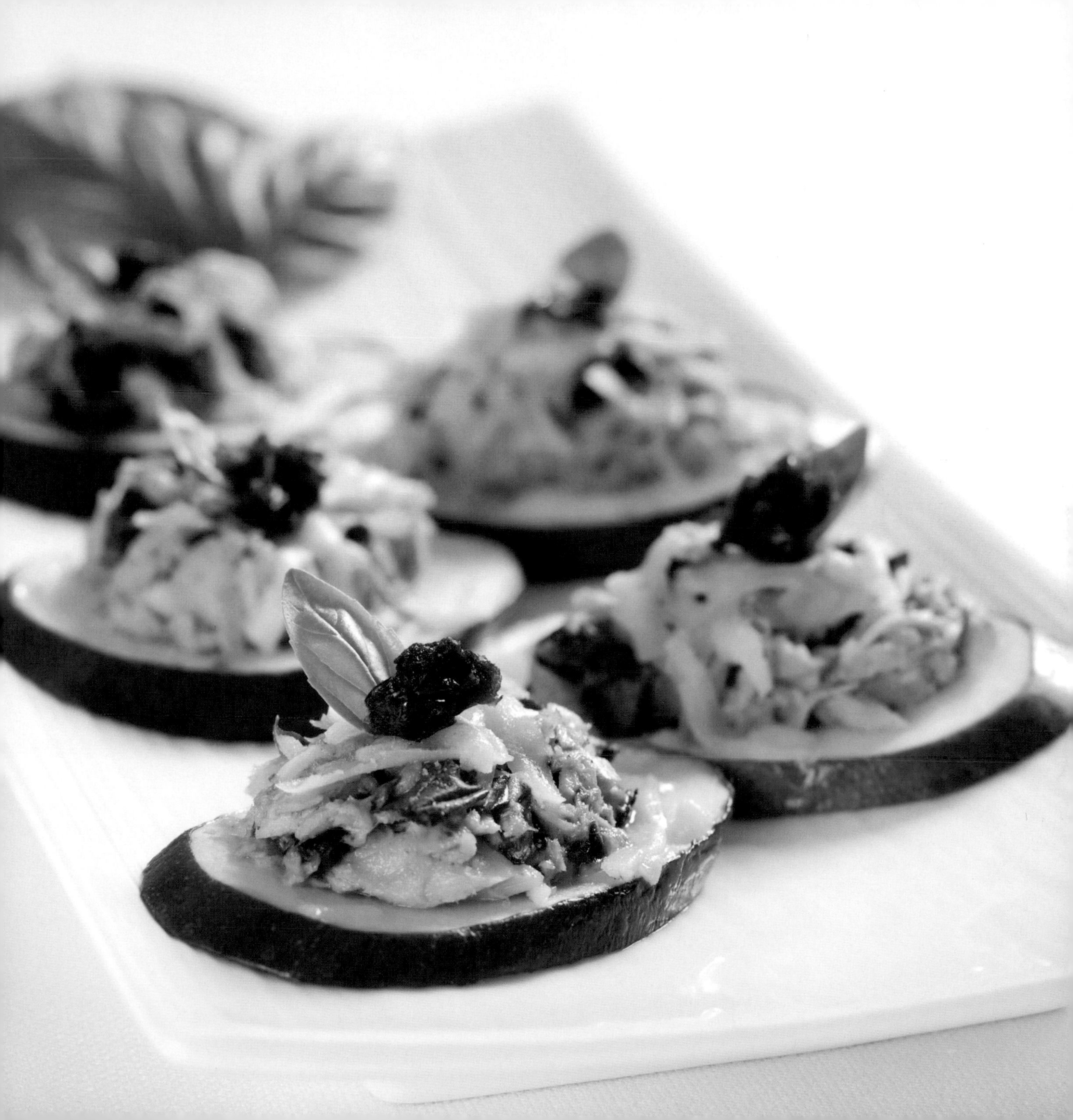

caramelized onion and balsamic cherry jam

SERVES 6 TO 8 | TOTAL TIME 50 MINUTES | ACTIVE TIME 50 MINUTES

This sophisticated "jam" is inspired by a Williams-Sonoma version I really enjoyed. This one, with dried cherries and sweet onion, is even tastier. Savoury and intense, the jam is fantastic as a dip or served with chicken or other grilled meats. Bring a jar as a hostess gift and you'll be one popular gal.

INGREDIENTS

3 tablespoons butter

3 large sweet onions, chopped into 1-inch-thick pieces

4 cloves garlic, halved

Dash of salt and freshly ground black pepper

⅓ cup granulated sugar

⅔ cup balsamic vinegar

½ cup dried cherries

1 cinnamon stick

METHOD

Melt butter in a large saucepan over medium-low heat. Add onions, garlic, salt and pepper. Sauté for 15 minutes, stirring frequently.

Stir in sugar; cook for 2 minutes. Add vinegar, cherries and cinnamon stick; cook for 30 minutes over low heat, stirring occasionally. Remove from heat and discard cinnamon stick.

TO SERVE

Scoop up warm or room-temperature jam with crusty bread cut into squares, or serve as a garnish with grilled meats..

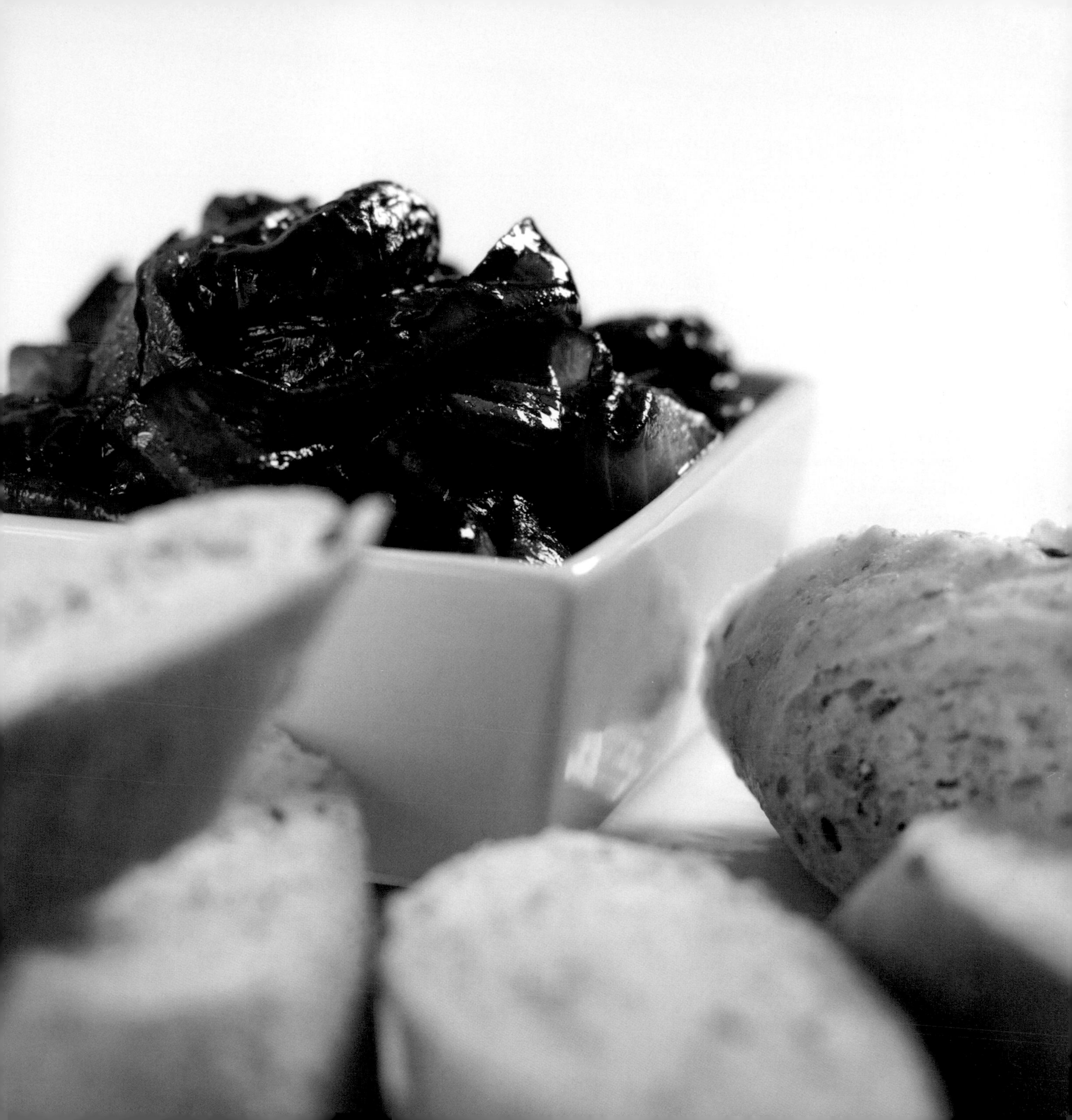

gourmet seven layer dip

SERVES 8 TO 10 | TOTAL TIME 40 MINUTES | ACTIVE TIME 25 MINUTES

If you're a fan of Mexican seven-layer dip (and who isn't?), you'll love this fresh, upscale and very delicious version. The roasted red pepper, artichoke hearts, Swiss cheese and cilantro make the flavour pop. I know you gourmet gals could make your own refried beans, but it takes such an awfully long time. So bring out the can opener and enjoy this dip hours sooner. Your friends will thank you for it.

INGREDIENTS

1 red pepper

1 (14-ounce) can refried beans

2 medium avocados

1 cup sour cream

1 (6-ounce) jar artichoke hearts

5 ounces Swiss or Gruyère cheese, shredded

½ cup chopped fresh cilantro

METHOD

To roast the red pepper, broil it directly on the oven rack under medium-high heat, turning occasionally, until the skin is blackened and blistery, about 10 to 15 minutes. Remove from oven and place in a paper bag for about 10 minutes to let cool and allow the skin to separate from the flesh.

Meanwhile, prepare the dip. Evenly spread refried beans into a large round or square serving platter. Cut avocados in half, remove pits and scoop flesh into a small bowl; mash with a fork until smooth. Spread avocado evenly over the beans. Spread sour cream over top the avocado. Chop artichoke hearts, discarding any tough pieces; arrange on sour cream. Finally, sprinkle cheese over top.

Remove the red pepper from the bag and gently slide the skin off. Remove the core and seeds. Chop the pepper into small pieces and sprinkle over the cheese layer. Finish dip with a sprinkle of cilantro.

TO SERVE

Serve with corn chips. If well covered, this dip keeps in the refrigerator for several days.

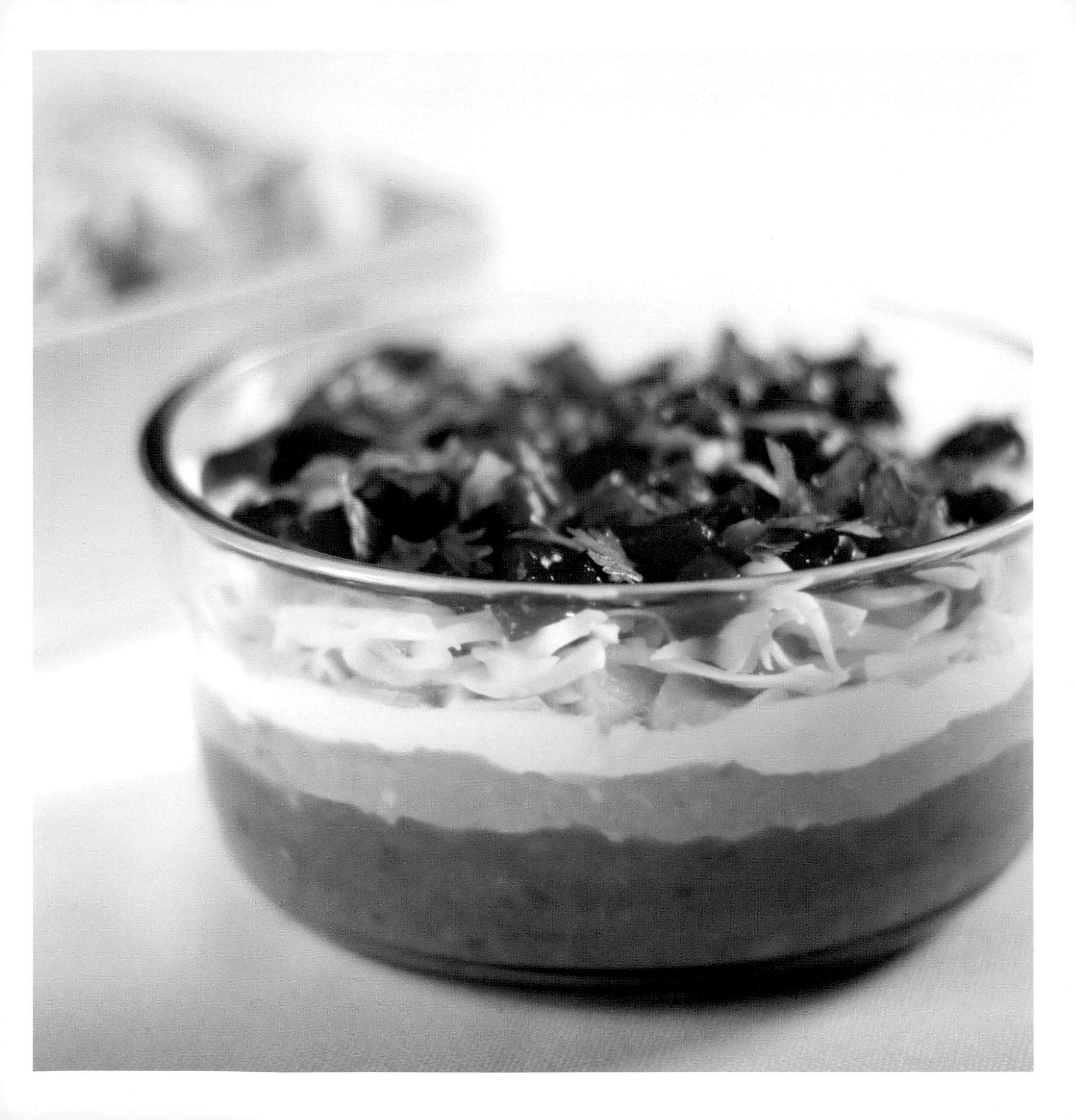

roasted garlic, sirloin meatball and toasted pita skewers

SERVES 6 TO 8 | TOTAL TIME 1 HOUR 40 MINUTES | ACTIVE TIME 40 MINUTES

Deconstruct your sandwich and get tremendous flavour in just one bite. Not only will the pregnant ladies love these skewers, so will your guy friends. They won't last long on the buffet table. Roasted garlic is mellow enough for even delicate tummies.

FOR SKEWERS

1 head garlic

Olive oil, for drizzling

3 to 4 Greek-style pitas

Kosher salt

12 to 16 bamboo skewers

MEATBALLS

2 tablespoons olive oil

½ cup onion, finely chopped

2 cloves garlic, minced

1 pound ground sirloin

½ cup dry bread crumbs

2 eggs

2 tablespoons soy sauce

½ teaspoon prepared horseradish

2 dashes of Worcestershire sauce

Salt and freshly ground black pepper

METHOD

Preheat oven to 375°F. Cut the top (about ½ inch) off the head of garlic and remove as much of the papery outer layers as you can. Drizzle garlic lightly with olive oil. Wrap in foil and place directly on middle rack in oven. Bake for 45 minutes.

Meanwhile, to make the meatballs, heat 1 teaspoon of the olive oil in a heavy-bottomed pan over medium heat. Add onions and cook until translucent, about 5 minutes. In a bowl, combine cooked onions, minced garlic, ground sirloin, bread crumbs, eggs, soy sauce, horseradish and Worcestershire sauce. Season with salt and ground pepper. Form mixture into 25 to 30 meatballs, each approximately 1½ inches in diameter. Place on a lightly oiled baking sheet and bake, along with the garlic, for 20 minutes.

When garlic is roasted, remove from the oven and unwrap. Let cool for a few minutes, then gently squeeze the pulp out of each clove; set aside.

Turn broiler to high. Brush pitas with remaining olive oil and cut into eighths. Place on a baking sheet, sprinkle with kosher salt and broil for 3 minutes. Turn over and broil for 2 more minutes.

TO SERVE

Assemble skewers, using 2 meatballs, 2 pita pieces and 2 garlic cloves for each, alternating ingredients as you go.

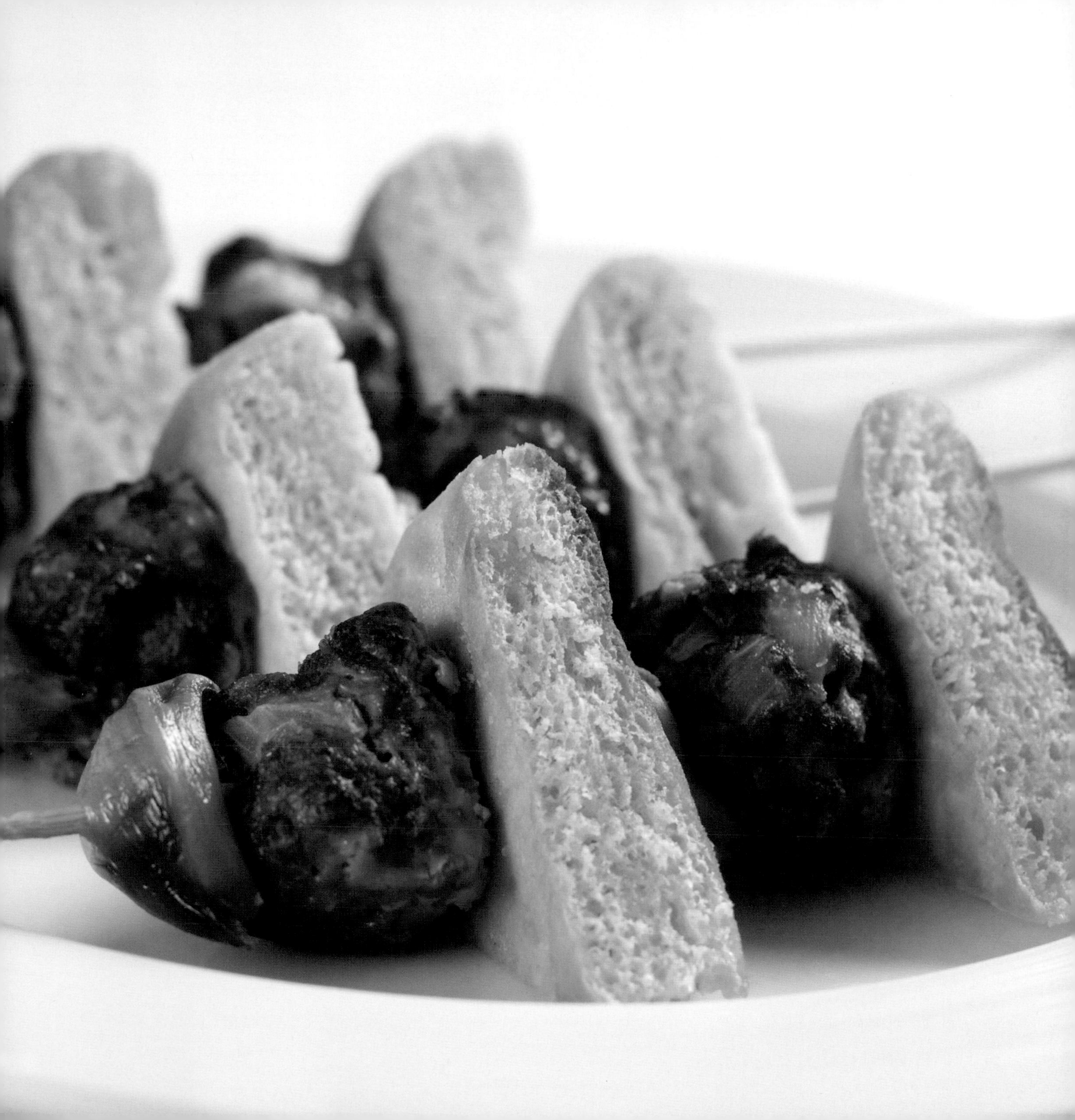

rustic sesame vegetable tart

SERVES 12 | TOTAL TIME 60 MINUTES | ACTIVE TIME 40 MINUTES

Incredibly satisfying, this rich, buttery tart is filled with sautéed vegetables. Like a pizza but without the cheese, this memorable appetizer will melt in your mouth. Rub your tummy as you eat it so that your baby can enjoy it too.

DOUGH

2½ cups all-purpose flour

½ cup butter, cubed

1 teaspoon salt

1 teaspoon granulated sugar

¾ cup cold water

FILLING

1 tablespoon olive oil

1 red onion, thinly sliced

1 red pepper, thinly sliced

1 zucchini, thinly sliced

Salt and freshly ground black pepper

1 tablespoon pure sesame oil

1 teaspoon sesame seeds

METHOD

To make the dough, in a food processor on low speed, combine flour, butter, salt and sugar. Continue to process as you add the water, ¼ cup at a time. Using your hands, shape the dough into a ball and flatten. Wrap in plastic wrap and refrigerate for 30 minutes.

Preheat oven to 375°F. Heat olive oil in a large saucepan over medium heat. Add onion, red pepper and zucchini. Season with salt and ground pepper. Sauté for 10 minutes, stirring occasionally. Remove from heat and sprinkle in sesame oil. Meanwhile, spread sesame seeds on a baking sheet and toast in oven for 3 to 5 minutes, until golden brown.

Flour a countertop or cutting board and roll the dough out into a large circle, approximately 15 inches in diameter. Place on an oiled baking sheet and spoon vegetable mixture into centre. Sprinkle with half of the toasted sesame seeds, fold in the edges of the dough and sprinkle with remaining sesame seeds. Bake for 20 minutes.

TO SERVE

Slice into 12 triangular slices. Serve warm.

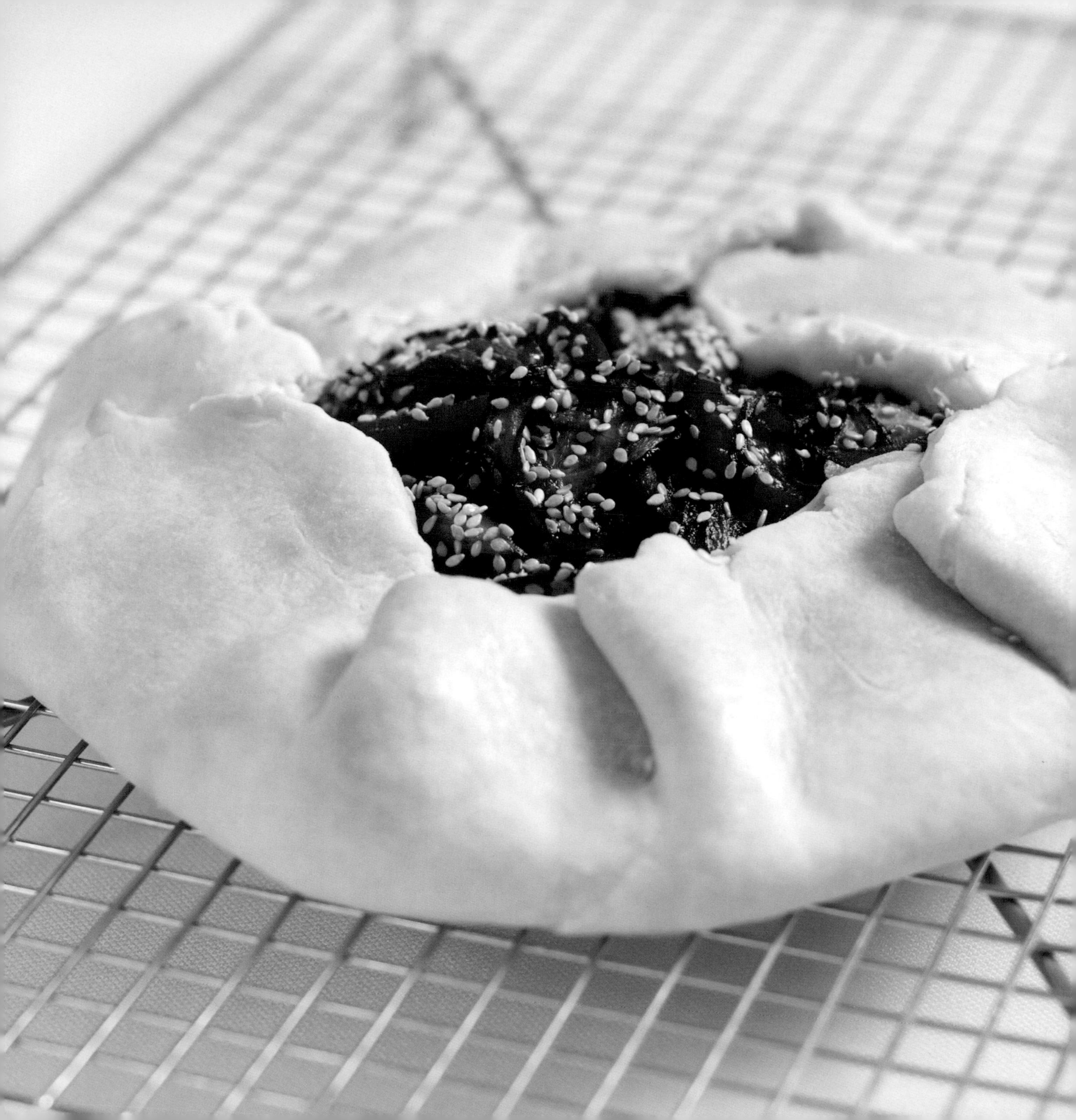

hazelnut, avocado and garlic whole-wheat crostinis

MAKES 12 TO 16 | TOTAL TIME 40 MINUTES | ACTIVE TIME 25 MINUTES

Garlic bread gets a major makeover with this fabulously tasty nibble. The smooth texture of the avocado and the crunch of the hazelnuts are a perfect match. Such a pretty presentation too, just like pregnant you.

INGREDIENTS

½ cup raw hazelnuts, skin on
¼ cup butter, softened
1 teaspoon fresh lemon juice
2 cloves garlic, crushed
1 whole-wheat French baguette
2 ripe avocados
½ teaspoon lemon zest

METHOD

Preheat oven to 350°F. Spread hazelnuts on a baking sheet and toast in oven for 15 minutes. Remove from oven and let cool slightly. Once hazelnuts are cool to the touch, using a towel or your fingers, rub off the skins. Using a mortar and pestle, coarsely grind the nuts.

Turn broiler to high. In a small bowl, combine butter, lemon juice and garlic. Cut bread at an angle into thick slices and spread with the lemon butter. Broil on a baking sheet for 4 minutes or until lightly browned. Remove skin and pit from avocados and discard; thinly slice avocado. Top baguette slices with avocado and crushed hazelnuts, and a sprinkling of lemon zest.

TO SERVE

Arrange crostinis on a platter and serve immediately.

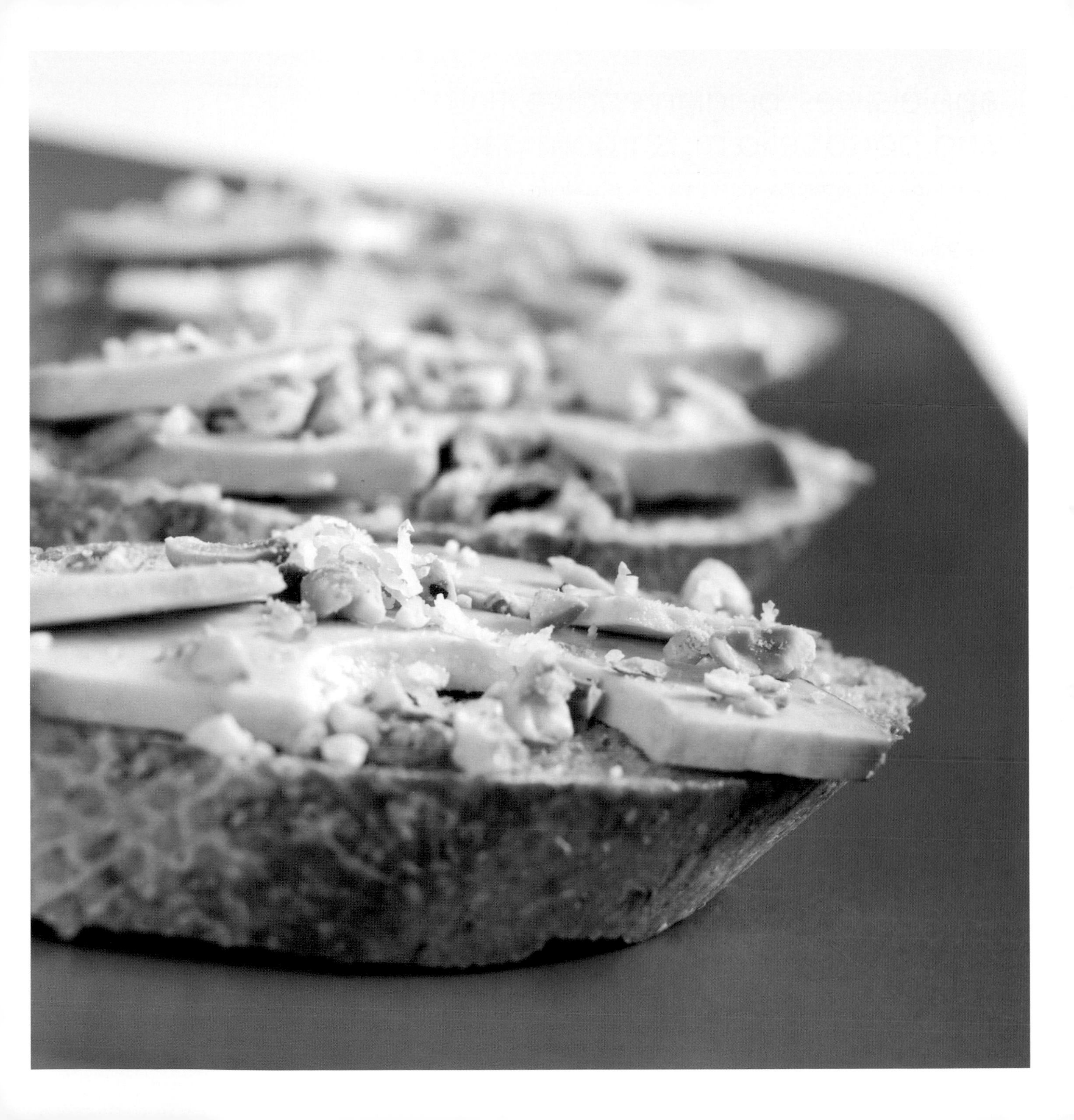

apple slices, belgian endive, flatbreads and portobello mushroom pâté

SERVES 6 TO 8 | TOTAL TIME 20 MINUTES | ACTIVE TIME 20 MINUTES

Traditional pâté is taboo for us moms-to-be, but I think this Portobello mushroom version is better anyway. The texture is meaty and the flavour is splendid. With tart crunchy apples, soft bread and tasty endive, you can keep scooping until you're full.

INGREDIENTS

2 tablespoons butter

1 small onion, chopped

1 clove garlic, chopped

2 large Portobello mushroom caps

1 teaspoon dried tarragon, plus a pinch for garnish

1 cup sliced almonds

2 tablespoons cream cheese

2 tablespoons fresh lemon juice

2 tablespoons soy sauce

Salt and freshly ground black pepper

1 to 2 red or green apples

1 head Belgian endive

METHOD

Thoroughly wash the mushroom caps. Scoop out the gills with a spoon and discard. Chop mushrooms. Melt butter in a frying pan over medium heat; add onion, garlic, mushrooms and tarragon. Sauté until vegetables are tender and golden. Transfer mushroom mixture to a food processor or to a bowl if using a hand blender. Add almonds, cream cheese, lemon juice and soy sauce, blending to combine. Season with salt and ground pepper.

Slice apples. Separate and rinse Belgian endive leaves.

TO SERVE

Spoon pâté into a small serving bowl and garnish with a light dusting of tarragon. Serve with sliced apples, Belgian endive, flatbread or crackers and breads of your choice, arranged on a platter around the dish of pâté.

The pâté can be prepared up to 2 days in advance. Serve cold or warm (heat in microwave).

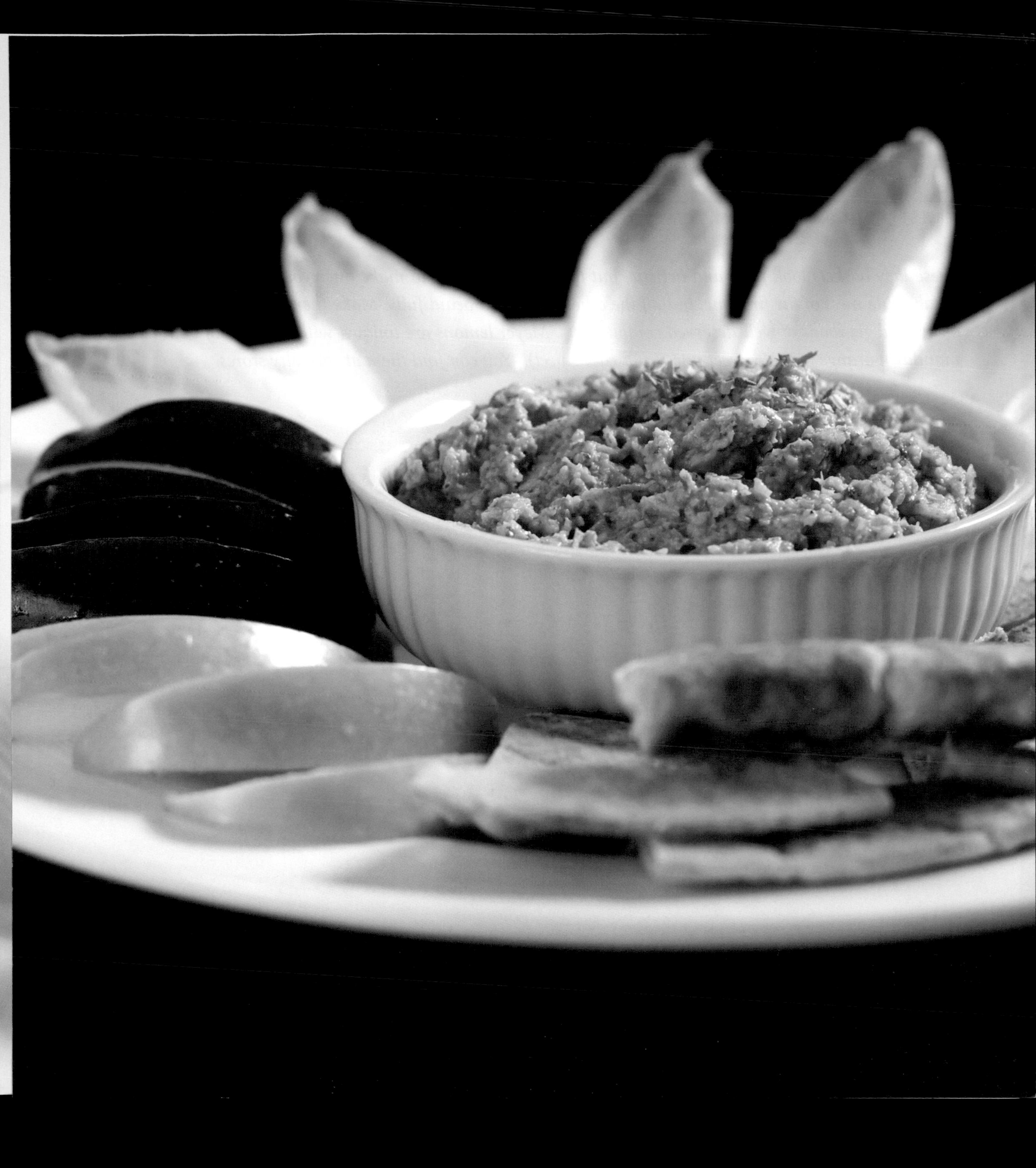

fresh tomato, basil and bocconcini skewers with lemon olive oil

MAKES 6 | TOTAL TIME 1 HOUR 30 MINUTES | ACTIVE TIME 20 MINUTES

This is a classic appetizer, but adding homemade lemon-infused oil makes it ultramodern and extra tasty. I can just picture the Take Home Chef coming to my house to help me make it. He's so handsome that I would whip up some fancy desserts to entice him to stay!

INGREDIENTS

¼ cup olive oil

Zest of 1 lemon

Juice from ¼ lemon

18 cherry tomatoes

12 small bocconcini (small fresh mozzarella balls)

12 fresh basil leaves

6 bamboo skewers

METHOD

Combine the olive oil, lemon zest and lemon juice; set aside for at least 1 hour to allow flavour to develop. Strain to remove the zest.

To assemble skewers, alternate between cherry tomatoes and bocconcini wrapped in a basil leaf. Repeat until each skewer has 3 tomatoes and 2 bocconcini.

TO SERVE

Artfully drizzle with the lemon-infused olive oil. Finish with a generous sprinkle of salt and freshly ground black pepper. Serve with crusty bread, if desired.

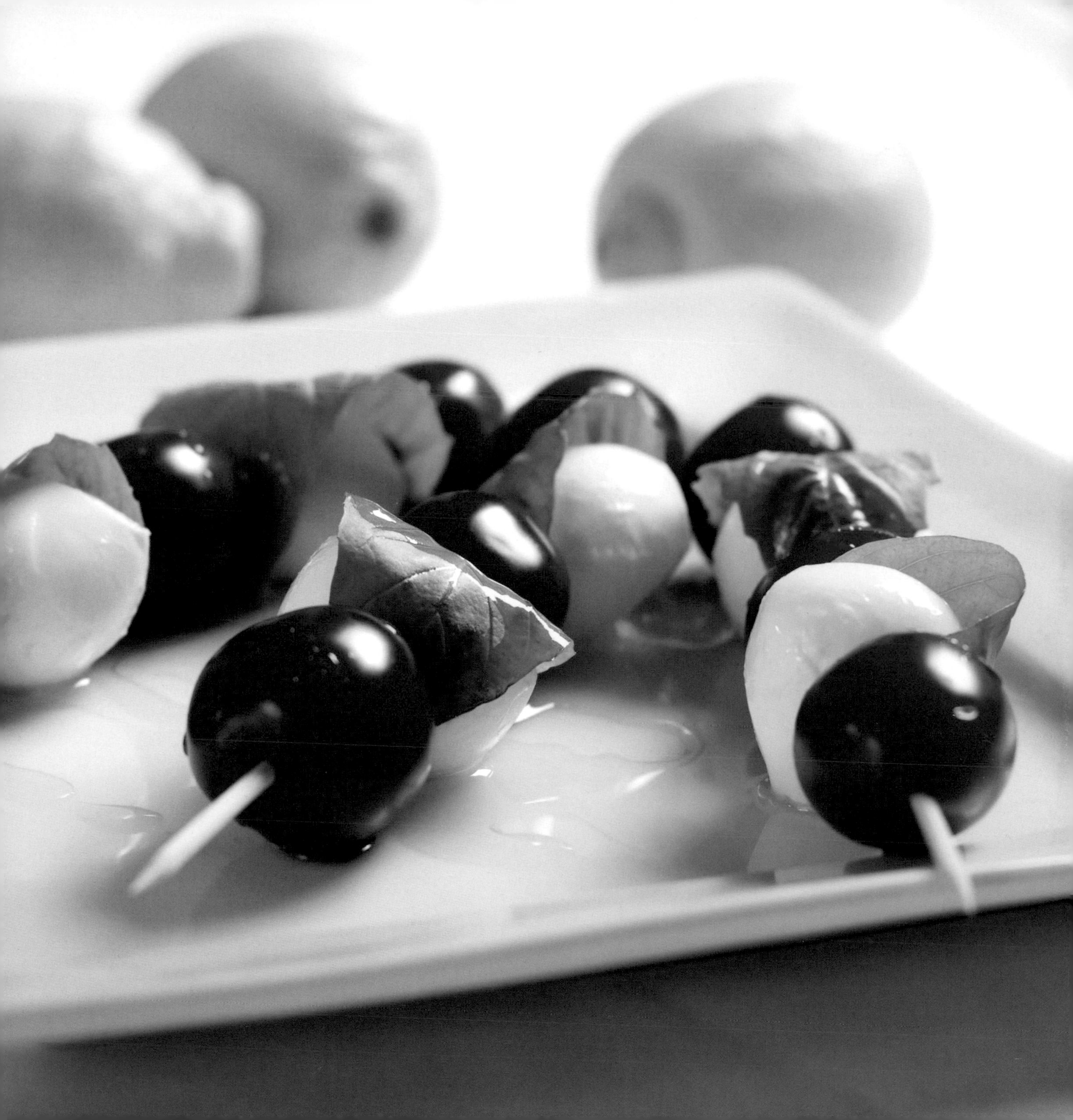

white cheddar with pear compote and walnuts

SERVES 4 | TOTAL TIME 40 MINUTES | ACTIVE TIME 25 MINUTES

This satisfying cheese dish is a great appetizer or dessert for those craving something substantial but not too sweet. The balsamic pear compote is so intensely flavourful (try using fig balsamic for even more flavour). Your baby suggests you have another bite!

INGREDIENTS

3 pears, peeled, cored and diced

½ cup loosely packed brown sugar

¼ cup halved walnuts

3 tablespoons good-quality balsamic vinegar

8 ¼-inch-thick slices white cheddar cheese

METHOD

In a saucepan, stir together pears, sugar, walnuts and balsamic vinegar. Cook for about 20 minutes over medium-low heat, stirring occasionally, until the pears are reduced and very tender. Cool for at least 15 minutes in the refrigerator before plating.

TO SERVE

On each plate, stack 2 slices of cheese. Spoon a generous amount of compote over top.

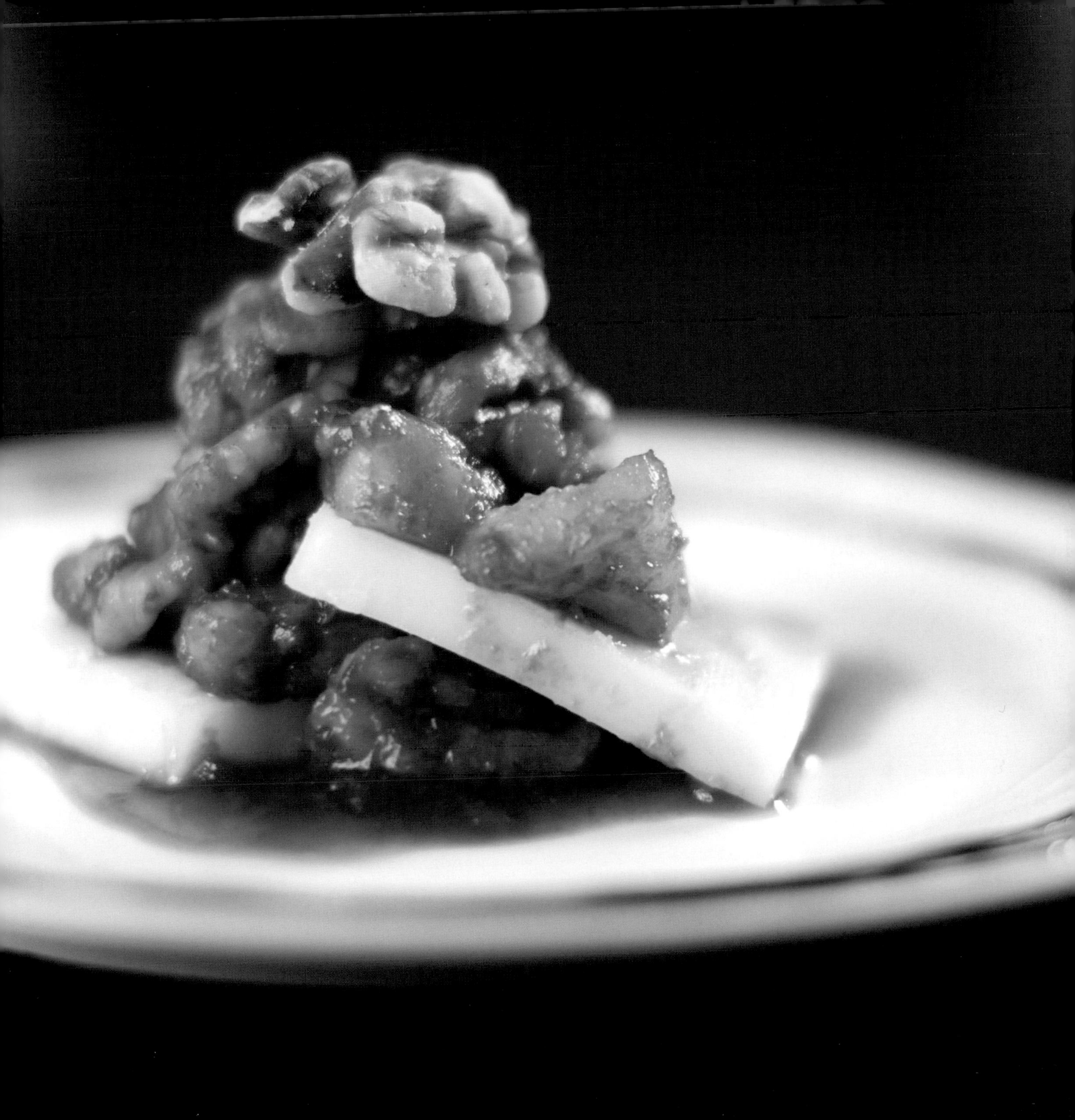

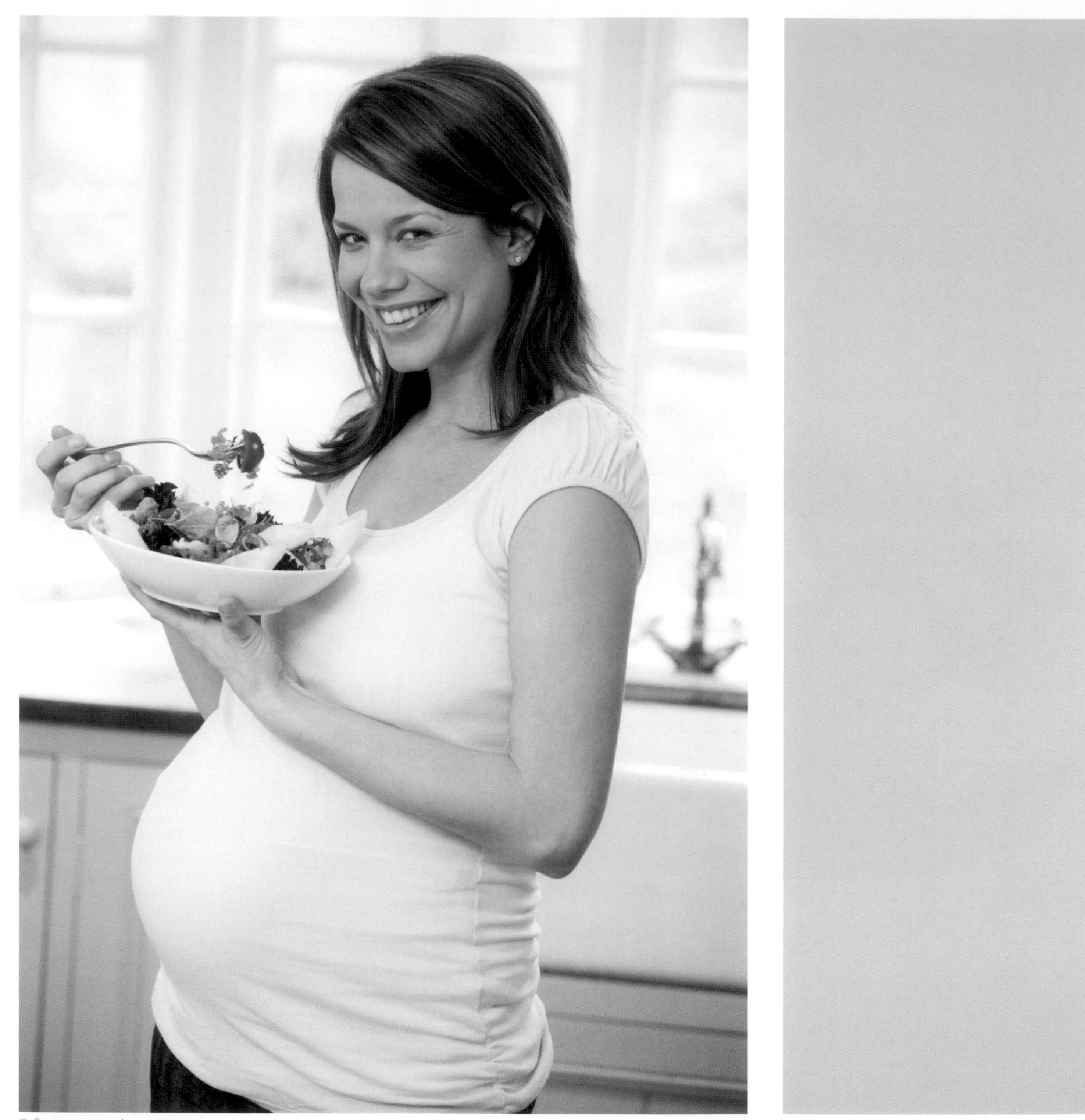

since your tummy might already feel full:

lighter fare

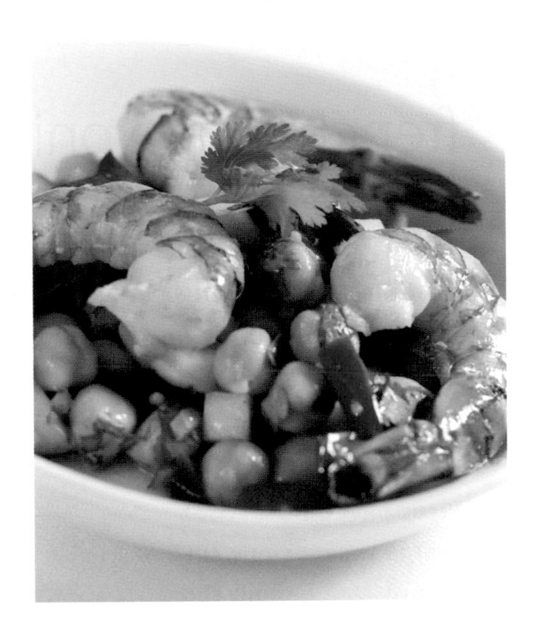

"Cooking is like love, it should be entered into with abandon or not at all."

~ *Harriet Van Horne*

butternut squash and carrot ginger soup with crème fraîche

SERVES 8 TO 10 | TOTAL TIME 1 HOUR | ACTIVE TIME 1 HOUR

If you're feeling a wee bit off, the ginger in this smooth and mellow soup will set your tummy right. It's an ideal lunch or dinner for a blustery or chilly day and full of wholesome flavour. The cilantro adds a delicate touch of spring.

CRÈME FRAÎCHE

1 cup sour cream, chilled

1 cup heavy (35% MF) cream, chilled

SOUP

2 tablespoons olive oil

½ large onion, chopped

4 cups chicken stock

1 pound carrots, peeled and chopped

1 large sweet potato, peeled and chopped

1 butternut squash, peeled and chopped

2 tablespoons chopped ginger

½ (10-ounce) can coconut milk

1 teaspoon curry powder

½ teaspoon ground cumin

½ teaspoon cinnamon

Salt and freshly ground black pepper

Fresh cilantro leaves, for garnish

METHOD

To make the crème fraîche, mix together the sour cream and heavy cream with a blender until thick, about 5 minutes. Refrigerate until ready to use.

Meanwhile, to make the soup, heat olive oil in a large pot over medium-high heat. Add onion and cook until golden and tender. Pour in chicken stock and bring to a boil. Add carrots, sweet potato and butternut squash; simmer, covered, for 25 to 30 minutes or until vegetable pieces are very tender and starting to fall apart. Add ginger, curry powder, cumin and cinnamon. Season with salt and ground pepper. Reduce heat to medium-low and cook for 5 to 10 minutes. Remove from heat and add coconut milk. Let soup cool somewhat, then, using a hand blender, purée in the pot, making sure to remove all lumps.

TO SERVE

Half fill bowls with soup and add a dollop of crème fraîche to each. Top with a sprig of cilantro. Serve with crusty bread and butter if desired.

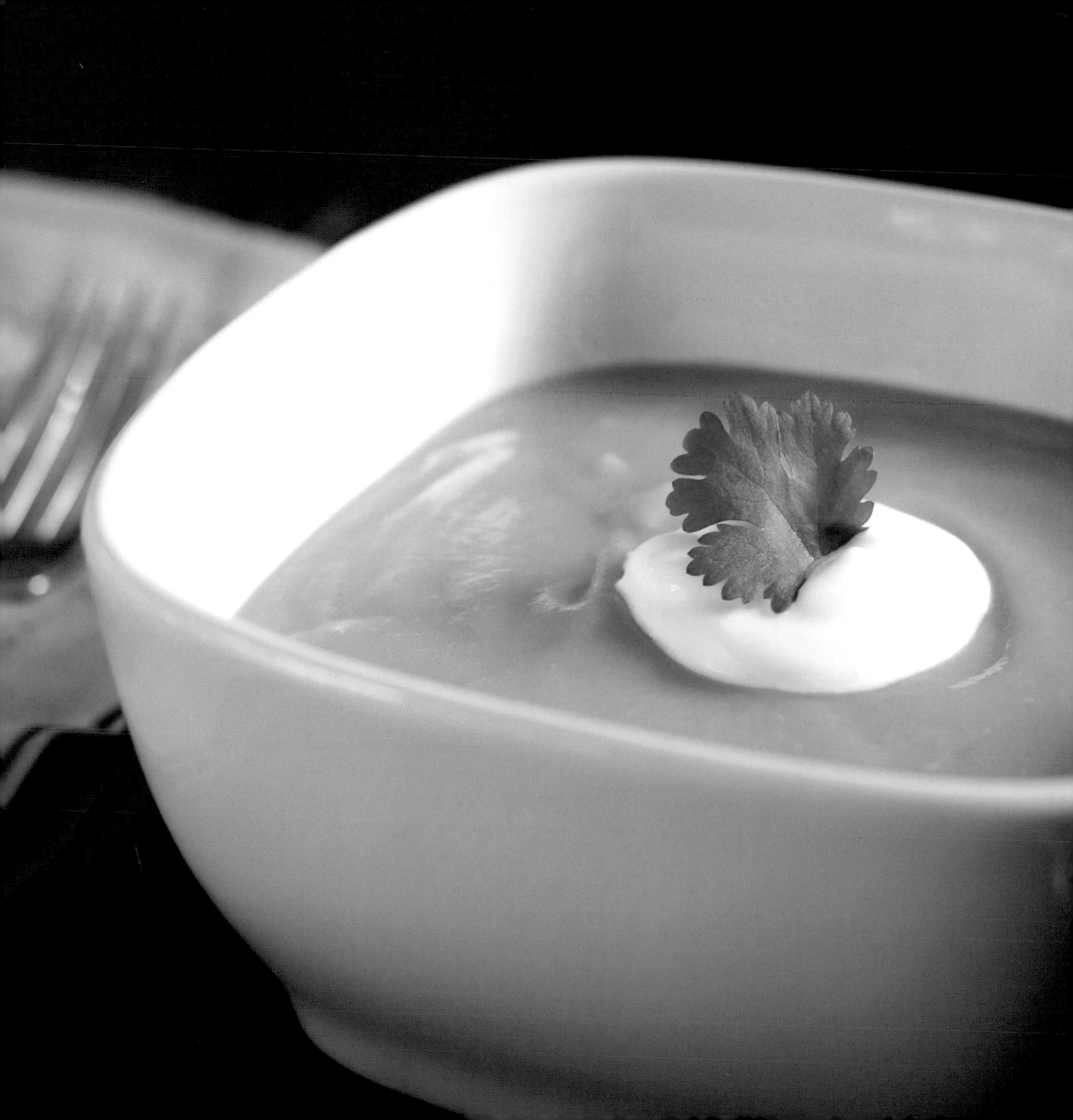

salmon, white asparagus and dill pea salad

SERVES 4 | TOTAL TIME 30 MINUTES | ACTIVE TIME 30 MINUTES

I love this dish as a cold salad when it's hot outside, and with warm salmon and asparagus otherwise. The dill peas really pop in this light and lively meal. Use green asparagus if you can't find white.

INGREDIENTS

1 pound spring salmon (or 4 medium fillets), skin on

Fresh lemon juice (approx 1 tablespoon)

Salt and freshly ground black pepper

2 tablespoons pine nuts

8 stalks white asparagus

½ cup plain yogurt

1½ cup fresh green peas

2 tablespoons finely chopped fresh dill

½ tablespoon prepared horseradish

½ shallot, minced

2 cups fresh mixed greens

1 carrot, grated

METHOD

Preheat oven to 350°F. Place salmon skin down on foil-lined baking sheet. Sprinkle with lemon juice, salt and ground pepper. Bake for 10 to 12 minutes or until fish flakes easily when tested with a fork. Remove and set aside to cool; remove and discard skin.

Spread pine nuts on a baking sheet and toast in the oven for 3 to 5 minutes or until golden brown.

Steam asparagus for 8 to 10 minutes, seasoning with dashes of lemon juice, salt and pepper. Set aside to cool.

In a small bowl, combine yogurt, peas, dill, horseradish and shallot. Season with ground pepper.

TO SERVE

Distribute greens among 4 individual serving plates. Top with dilled peas, salmon, asparagus, grated carrot and toasted pine nuts.

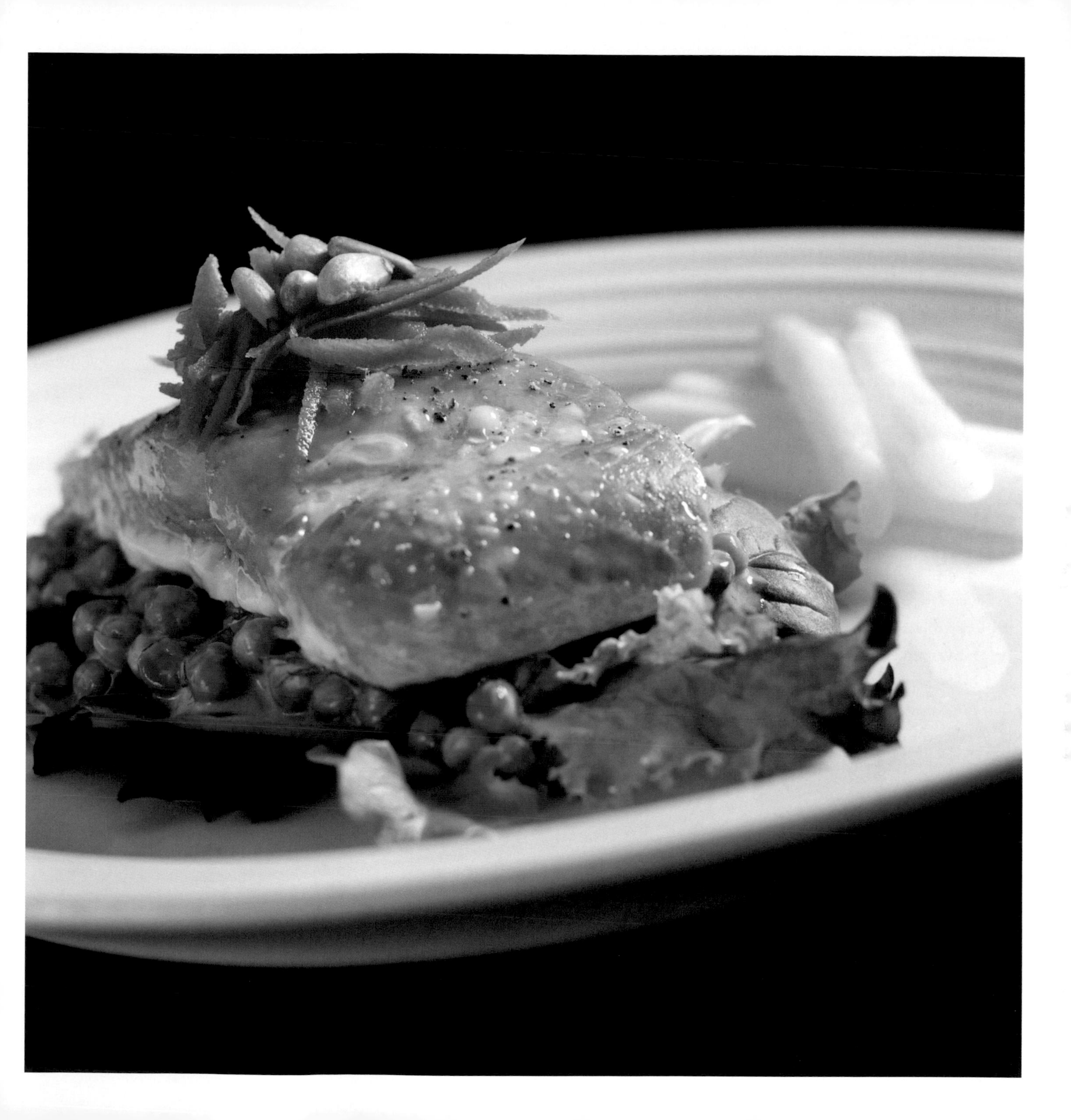

lemongrass tiger prawn and chickpea salad

SERVES 4 | TOTAL TIME 25 MINUTES | ACTIVE TIME 25 MINUTES

Aromatic lemongrass lends a fresh quality to this dish of juicy, plump prawns and earthy chickpeas. Sit down and relax with this simple yet elegant meal, and let it nourish you to the core.

SALAD

1 (19-ounce) can chickpeas, drained and rinsed

½ cup diced zucchini

¼ cup chopped red pepper

¼ cup chopped fresh cilantro

1 tablespoon olive oil

12 jumbo tiger prawns, peeled and deveined, tails on

DRESSING

¼ cup olive oil

2 tablespoons champagne vinegar

1 tablespoon minced shallot

1 tablespoon grated lemongrass

½ tablespoon fresh lemon juice

2 cloves garlic, crushed

Salt and freshly ground black pepper

METHOD

In a large bowl, toss chickpeas with the zucchini, red pepper and cilantro.

To make the dressing, combine the olive oil, vinegar, shallot, lemongrass, lemon juice and half of the garlic. Pour over salad and toss to coat. Season with salt and ground pepper.

Heat 1 tablespoon of olive oil in a large saucepan over medium heat. Add the remaining garlic and cook for 1 minute. Add prawns and cook for about 1 minute per side, until pink.

TO SERVE

Spoon salad into individual bowls or plates. Top with 3 prawns per serving.

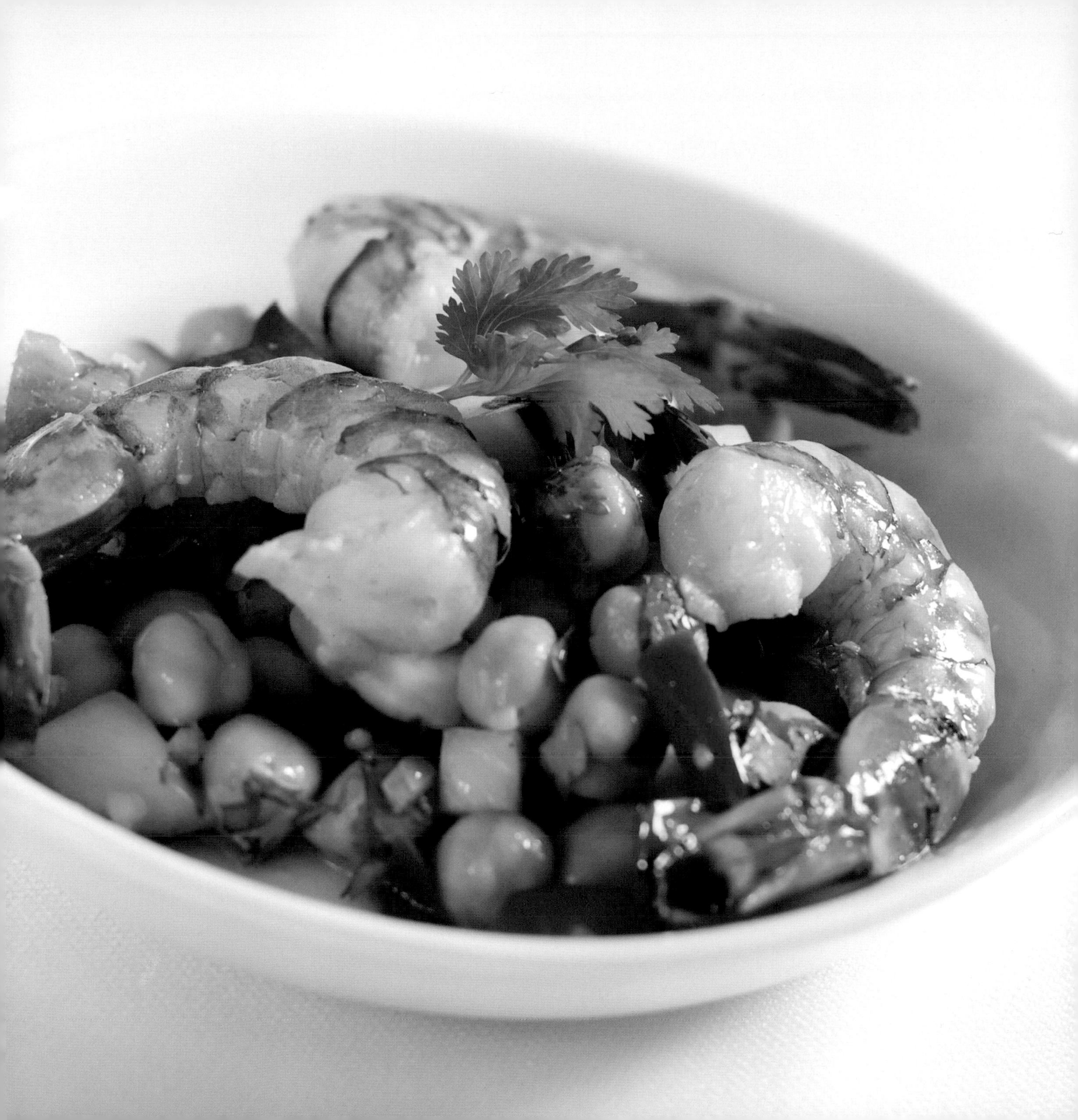

sesame cashew red cabbage noodle salad

SERVES 4 | TOTAL TIME 30 MINUTES | ACTIVE TIME 20 MINUTES

Nutty and crunchy, this beautifully presented salad could be a menu item at any fine restaurant. If you're in a salad rut, shake things up with this splendid dish. It's a colourful and exciting starter for dinner with your sweetie, or when entertaining several guests.

SALAD

1 cup extra-fine egg noodles

2 teaspoons sesame oil

⅔ cup cashews

2 tablespoons sesame seeds

1 small bunch baby spinach, stems removed

1 avocado, pitted, peeled and thinly sliced

¼ red cabbage, finely chopped

1 carrot, shredded

1 small tomato, diced

DRESSING

6 tablespoons olive oil

2 tablespoons champagne vinegar

1 tablespoon fresh lemon juice

1 clove garlic, minced

½ shallot, minced

Dash of salt and freshly ground black pepper

METHOD

Cook egg noodles according to package instructions. Drain and toss with sesame oil in a bowl. Chill in the refrigerator.

Meanwhile, in a bowl, whisk together dressing ingredients; set aside.

Preheat oven to 400°F. Spread cashews on a baking sheet and toast in oven for 3 to 4 minutes. Remove and transfer to a bowl. Spread sesame seeds on baking sheet and toast for 3 to 4 minutes, until golden.

Rinse the spinach well; pat dry. Distribute among 4 dinner plates, arranging in the centre of each. Fan avocado slices around each serving of spinach. Top with cooled egg noodles, then cabbage, constructing a loose pyramid. Finally, top spinach with carrot, tomato and toasted cashews.

TO SERVE

Sprinkle toasted sesame seeds liberally over each salad; drizzle with dressing.

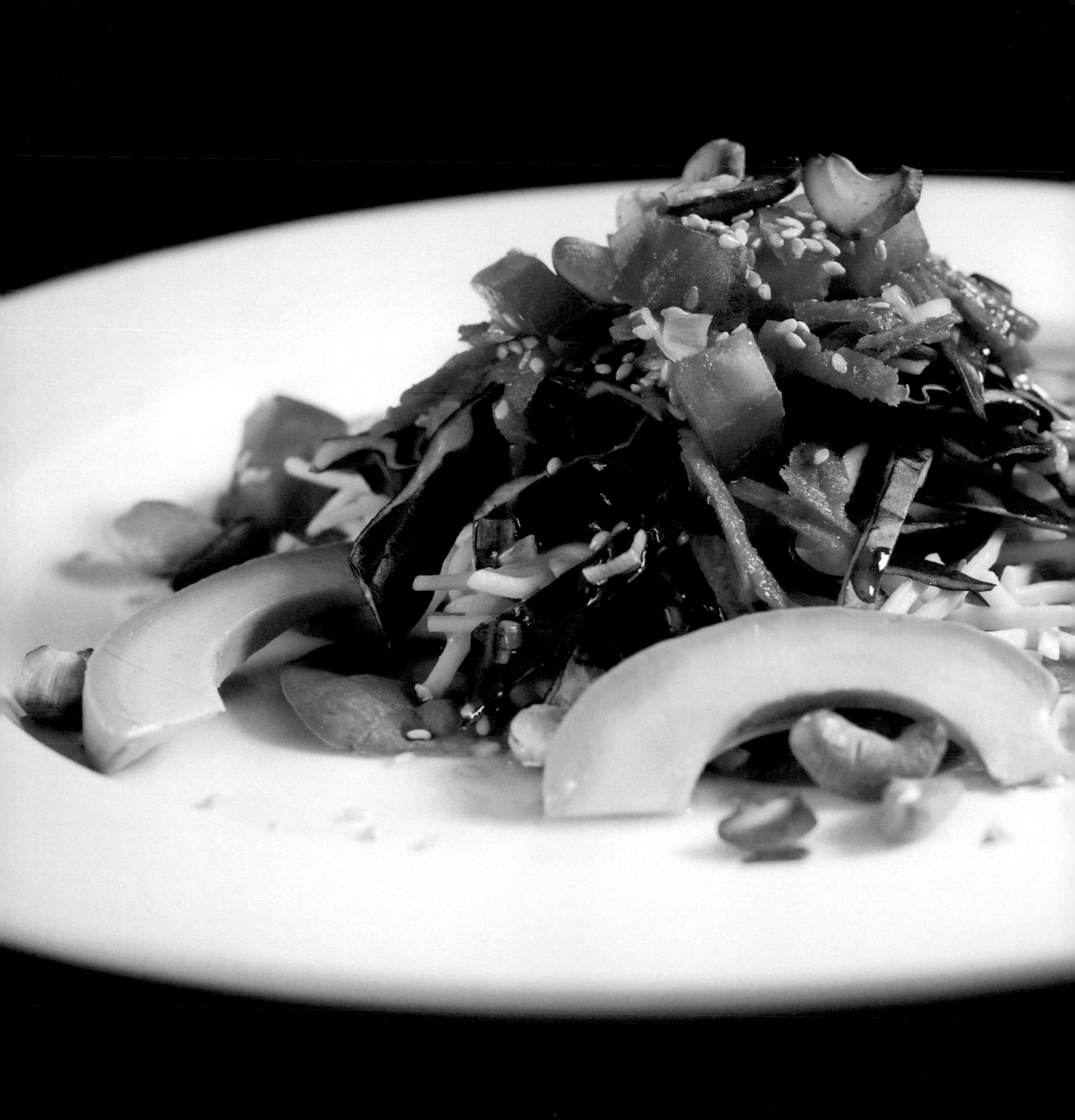

spiced caramelized cauliflower and candied curry pecan salad

SERVES 4 | TOTAL TIME 1 HOUR 40 MINUTES | ACTIVE TIME 30 MINUTES

Imagine you're on the TV competition Iron Chef, and the secret ingredient is … cauliflower! You'll be so pleased to have this sassy and splendid dish up your sleeve. You may think pecans and cauliflower are a quirky pairing, but it really works.

PECANS

2 cups pecans (pieces or halves)

1 egg white

¼ cup granulated sugar

2 teaspoons curry powder

1 teaspoon salt

CAULIFLOWER

1 head cauliflower, cut into sliced florets

3 tablespoons melted butter

1 tablespoon brown sugar

1 teaspoon paprika

½ teaspoon cinnamon

½ teaspoon ground cumin

Salt and freshly ground black pepper

Baby spinach leaves, for garnish (optional)

METHOD

To make the candied pecans, preheat oven to 250°F. Spread pecans on a baking sheet and toast in oven for about 10 minutes, until warm and fragrant. Meanwhile, in a bowl, whisk egg white. Add toasted pecans, granulated sugar, curry powder and salt. Mix well, then transfer to a oiled baking sheet. Spread pecans in a single layer and bake for 60 minutes.

Meanwhile, to prepare the cauliflower, in a large bowl, combine cauliflower, melted butter, brown sugar, paprika, cinnamon and cumin. Season with salt and ground pepper. Toss to coat.

When pecans are baked, remove from oven and increase temperature to 500°F. Place cauliflower on a baking sheet in a single layer and bake for 18 to 20 minutes.

TO SERVE

Serve cauliflower warm, tossed with the candied curry pecans. Garnish with baby spinach leaves (if using).

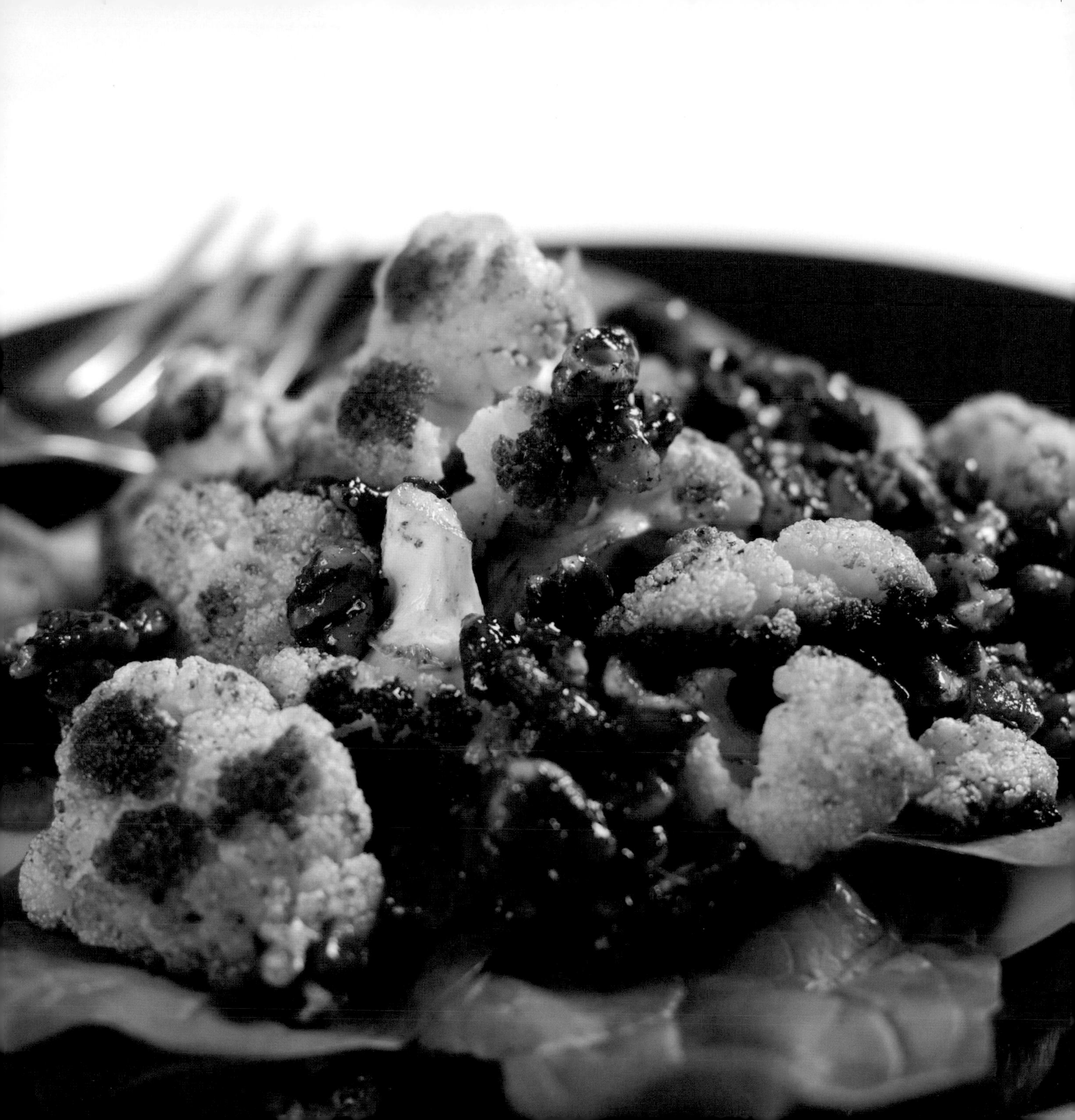

roasted balsamic vegetable panini with roasted garlic aioli

SERVES 8 | TOTAL TIME 1 HOUR 30 MINUTES | ACTIVE TIME 30 MINUTES

These delightful roasted vegetables are a staple in my home. I make big batches and serve them in appetizer platters, in rolls, wraps, salads and pasta dishes, and as side dishes. You're sure to love them in a panini-style sandwich with roasted garlic aioli, which is perfectly safe for pregnant ladies to eat.

GARLIC AIOLI

1 head garlic

4 heaping tablespoons low-fat mayonnaise

Salt and freshly ground black pepper

VEGETABLE PANINI

4 cloves garlic, quartered

1 red pepper, sliced ½ inch thick

1 green pepper, sliced ½ inch thick

1 red onion, sliced 1 inch thick

1 zucchini, sliced ½ inch thick

1 eggplant, sliced 1 inch thick

1 cup mushrooms, halved

½ cup olive oil

½ cup balsamic vinegar

1 tablespoon each dried rosemary, oregano and thyme

Salt and freshly ground black pepper

16 slices panini-style flatbread or large French bread

24 slices mozzarella cheese

METHOD

Preheat oven to 375°F. Cut the top (about ½ inch) off the head of garlic and remove as much of the papery outer layers as you can. Drizzle gently with olive oil. Wrap in foil. Bake directly on middle rack in oven for about 45 minutes.

Remove garlic and turn broiler to high. Place vegetables in a large container with a lid. Add vinegar, olive oil, rosemary, oregano and thyme. Season with salt and ground pepper. Toss vegetables to evenly coat. Spread in a single layer on a baking sheet and roast in the oven until fragrant and tender, about 20 to 25 minutes.

Let garlic cool for a few minutes, unwrap from foil then gently squeeze pulp out of each garlic clove and into a small bowl. Using a fork, mash garlic pulp well. Add mayonnaise, stirring gently to combine. Season with salt and ground pepper.

Preheat panini press or indoor grill. Spread garlic aioli on bread slices, then add layers of cheese and roasted vegetables. Press until bread is warm and cheese is melted.

TO SERVE

Cut each panini in half and serve individually.

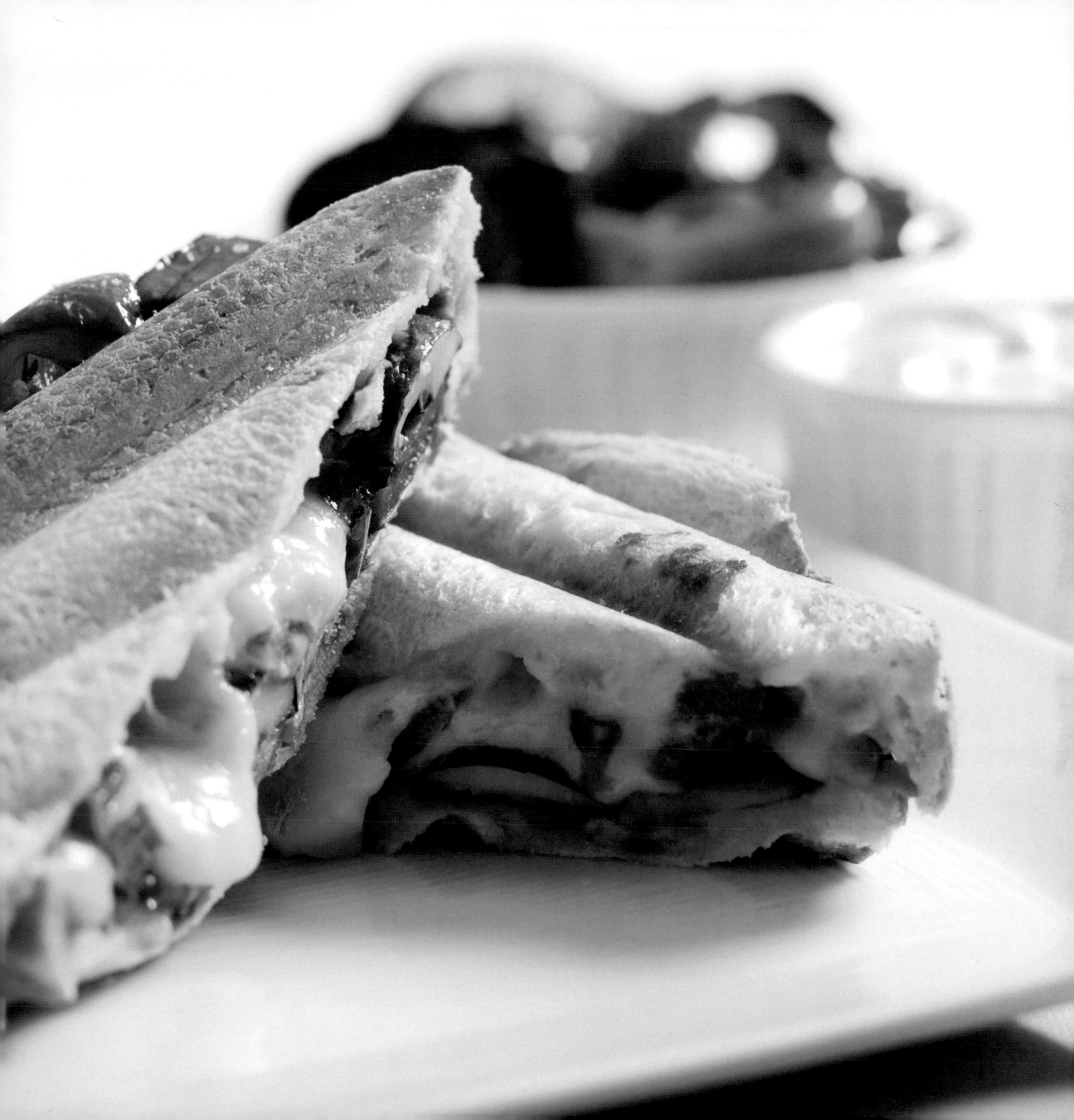

grilled pear and thai basil sandwich

SERVES 2 | TOTAL TIME 10 MINUTES | ACTIVE TIME 5 MINUTES

Grilled sandwiches are so classic and comforting, so we might as well give them a gourmet twist! The pear and Thai basil give this a fresh, bright flavour and make it extra special. These flavours will stand out beautifully and fulfill any cravings for cheesy, crispy or savoury foods. Thai basil is available at Asian markets and large grocery stores.

INGREDIENTS

10 fresh Thai basil leaves

1 pear, skin on, sliced very thinly

10 to 20 thin slices aged white cheddar cheese

4 slices sourdough bread

2 tablespoons butter

METHOD

Stack and roll the basil leaves; slice into thin strips. Heat a large pan over medium heat.

Layer one-quarter of the cheese on a slice of bread; top with half of the pear and another one-quarter of the cheese. Sprinkle with half of the basil. Top with a slice of bread. Repeat with the remaining ingredients to make a second sandwich. Thinly butter both slices of bread on one side; grill both sides until golden brown.

TO SERVE

Remove from pan and let stand for 1 to 2 minutes. Slice into halves and serve.

toasted three-cheese sandwich on homemade dill onion bread

SERVES 2 | TOTAL TIME 1 HOUR | ACTIVE TIME 30 MINUTES

My husband's dear granny passed down this recipe for dill bread. You don't need a breadmaker to prepare these fresh and fragrant loaves. Here, thick slices are grilled crisp with an ooey, gooey blend of glistening cheeses. Granny would be proud! You'll have plenty of leftover bread with this recipe, and you can serve it with soups and salads, or make other types of sandwiches (salmon is particularly tasty on dill bread). It also freezes well.

BREAD

1 tablespoon active dry yeast

½ cup warm water

2¼ teaspoon granulated sugar

1 small onion, finely chopped

1 egg

1 cup sour cream

4 tablespoons chopped fresh dill

1 tablespoon margarine, softened

1 teaspoon chopped fresh basil

1 teaspoon salt

3 cups all-purpose flour

EGG WASH

1 egg yolk

1 tablespoon water

FILLING

¼ cup shredded cheddar cheese

¼ cup shredded Swiss cheese

¼ cup grated Parmesan cheese

METHOD

Add yeast to warm water and ¼ teaspoon of the sugar; cover and let stand for about 10 minutes. Stir in the onion, egg, sour cream, dill, margarine, basil and salt. Stir in 2½ cups of the flour. Turn dough onto a flour-dusted surface and knead for 10 minutes, gradually adding the remaining ½ cup of flour (or more) as necessary if dough is too moist.

Let the dough rise in a large bowl in a warm, draft-free place until it at least doubles in size. Shape into 2 long loaves and place on a well-oiled baking sheet. Let rise for 20 minutes in a warm, draft-free place. In a small bowl, combine egg yolk and water. Brush loaves with the egg wash and bake at 350°F for 25 minutes.

Cut 4 slices of bread. Sprinkle each with the cheeses. Place open-faced under broiler (set on high) until cheese is melted and bubbly.

TO SERVE

Serve whole on individual plates.

chicken rosemary horseradish cream wrap

SERVES 2 | TOTAL TIME 20 MINUTES | ACTIVE TIME 20 MINUTES

Wraps are great meals for expectant moms, as you can stuff them full of so much fine food. Chicken, bacon and spinach are zested up with rosemary and horseradish cream in this superb dish. It'll keep you happy until it's time to get your blanket and wrap yourself up tight.

INGREDIENTS

3 strips bacon

1 boneless, skinless chicken breast

3 tablespoons sour cream

1 tablespoon prepared horseradish

1 tablespoon fresh lemon juice

½ teaspoon freshly ground black pepper

¼ teaspoon dried rosemary

1 tomato

2 tortillas

½ cup chopped fresh spinach

¼ cup shredded Monterey Jack cheese

METHOD

Using kitchen scissors, cut bacon into small pieces. In a large frying pan, cook bacon over medium heat until crisp. Remove and blot on paper towel to remove excess grease. Drain off any excess bacon grease from pan and return to heat. Brown chicken breast on both sides, about 2 to 3 minutes per side. Remove from pan and cut into thin slices, then return to pan to fully cook, turning as necessary.

Meanwhile, in a small bowl, combine sour cream, horseradish, lemon juice, black pepper and rosemary. Finely chop tomato, discarding any excess seeds and liquids.

In the centre of each wrap, mound chicken, bacon, tomato, spinach and cheese; top with horseradish sauce and roll up.

TO SERVE

Use 2 cocktail toothpicks to hold each wrap together; cut each in half and serve.

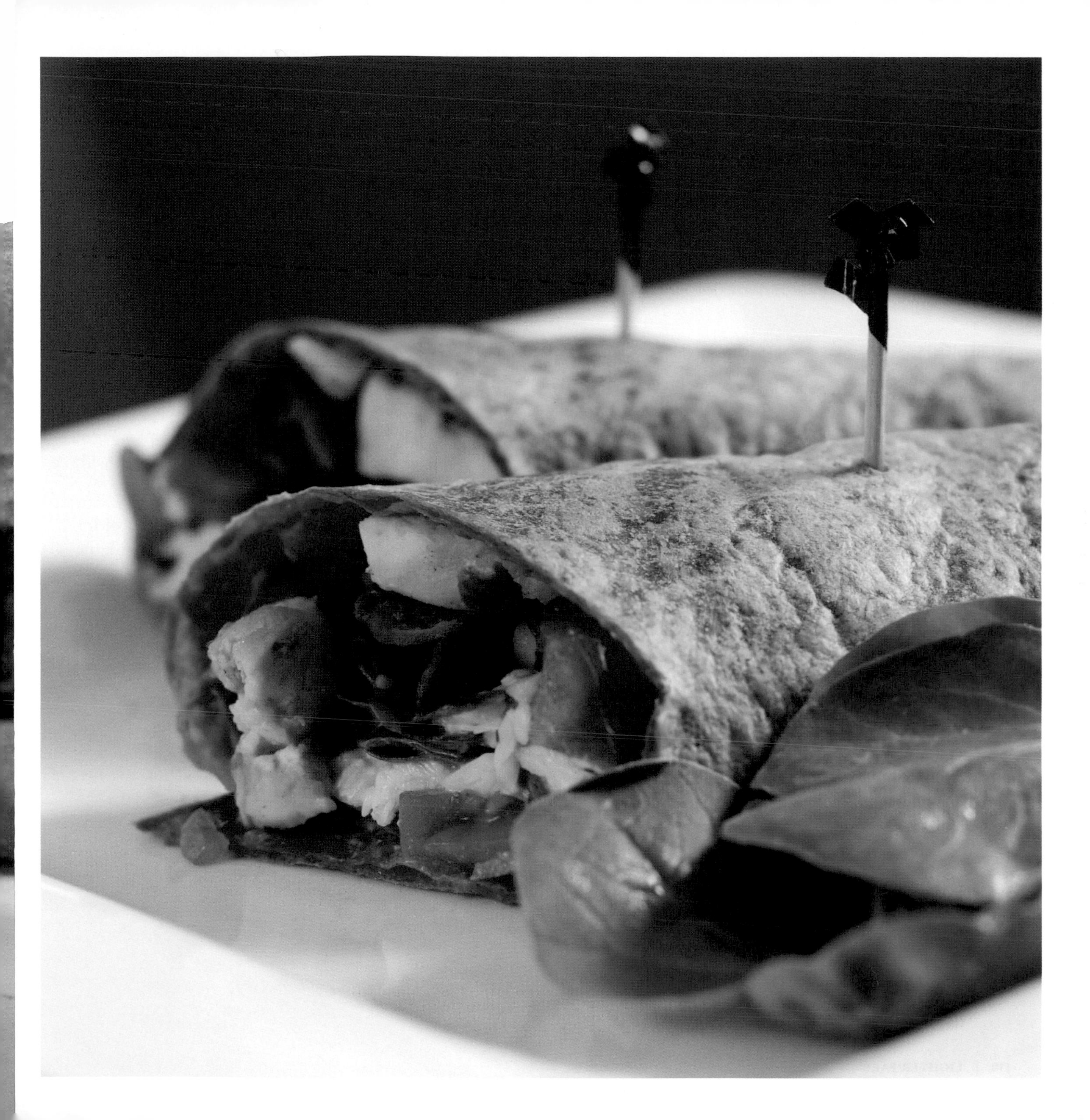

mild curry chicken pizza on naan

SERVES 4 | TOTAL TIME 20 MINUTES | ACTIVE TIME 20 MINUTES

I love the complex and enchanting flavours of Indian food. This easy and satisfying pizza made with naan, an Indian bread, will whisper its exotic music while you create and eat it. It's not too spicy, so even moms-to-be with delicate tummies or palates will love it.

INGREDIENTS

1 teaspoon vegetable oil

2 boneless, skinless chicken breasts

¼ red onion, thinly sliced

1 clove garlic, finely chopped

3 tablespoons tomato paste

1 tablespoon mild Indian red curry paste

4 pieces naan

½ cup fresh spinach, finely chopped

3½ ounces Monterey Jack cheese, shredded

Freshly ground black pepper

METHOD

Turn broiler to high. Heat vegetable oil in a large frying pan over medium heat. Add chicken, browning one side, about 2 to 3 minutes. Flip chicken, add onion and garlic to pan and continue cooking to brown other side of chicken. Remove chicken from pan and cut into thin slices, then return to pan to fully cook, turning as needed.

In a small bowl, combine tomato paste and curry paste; spread on naan. Top naan with chicken-onion mixture, spinach and cheese. Broil on a baking sheet for 5 minutes or until cheese is melted and bubbling.

TO SERVE

Cut each naan pizza into 4 pieces and sprinkle with ground pepper. Eat with a knife and fork or with your fingers.

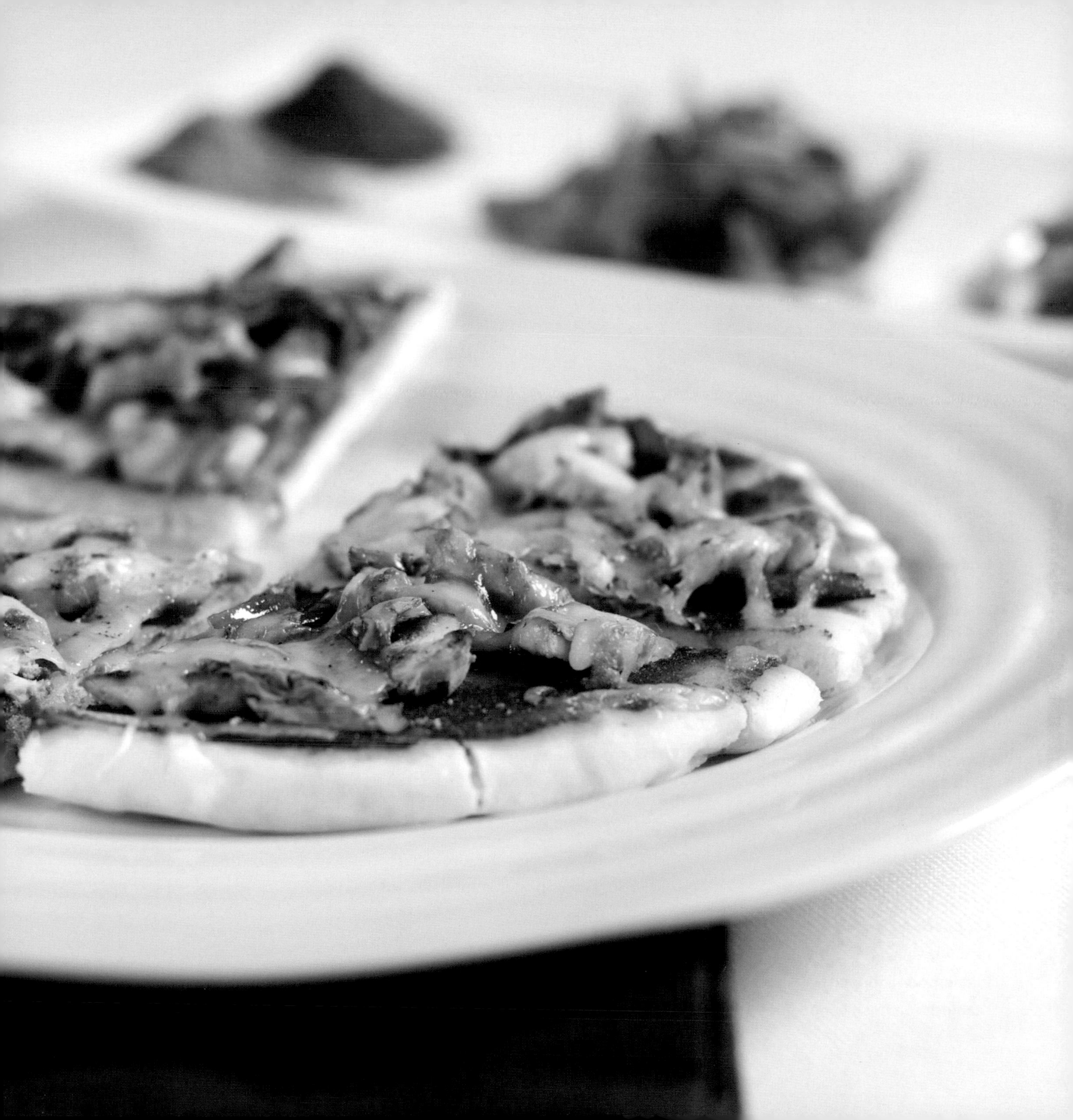

succulent crab cakes with tarragon sour cream

SERVES 4 | TOTAL TIME 1 HOUR 30 MINUTES | ACTIVE TIME 30 MINUTES

These moist and tender crab cakes pair beautifully with fresh and lively tarragon cream. Don't bother cooking whole crabs to make this delectable dish; just buy fresh crabmeat from your seafood shop or grocer. I know you pregnant gals have better things to do than crack crab shells!

CRAB CAKES

1 tablespoon butter

1 clove garlic, chopped

½ large onion, chopped

¼ red pepper, minced

1 egg

2 tablespoons mayonnaise

1 tablespoon each Dijon mustard and fresh lemon juice

2 dashes each Worcestershire sauce and hot sauce (such as Tabasco)

1 pound crabmeat (shell removed)

1 cup panko (Japanese bread crumbs)

1 tablespoon each chopped fresh mint and tarragon

Dash of salt and freshly ground black pepper

2 tablespoons olive oil

4 fresh mint sprigs, for garnish (optional)

TARRAGON SOUR CREAM

1 cup sour cream

1 shallot, minced

1 tablespoon chopped fresh tarragon

1 tablespoon fresh lemon juice

METHOD

Melt butter in a large frying pan over medium heat. Add garlic, onion and red pepper; cook for 5 minutes or until onion is translucent. Transfer to a small bowl and set aside.

In a large mixing bowl, whisk together egg, mayonnaise, mustard, lemon juice, Worcestershire sauce and hot sauce. Add crabmeat, panko, mint, tarragon, salt, pepper and onion mixture. Using a wooden spoon, stir to mix.

Using your hands, form the crab mixture into 8 patties. Place on a waxed paper–lined plate, cover and refrigerate for about 45 minutes to allow crab cakes to set.

Meanwhile, prepare the tarragon sour cream. In a bowl, combine sour cream, shallot, tarragon and lemon juice. Cover and chill in the refrigerator until ready to serve crab cakes.

Once crab cakes have set, heat 1 tablespoon of the olive oil in each of 2 large frying pans over medium-low heat. Fry crab cakes for 5 minutes, then gently flip each over and cook for another 5 minutes, until crisp and hot through.

TO SERVE

Serve 2 crab cakes per person, each topped with a dollop of tarragon sour cream. Garnish with a sprig of mint if desired.

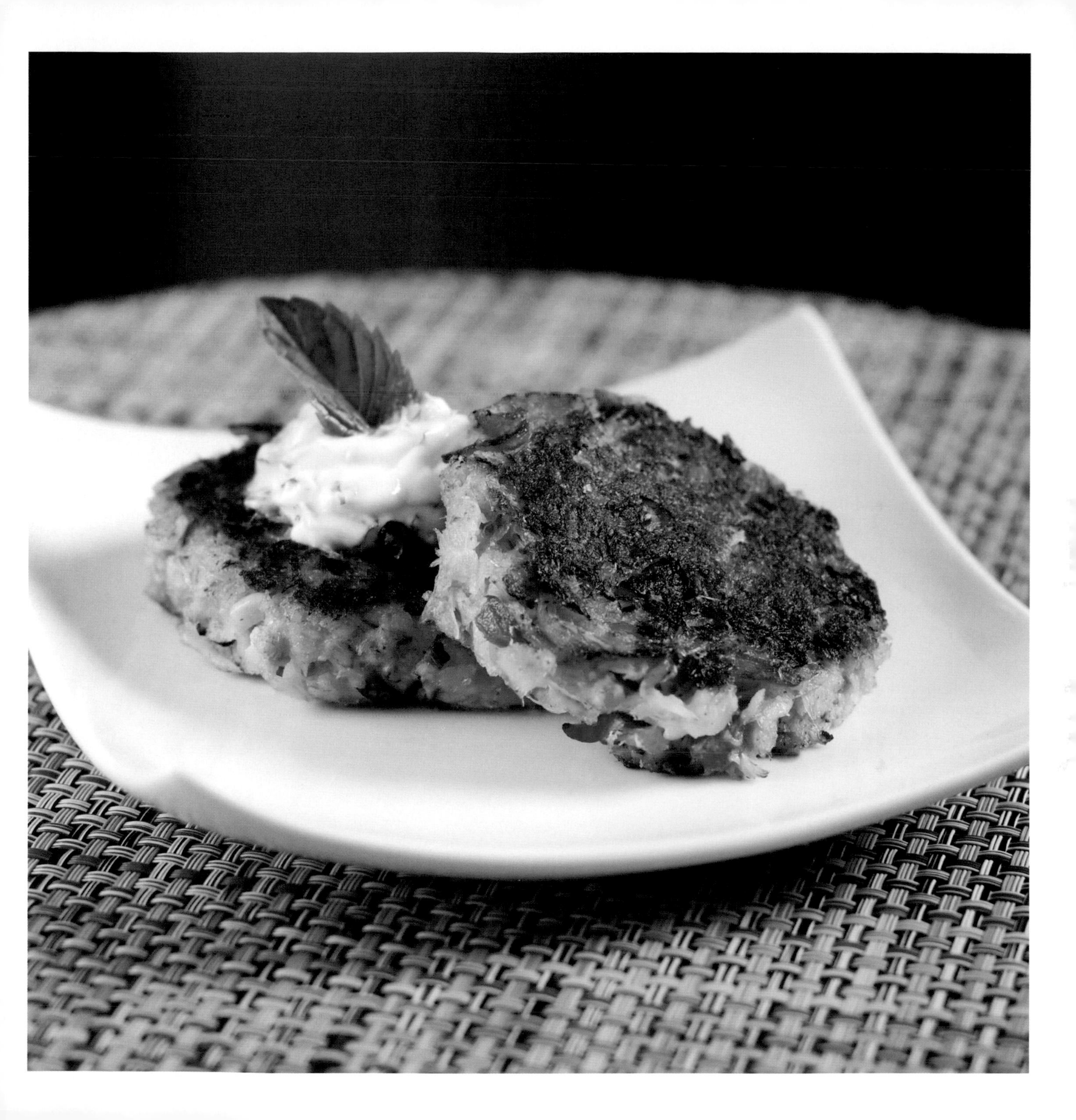

panko-crusted stuffed grilled portobello

SERVES 4 | TOTAL TIME 25 MINUTES | ACTIVE TIME 25 MINUTES

An outstanding blend of texture and flavour, this grand vegetarian Portobello has a meaty base, simple filling, light and crisp panko topping and an unexpected kiss of ginger. Gourmet gals everywhere are enjoying Japanese panko in new ways.

INGREDIENTS

1 teaspoon olive oil, plus extra for brushing

1 clove garlic, chopped

1 handful fresh spinach leaves, chopped (plus additional leaves for garnish)

½ red pepper, chopped

1 teaspoon freshly grated ginger

2 tablespoons soy sauce

4 large Portobello mushrooms caps

6 tablespoons ricotta cheese

4 tablespoons panko (Japanese bread crumbs)

METHOD

Preheat the barbecue or indoor grill to medium-high. Heat olive oil in a frying pan over medium heat. Cook garlic, spinach, red pepper and ginger with the soy sauce for 3 to 4 minutes, until tender. Thoroughly wash the mushroom caps. Scoop out the gills with a spoon and discard. Lightly brush the mushroom with olive oil; grill for 2 to 3 minutes each side if using a barbecue, or with the lid down if using an indoor grill.

In a bowl, mix the sautéed vegetables with the ricotta. Scoop mixture into the mushroom cap; sprinkle with panko. Warm under the broiler (set at high) for about 5 minutes or until the panko is golden brown and crisp.

TO SERVE

Serve on individual plates and garnish with fresh spinach leaves.

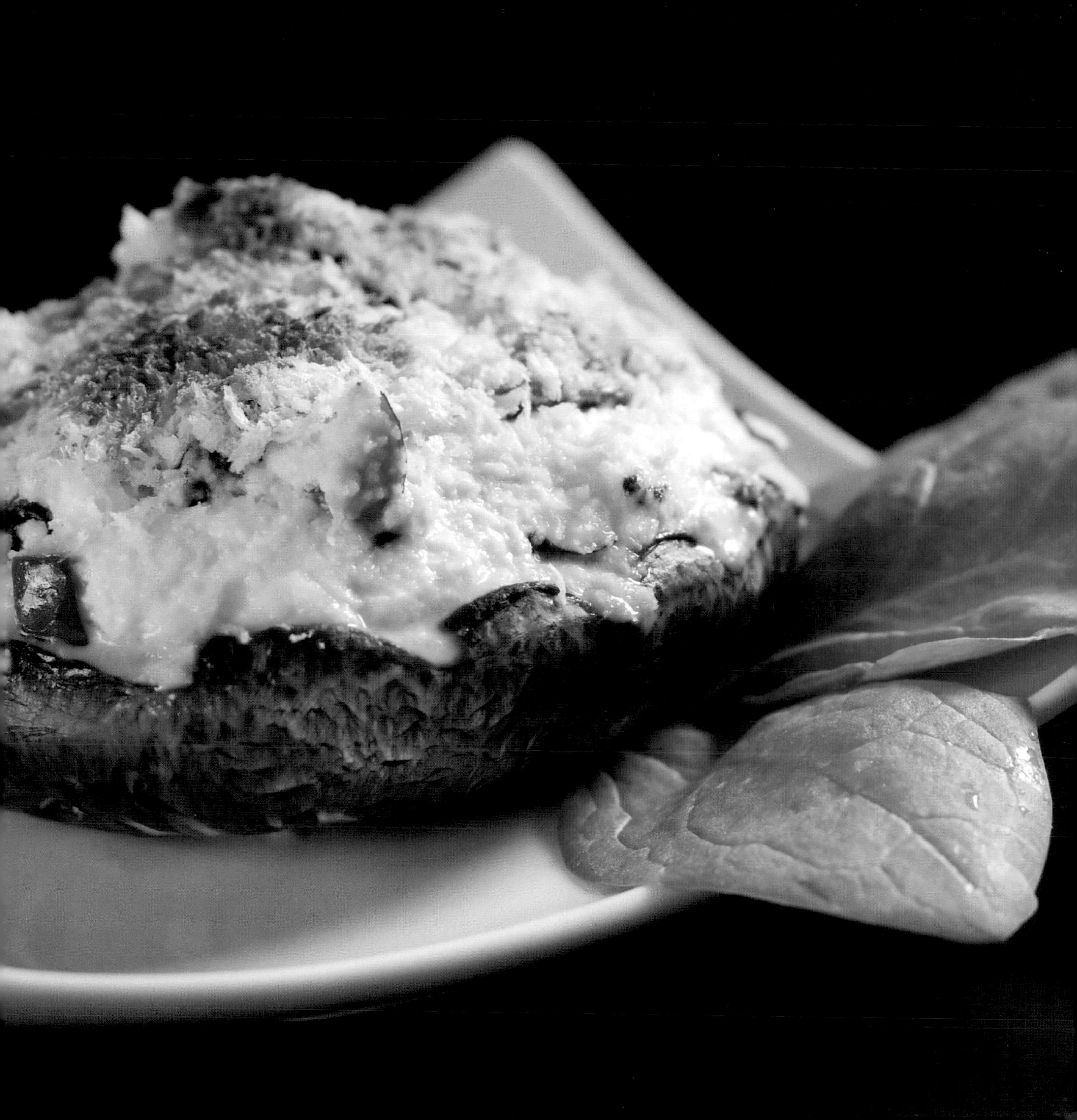

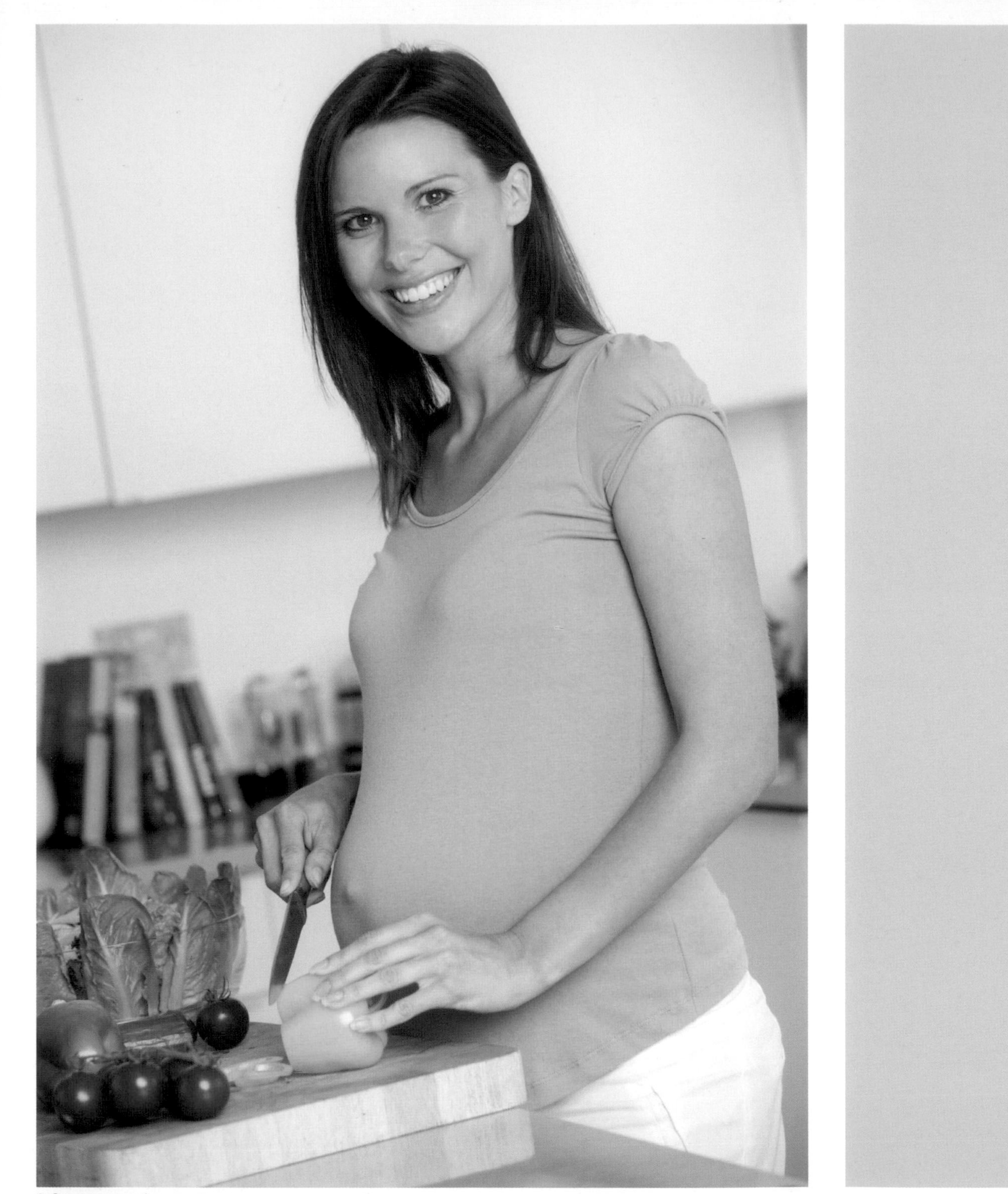

delicious food to nourish your body and soul:

entrées

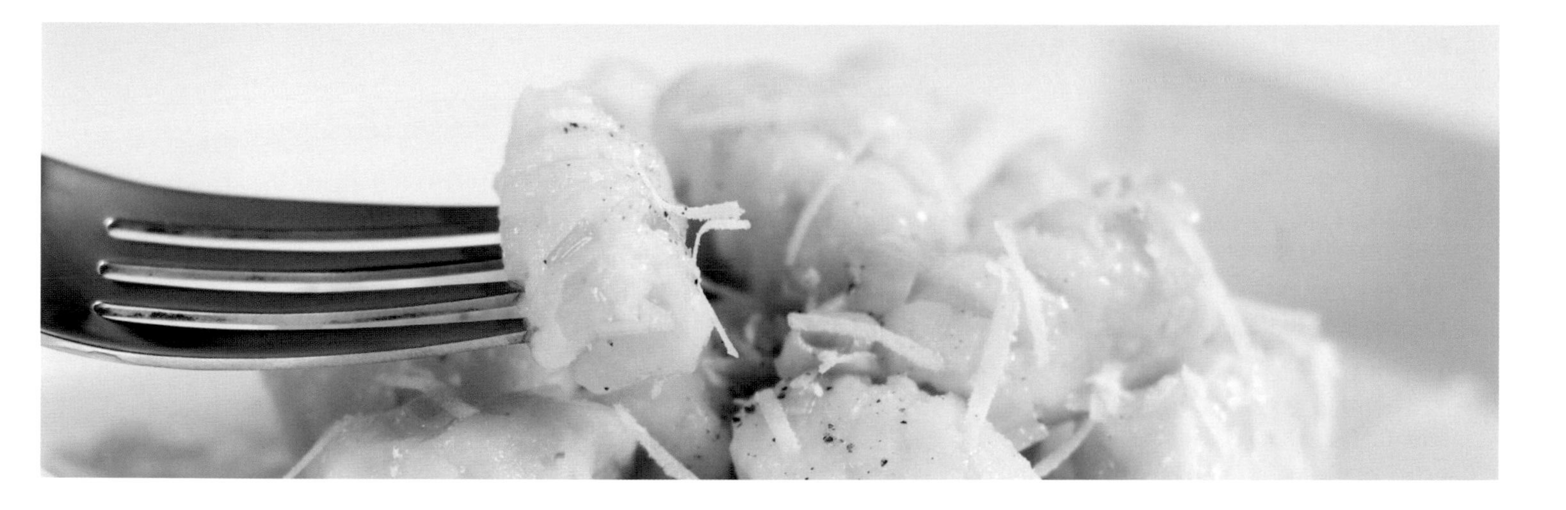

"Life is a combination of magic and pasta."

~ Frederico Fellini

sautéed sablefish with eggplant caviar

SERVES 4 | TOTAL TIME 1 HOUR 20 MINUTES | ACTIVE TIME 40 MINUTES

Wow! This special fish is just delicious (and safe to eat while pregnant). It has a silky, buttery texture and is so simple to prepare. Don't be fooled by the word "caviar" — this recipe doesn't contain any fish eggs and isn't salty or slimy either. Based on a traditional recipe but with a gourmet twist, the eggplant becomes a warm and delicious side that pairs perfectly with the sablefish. Use any leftovers as a dip for warm pita bread. This melt-in-your-mouth meal is sure to impress.

CAVIAR

1 head garlic

2 tablespoons olive oil, plus extra for drizzling

2 large eggplants

1 tablespoon balsamic vinegar

1 shallot

1 cup chopped fresh basil, cilantro and dill (equal parts of each)

Salt and freshly ground black pepper

FISH

½ lemon

4 fresh sablefish fillets, skin on

Salt and freshly ground black pepper

2 tablespoons flour

1 tablespoon olive oil

2 stalks green onion, cut lengthwise into thin strips, for garnish

METHOD

Preheat oven to 375°F. Cut the top (about ½ inch) off the garlic head and remove as much of the papery outer layers as you can. Drizzle gently with olive oil. Wrap in foil. Cut the eggplants in quarters lengthwise and wrap each piece individually in foil. Bake the eggplants and garlic the on middle rack in oven for about 45 minutes. The eggplants should be tender when done — if not, leave them in a bit longer. Remove from oven, unwrap the foil and set aside until cool to the touch.

Using a sharp knife, remove the skin from the eggplants and discard. Transfer the eggplants to a food processor. Squeeze the pulp out of each garlic clove and add to food processor. Add the 2 tablespoons of olive oil, vinegar and herbs and process to blend well. Taste the mixture, seasoning with salt and ground pepper. Set aside.

To prepare the fish, squeeze the juice from half of a lemon over the fillets; lightly season with salt and pepper. Lightly dust the non-skin side of the fillets with flour. Heat a non-stick frying pan over medium heat for several minutes until hot. Add olive oil. Place the fillets in the pan, skin-side down. Sear for 2 to 3 minutes; flip and cook for another 1 to 2 minutes. The fish will be juicy and flaky when cooked — don't overcook or it will dry out.

TO SERVE

Place fish alongside a small scoop of eggplant caviar mixture and garnish with green onion.

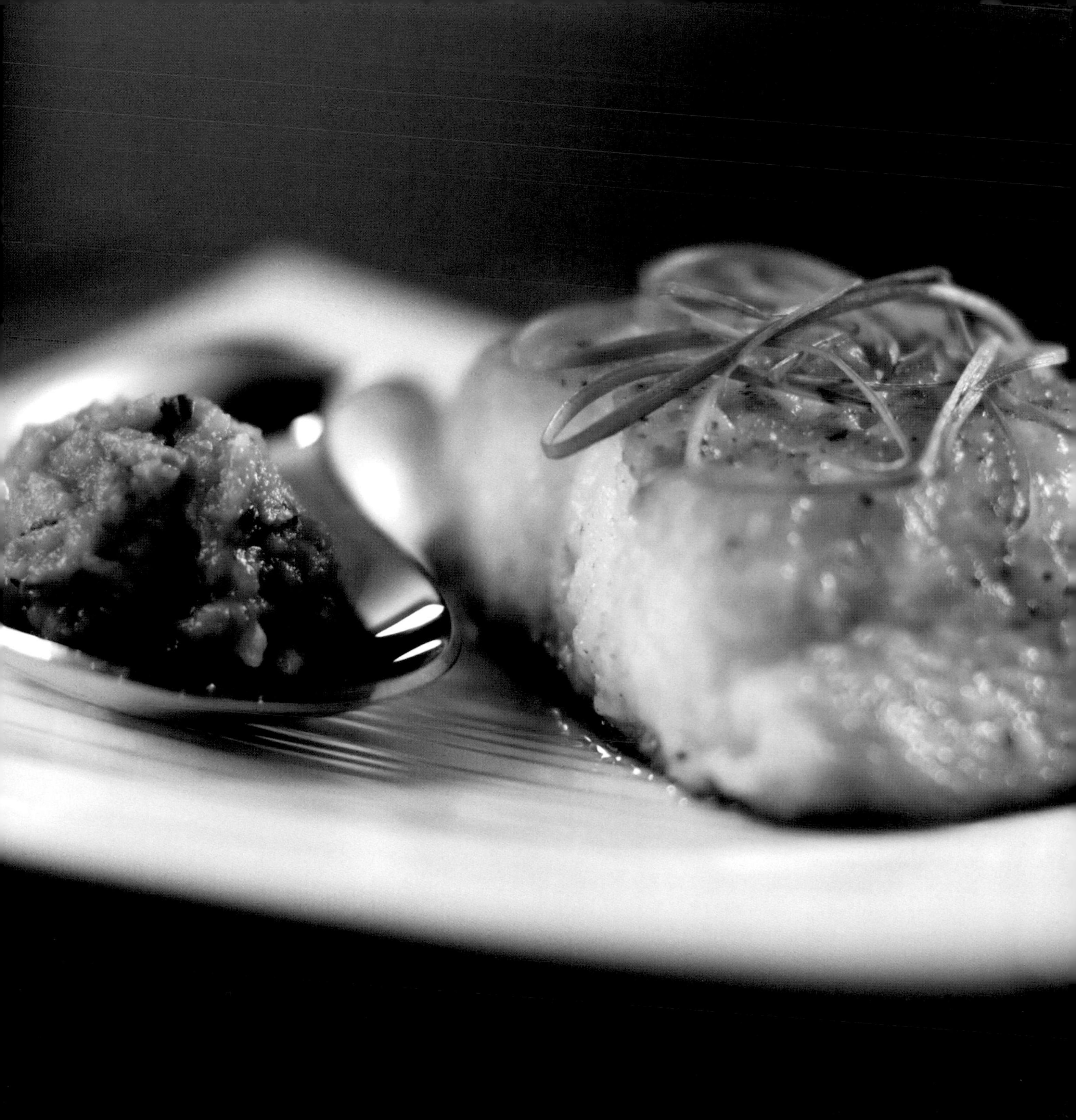

chocolate sesame salmon with steamed broccoli

SERVES 4 | TOTAL TIME 40 MINUTES | ACTIVE TIME 40 MINUTES

You need only add a small amount of smooth dark chocolate to this divinely flavoured sauce. Garlic, ginger, sweet soy and sesame balance out the rich decadence. This is a spectacular and modern approach to a pregnant gal's favourite fish.

INGREDIENTS

4 fresh salmon fillets

2 squares dark chocolate

2 cloves garlic, finely chopped

½ cup milk

½ cup sweet soy sauce

¼ cup sesame oil

2 tablespoons soy sauce

2 tablespoons honey

1 tablespoon ginger, finely chopped

Dash of Worcestershire sauce

Dash of chili oil

1 teaspoon cornstarch stirred in 1 tablespoon water

¼ cup sesame seeds, toasted, for garnish

2 cups broccoli florets

METHOD

Preheat oven to 425°F. Place salmon skin-side down on a baking sheet. To a saucepan, add all ingredients except cornstarch, sesame seeds and broccoli; cook over medium heat for 10 minutes, until bubbling. Reduce heat to low. Whisk cornstarch mixture into sauce to thicken and cook for another 2 to 3 minutes. Pour a few spoonfuls of the sauce over the salmon. Bake salmon for 12 to 15 minutes, depending on thickness of the fillets. Continue warming the remaining sauce over low heat until ready to serve.

Meanwhile, preheat toaster oven and toast sesame seeds on a tray for a few minutes until golden (or toast in oven along with fish). Watch carefully to ensure they don't burn.

Steam broccoli in a steamer basket over boiling water for 3 to 4 minutes or until bright green.

TO SERVE

Arrange salmon fillets on individual plates and spoon several spoonfuls of sauce over top. Sprinkle generously with toasted sesame seeds and serve with broccoli on the side.

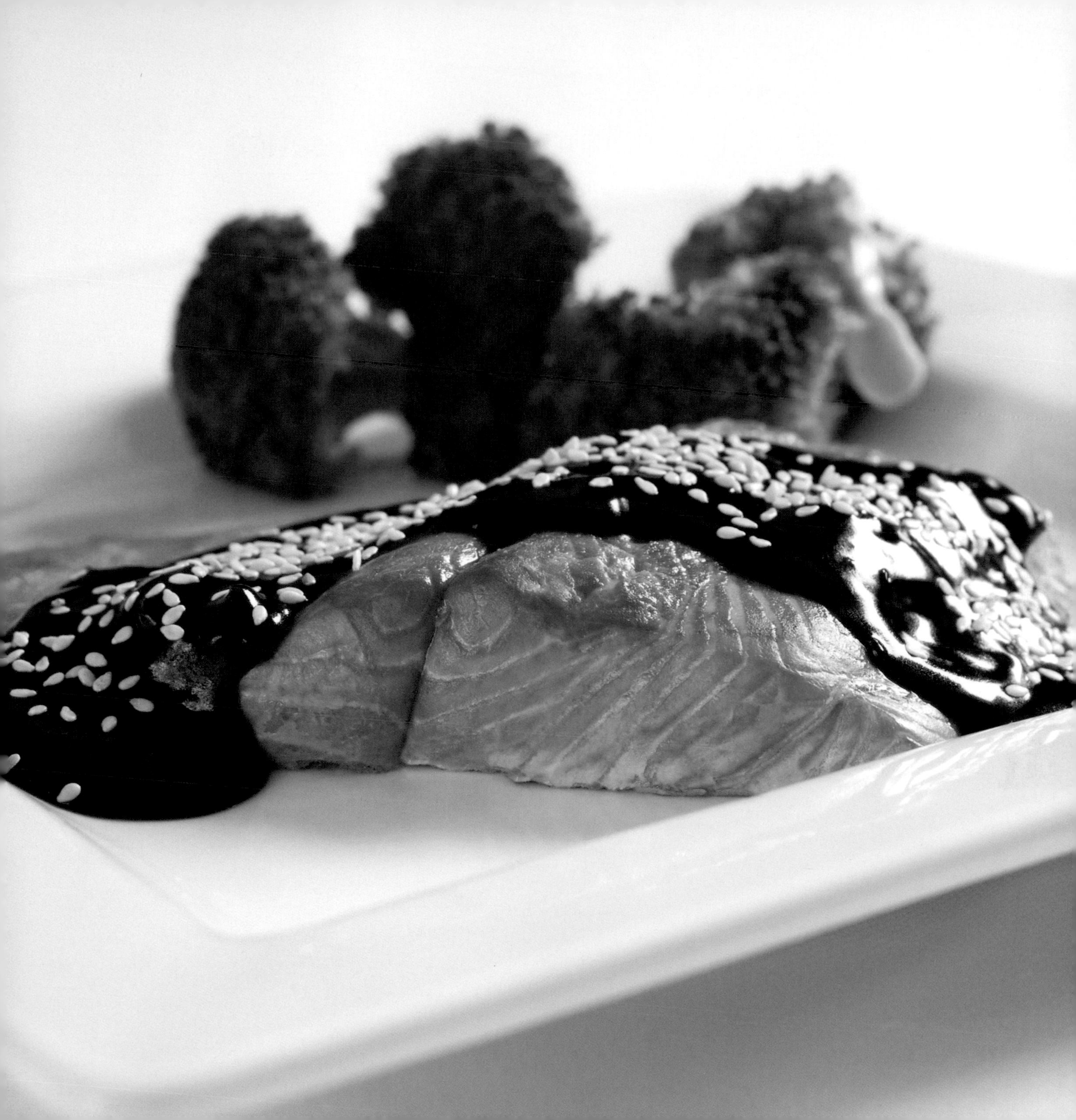

tilapia fillets with coconut curry cream sauce

SERVES 4 | TOTAL TIME 2 HOURS | ACTIVE TIME 30 MINUTES

Mild and pleasantly flavourful, this gorgeous curried tomato sauce enhances the taste of this light, flaky fish. It is a simple and ultimately satisfying meal. Take a trip to your local seafood shop to get inspiration for other unique and pregnancy-friendly fish dishes.

INGREDIENTS

1 (15-ounce) can diced tomatoes, liquid reserved

1 cup plain yogurt

½ cup coconut milk

2 tablespoons Indian red curry paste

1 teaspoon cornstarch stirred in 1 tablespoon of water

4 fillets tilapia

METHOD

In a saucepan, combine tomatoes and their liquid, yogurt, coconut milk and curry paste. Pour one-third of the mixture over fish fillets in a casserole dish and marinate, covered, for at least 1 hour in the refrigerator.

Preheat oven to 400°F. Bake fillets for 10 to 12 minutes or until fish flakes easily when tested with a fork. Meanwhile, add cornstarch mixture to sauce and cook over medium heat, stirring frequently until sauce has thickened. Reduce heat if sauce begins to boil.

TO SERVE

Serve 1 fillet per plate with a generous blanket of curry cream sauce. Serve with thick slices of crusty bread.

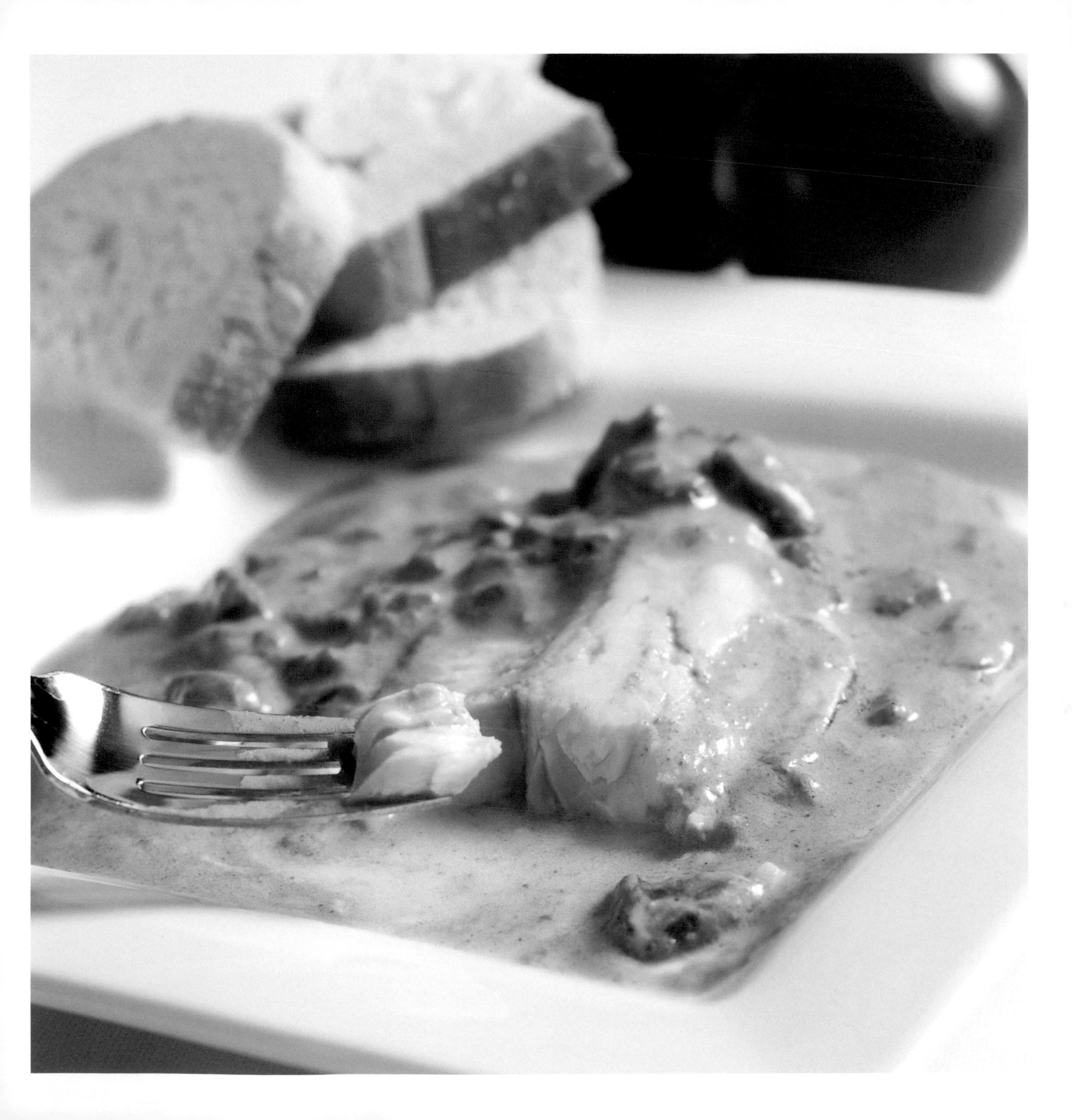

seared scallops with cilantro honey pesto and baby arugula salad

SERVES 4 | TOTAL TIME 25 MINUTES | ACTIVE TIME 25 MINUTES

Serve this dish of delicate, fresh scallops with quirky, lively pesto when you want to knock the socks off your sweetie. You'll feel like you're dining at the finest restaurant in the city. Perhaps other clothes will also get knocked off after this meal!

INGREDIENTS

⅓ cup pine nuts

⅓ cup olive oil plus 2 tablespoons

1 medium bunch fresh cilantro

1 small bunch fresh basil, coarsely chopped

3½ ounces Romano or Parmesan cheese (not pre-grated)

1 clove garlic

2 tablespoons honey

Salt and freshly ground black pepper

12 large (or 16 medium) fresh scallops

2 bunches baby arugula

¼ red onion, very finely sliced

METHOD

To make the pesto, in a frying pan over medium-high heat, toast pine nuts in 1 tablespoon of the olive oil for about 3 to 4 minutes, until golden. Remove the base of the stems from the cilantro; chop the leaves coarsely and place in a blender. Add the pine nuts and basil. Grate two-thirds of the cheese and add to the blender. Add the garlic, honey and ⅓ cup of the olive oil, blending until smooth. Season with salt and ground pepper.

Spoon pesto onto serving dishes in 3 to 4 evenly spaced circles (depending on number of scallops per plate); the circles should be slightly larger than the scallops.

Heat the remaining 1 tablespoon of olive oil in a frying pan over medium-high heat. Lightly salt and pepper the scallops. When the pan is very hot, sear the scallops, flipping over after 2 to 3 minutes (or when nicely browned). Cook for another 2 to 3 minutes. Do not overcook — the scallops should be tender and appear slightly pearly inside.

TO SERVE

Place scallops atop pesto circles. Arrange baby arugula, red onion slices and the remaining cheese, grated, on each plate beside the scallops.

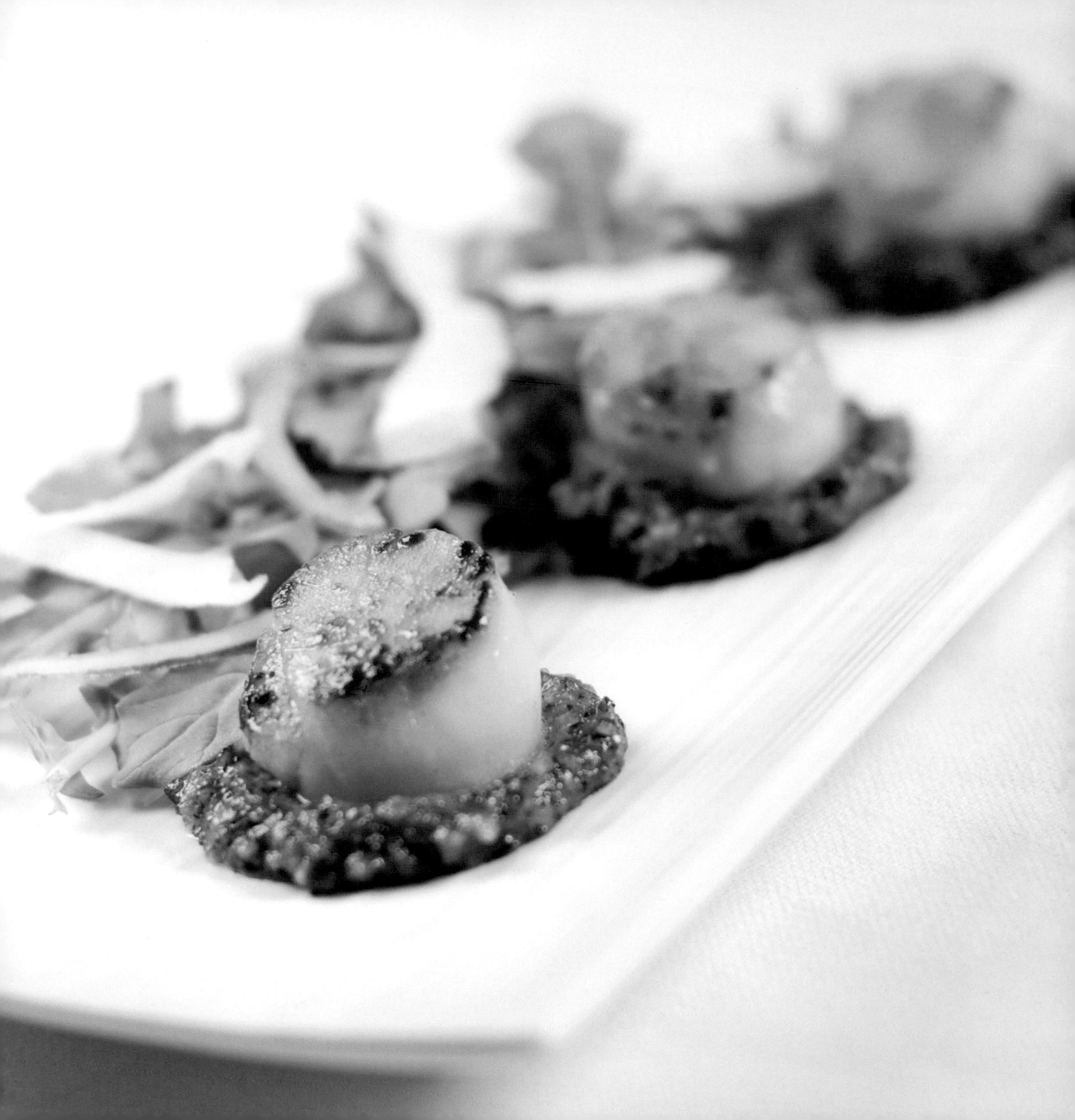

garlic shrimp and feta linguine

SERVES 4 | TOTAL TIME 25 MINUTES | ACTIVE TIME 25 MINUTES

My sister, Angie Brennand, in Toronto makes this zesty, garlicky seafood dish, which is perfectly safe to eat during pregnancy as long as you select pasteurized feta. Be sure to check, as many brands are not pasteurized. Also be sure to brush your teeth before kissing your sweetie!

INGREDIENTS

2 tablespoons olive oil

1 small white onion, diced

24 large shrimp, peeled, deveined, tail removed

16 ounces fresh linguine

4 large cloves garlic, crushed

1 (28-ounce) can diced tomatoes, drained

3½ ounces pasteurized feta cheese (cubed)

Freshly ground black pepper

METHOD

In a large pot over high heat, bring 8 cups of water to a boil. Cook linguine according to instructions on the package.

Meanwhile, heat olive oil in a large frying pan over medium heat. Add onion; cook until translucent, about 3 to 4 minutes. Add shrimp; cook until pink, about 2 to 3 minuutes. Remove shrimp and set aside. Add garlic and tomatoes to pan; cook over medium-high heat until most of the liquid is evaporated. Add feta. Reduce heat to medium, stirring until the cheese blends into the sauce. Season with ground pepper.

TO SERVE

Plate pasta topped with the sauce and shrimp.

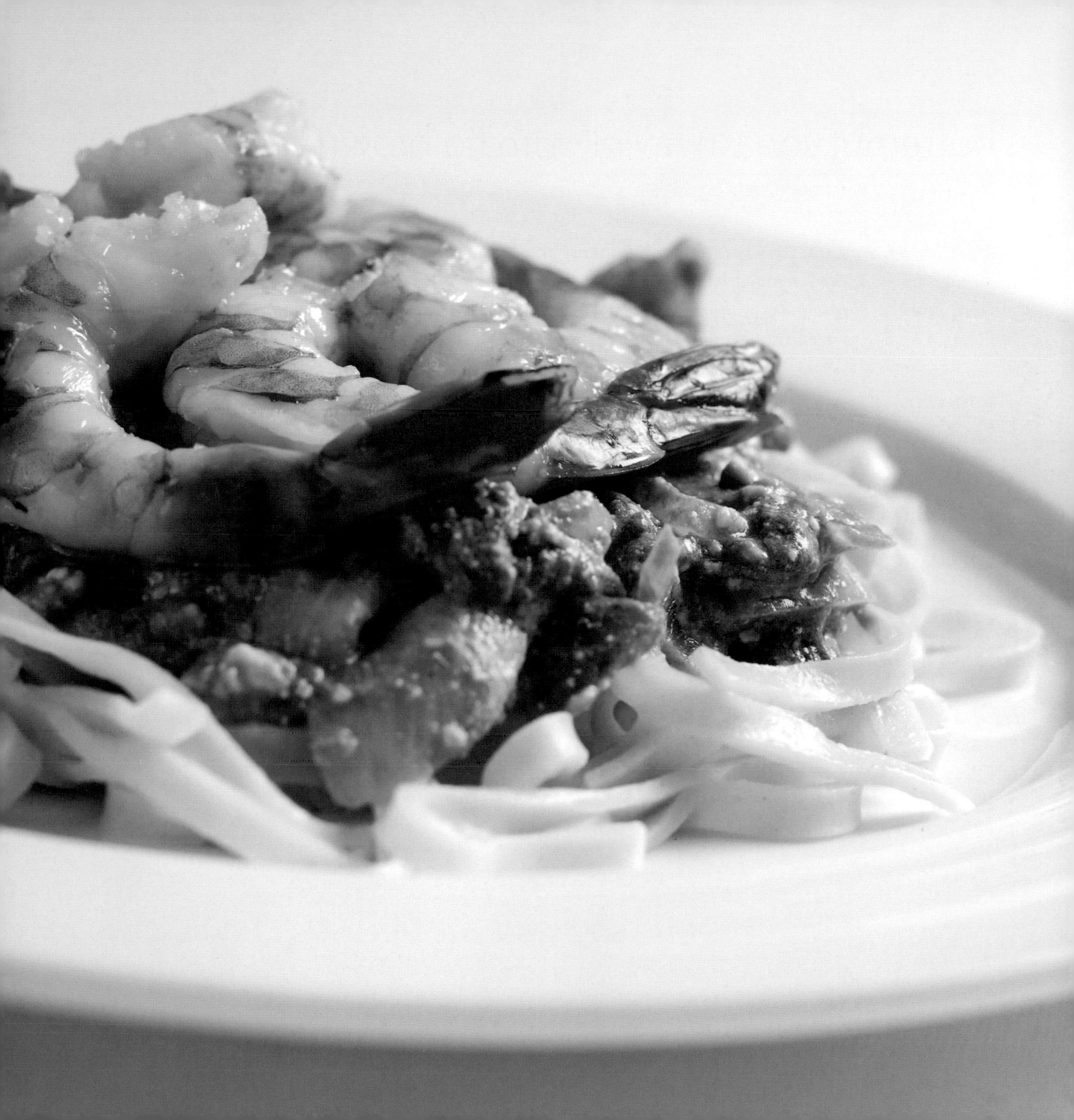

butternut squash ravioli with fig brown butter sauce

SERVES 4 | TOTAL TIME 15 MINUTES | ACTIVE TIME 15 MINUTES

My husband claims he could eat this meal almost every day. The subtle fig flavour in this remarkable pasta dish comes from the flavoured balsamic vinegar. You can find it at any specialty store or large supermarket. Don't bother trying to make your own ravioli — buy some fresh and spend the extra time pampering yourself or taking a nap! This dish is simple to make but tastes exquisite.

INGREDIENTS

2 shallots

¼ cup butter

⅓ cup fig balsamic vinegar

14 ounces fresh butternut squash ravioli

3½ ounces Parmesan cheese

METHOD

In a large pot, bring 8 cups of water to a boil. Meanwhile, peel shallots; slice into thin rings. In a small saucepan, melt the butter over medium heat; add shallots. Cook until tender, about 3 to 4 minutes. Add the vinegar, stirring well to incorporate. Continue to stir, gently, until sauce is slightly reduced and thickened, about 4 to 5 minutes. Add ravioli to boiling water; cook for 4 to 5 minutes until done.

TO SERVE

Serve ravioli with sauce over top. Finish with a sprinkling of grated cheese.

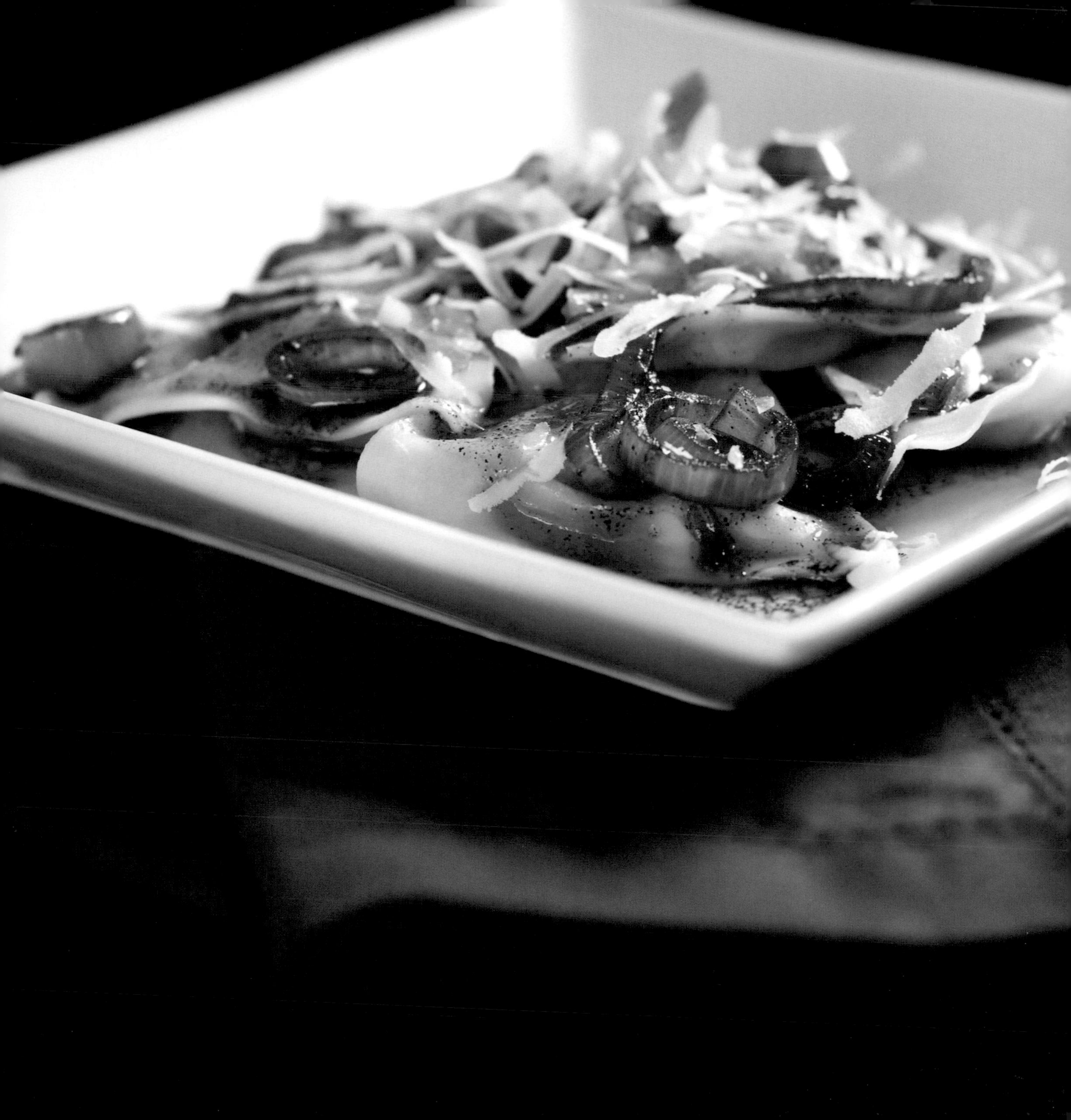

eggplant and spinach lasagna with béchamel sauce

SERVES 8 TO 12 | TOTAL TIME 1 HOUR 30 MINUTES | ACTIVE TIME 45 MINUTES

Creamy and comforting, yet far more elegant than regular lasagna, this dish will surely be a favourite. If you're cooking for just two, you'll have plenty of leftovers, so your workmates can drool over your gourmet cooking at lunchtime.

INGREDIENTS

2 large eggplants

Olive oil for brushing (approx 2 tablespoons)

Kosher salt

5 cloves garlic, minced

3 tablespoons butter

5 tablespoons all-purpose flour

5 cups milk

1 bay leaf

1½ teaspoon salt

Dash of freshly ground black pepper

1 teaspoon olive oil

½ onion, diced

1 pound lean ground beef

1 cup chopped fresh spinach

1 pkg oven-ready lasagna noodles

2 cups ricotta cheese

3 cups shredded mozzarella cheese

METHOD

Preheat oven to 450°F. Slice eggplants into ½-inch-thick rounds. Brush slices on both sides with olive oil. Spread on a baking tray; sprinkle kosher salt over top. Bake for 20 to 25 minutes, turning after 10 minutes. Remove and reduce temperature to 425°F.

Meanwhile, in a saucepan over medium-low heat, cook one-quarter of the garlic in butter for 1 minute. Stir in flour and cook for 3 minutes, whisking continuously. Whisk in milk gradually. Add bay leaf, 1 teaspoon of the salt and the ground pepper. Increase heat to high and cook until milk scalds; then reduce heat and simmer for 15 minutes or until liquid has reduced to about 4 cups. Discard bay leaf and set sauce aside.

Heat 1 teaspoon of the olive oil in a saucepan over medium heat. Add onion and the remaining garlic; cook for 1 to 2 minutes. Add beef and the remaining ½ teaspoon of salt; cook until browned. Add spinach and cook for 2 minutes or until dark green and starting to wilt.

Lightly oil a 13- × 9-inch baking dish. To assemble lasagna, spread one-quarter of the sauce over the bottom of the baking dish. Top with a layer of noodles. Cover with 1 cup of the ricotta, then 1 cup of the mozzarella, half of the eggplant, one-quarter of the sauce and all of the meat. Add another one-quarter of the sauce, a layer of noodles and the remaining ricotta and eggplant. Top with the remaining sauce and mozzarella. Cover with foil and bake for 30 minutes. Remove foil and bake an additional 10 minutes.

TO SERVE

Cut lasagna into squares and serve hot on individual plates.

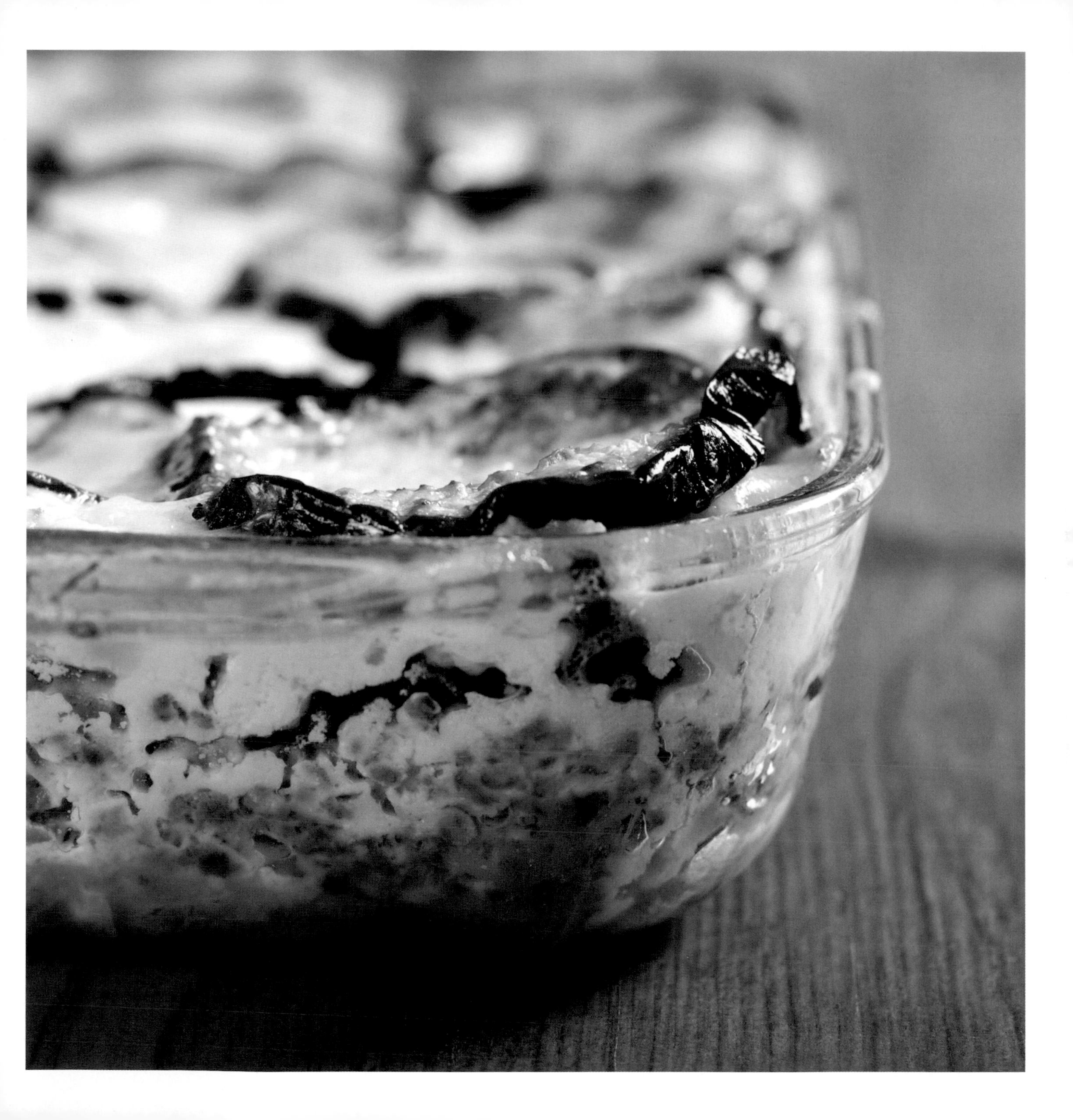

gnocchi with truffle butter sauce

SERVES 4 | TOTAL TIME 1 HOUR | ACTIVE TIME 1 HOUR

Long considered an aphrodisiac, truffle oil flavours both the gnocchi and simple butter sauce in this remarkable dish. Set the table, put on some music, light the candles … and I doubt you'll be able to keep your hands off each other! Enjoy dinner and your romantic evening.

GNOCCHI

1 pound Yukon gold potatoes

1 cup all-purpose flour

1 teaspoon salt

1 egg

1 tablespoon truffle oil

SAUCE

3 tablespoons butter

¼ cup chopped leek

1 clove garlic, minced

Salt and freshly ground black pepper

1 tablespoon truffle oil

METHOD

In a large pot, bring 8 to 10 cups of water to a boil. Peel potatoes and cut each into eight chunks. Boil for 10 minutes or until tender. Drain and mash. Stir in flour and salt. Add egg and truffle oil and stir until just combined.

Refill the pot with fresh water and bring to a boil. Turn potato mixture onto a floured board and knead until smooth. Roll dough into thin ropes and cut into 1-inch-long pieces. With the back of a fork, gently roll each piece across the tines to create grooves. Drop gnocchi into the boiling water, in batches of about 10. Remove when they float to the top, about 4 minutes.

To make the sauce, melt the butter in a saucepan over medium-low heat. Add the leek and garlic; season with salt and ground pepper. Sauté for 4 to 5 minutes. Stir in truffle oil.

TO SERVE

Serve gnocchi on individual plates and drizzle sauce over top.

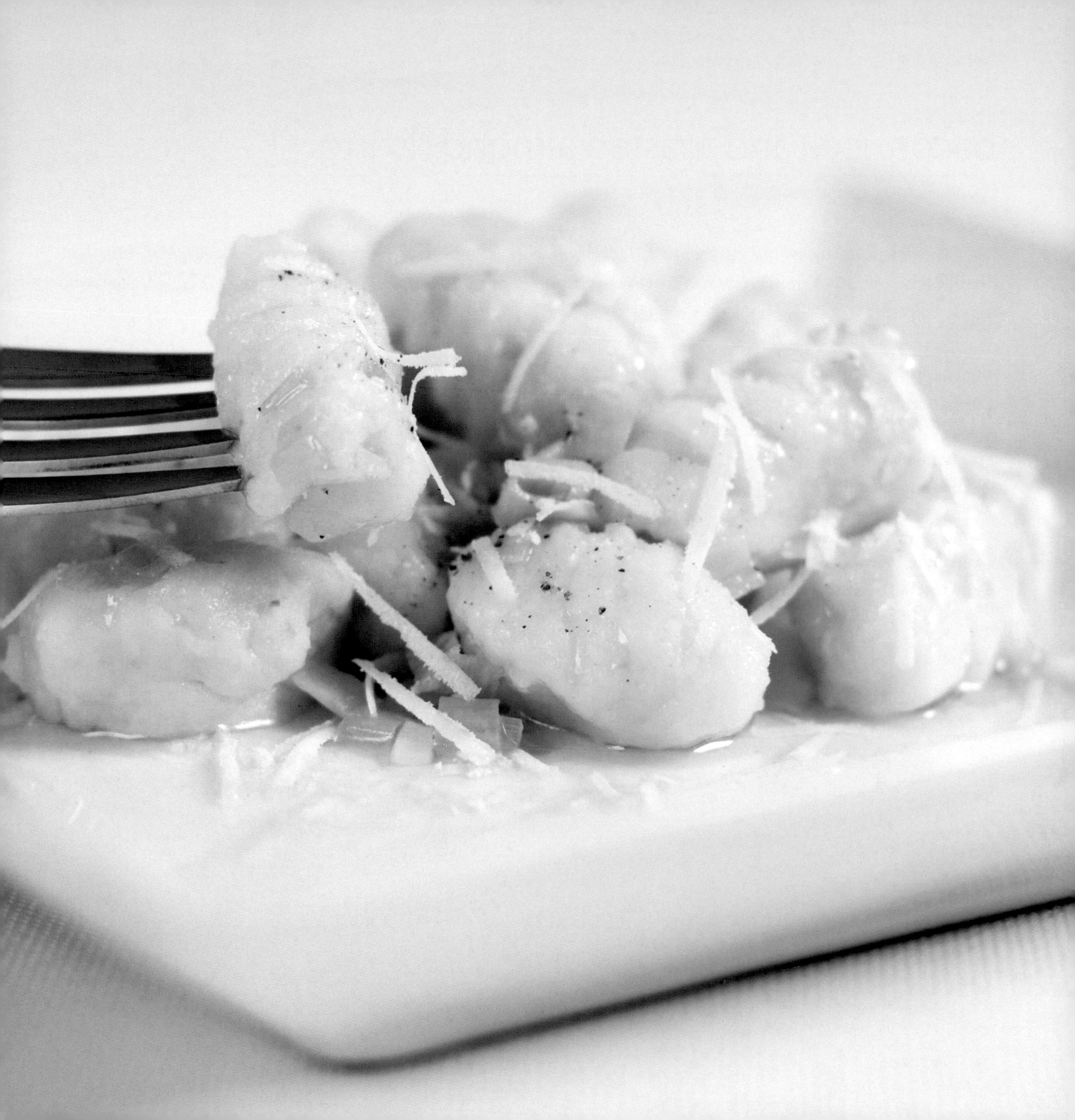

bacon, leek and toasted almond risotto

SERVES 4 | TOTAL TIME 40 MINUTES | ACTIVE TIME 40 MINUTES

Chef Gordon Ramsay would be proud! I don't think there's been a pregnant chef on Hell's Kitchen, but that doesn't mean we can't make a risotto worthy of his fine dining standards. The combination of bacon, leek and toasted almond is divine.

INGREDIENTS

6 strips bacon

3 leeks

2 tablespoons olive oil

1½ cups arborio rice

5½ cups low-sodium chicken stock, warmed

⅓ cup grated Parmesan cheese

⅓ cup toasted slivered almonds

METHOD

Using kitchen shears, cut bacon into small pieces. Finely chop leeks, white and pale green parts only. In a large pot over medium-high, cook bacon to desired doneness. Add leeks for the last minute of cooking time. Remove bacon and leeks and set aside.

Reduce heat to medium and add olive oil and rice, stirring continuously for 2 minutes. Add 1½ cups of the chicken stock. Stir well; then cook for 5 minutes or until stock is absorbed, stirring occasionally. Repeat, adding 1 cup of stock every 5 minutes until stock is absorbed. (This process will take about 25 minutes.) With the last cup of stock, add the bacon and leeks.

TO SERVE

Top with Parmesan and toasted almonds. Serve immediately.

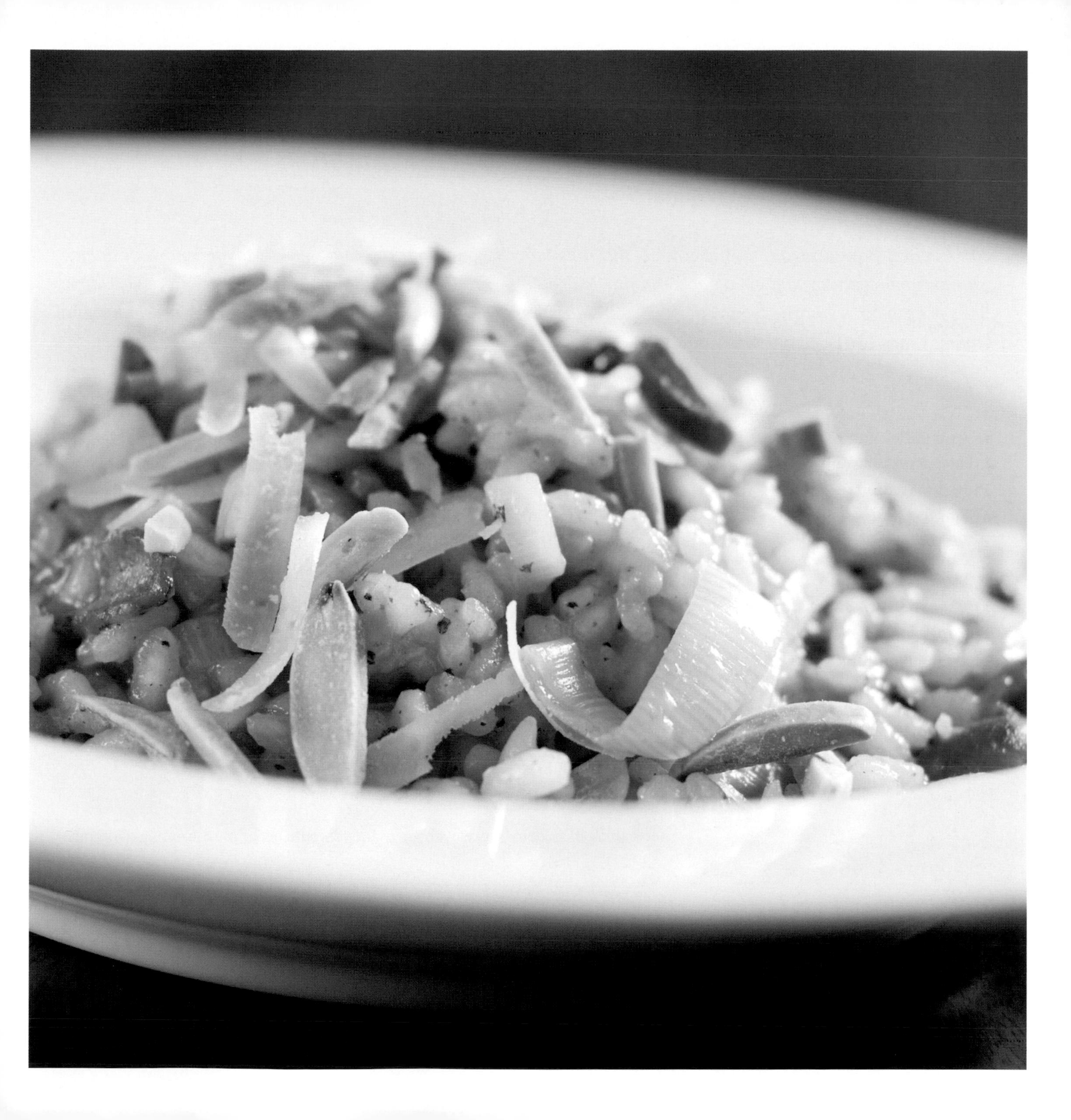

rosemary garlic roast beef

SERVES 4 TO 6 | TOTAL TIME 3 HOURS | ACTIVE TIME 20 MINUTES

Like the Beef Bourguingon in Julie & Julia, *this roast may become your signature dish. Maybe you want to blog your entire pregnancy and get a book and movie deal? Pregnant gals should dine on the outer, more well-done slices of beef, but your guests may prefer the middle slices. Pair this meal with Tempura Beets, Mushrooms and Onions (page 156).*

ROAST

2 cloves garlic, finely chopped

2 tablespoons olive oil

2 teaspoons dried rosemary

4 pounds standing beef rib roast, at room temperature

GRAVY

1 teaspoon paprika

1½ cups water

1 beef bouillon cube

2 tablespoons all-purpose flour

METHOD

Preheat oven to 450°F. Using a mortar and pestle, grind together garlic, rosemary and olive oil; spread all over roast. Cook roast in a roasting pan, uncovered, on the middle rack in oven for 15 minutes. Reduce temperature to 325°F and cook for 18 to 20 minutes per pound, or until a meat thermometer inserted into the thickest part of the roast reads 140°F to 145°F (medium doneness). Remove roast from pan and tent with foil for 15 minutes. Reserve roast drippings.

To make the gravy, skim excess fat off the roast drippings and discard. Place the roasting pan on the stovetop over medium-high heat for 5 to 10 minutes to reduce drippings, stirring often and deglazing the pan by scraping up browned bits of beef left on the bottom. Stir in paprika; add ½ cup of the water and bouillon cube, stirring to combine. In a sealed container, shake flour and the remaining 1 cup of water to blend. Gradually add flour mixture to gravy, adding only enough to achieve desired thickness, stirring vigorously to prevent lumps.

TO SERVE

Serve thick slices of roast beef with gravy and tempura beets, mushrooms and onions.

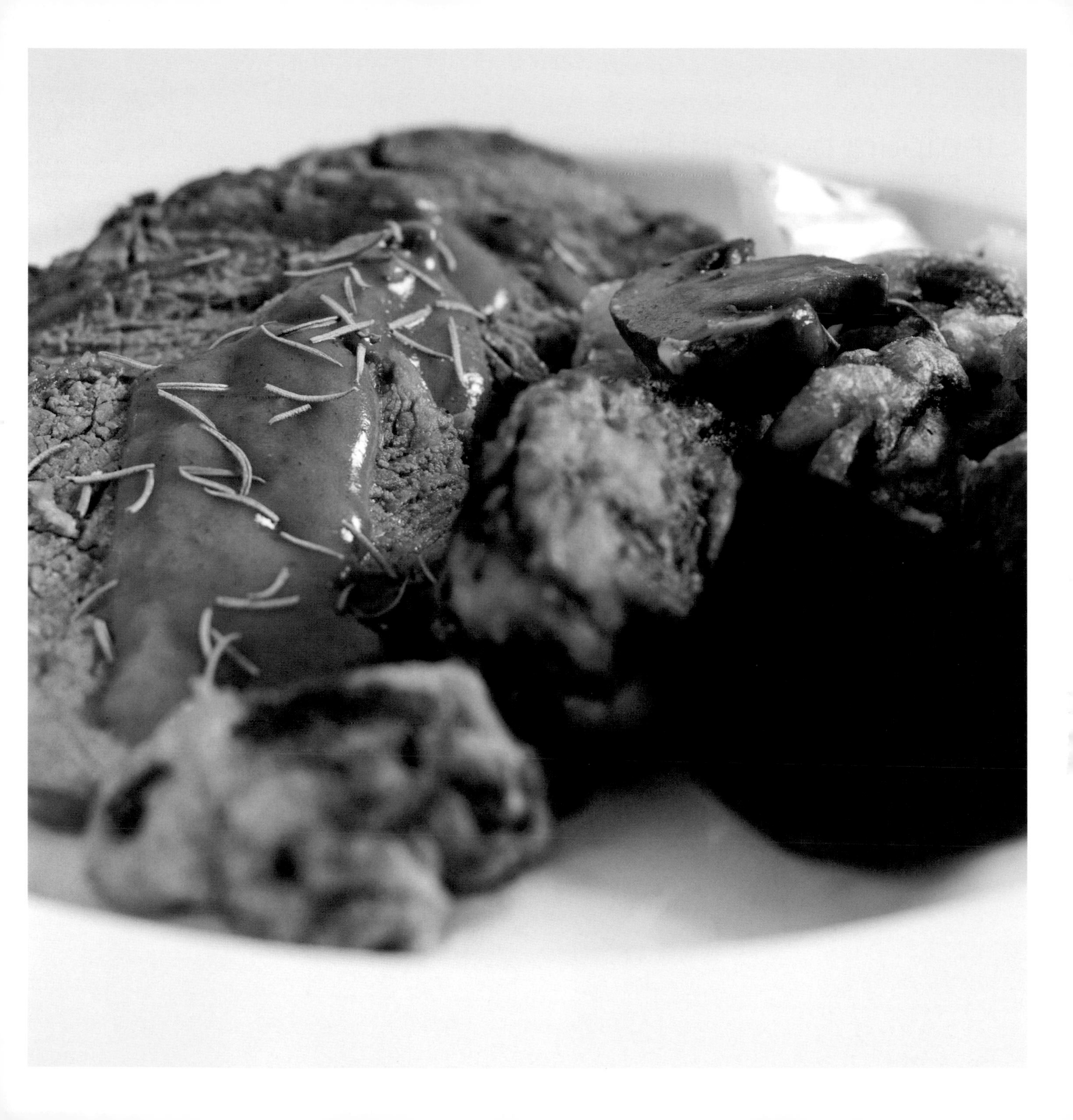

tempura beets, mushrooms and onions

SERVES 4 TO 6 | TOTAL TIME 1 HOUR | ACTIVE TIME 20 MINUTES

This dish accompanies the Rosemary Garlic Roast Beef (page 154), but feel free to also serve it with anything else you fancy. It is unexpected and so satisfying. For a variety of flavours and textures, batter only two-thirds of the vegetables.

INGREDIENTS

3 large beets

1 tablespoon olive oil

1 onion, coarsely chopped

6 mushrooms, cut in eighths

Salt and freshly ground black pepper

1 to 2 cups vegetable oil

1 (5-ounce) pkg tempura batter mix

METHOD

Boil whole, unpeeled beets in a large saucepan for 35 to 45 minutes, topping up with water if it gets too low. Beets are done when a fork pierces them easily. Rinse beets in cold water. Scrape off skin with a spoon and cut each beet into 8 to 12 wedges.

Heat the olive oil in a large saucepan over medium heat. Add the onion and cook until translucent. Add the mushrooms; cook until tender. Season with salt and ground pepper. Remove from heat.

Pour vegetable oil into a medium saucepan to 1 inch deep and warm over medium heat. Follow instructions on tempura batter mix package to achieve a thick batter. Test oil temperature by dropping in a small amount of batter — it should start to fry and brown if oil is hot enough. Dip some of the beets, onions and mushrooms in the batter, coating completely. Drop all of the vegetables into the hot oil (in batches if necessary) and cook for 1 minute, turning to cook all sides. Remove and blot excess oil on paper towel.

TO SERVE

Serve immediately.

apple and anjou pear beef with smashed yams

SERVES 4 | TOTAL TIME AT LEAST 5 HOURS 30 MINUTES | ACTIVE TIME 30 MINUTES

Exceptionally tender, this beef dish is a great reminder of why a slow cooker is such a great piece of kitchen equipment for a mom-to-be. The beef will be cooked-through, juicy and succulent. The apples and pears add flair to this stick-to-your ribs meal.

BEEF

2 to 3 pounds boneless beef roast

1 large sweet onion, sliced

2 cloves garlic, sliced

2 large apples, peeled, cored and sliced

2 large Anjou pears, peeled, cored and sliced

1 cup water

2 tablespoons soy sauce

2 tablespoons olive oil

1 tablespoon cornstarch

Salt and freshly ground black pepper

YAMS

2 large yams

¼ cup milk

2 tablespoons butter

2 tablespoons brown sugar

Salt and freshly ground black pepper

METHOD

Heat olive oil in a large pan over medium high heat; brown roast on all sides. Transfer beef to a slow cooker (cut in half, if necessary, to fit) and add onion, garlic, half of the apples and pears, water, soy sauce, olive oil and cornstarch. Season with salt and ground pepper. Cook for 5 to 6 hours on low or until meat is tender. In the last 30 to 45 minutes of cooking time, add the remaining apples and pears to the slow cooker.

Begin preparing yams. Fill a large pot with water and bring to a boil. Peel and chop yams into small cubes. Add to water and boil for 8 to 10 minutes or until tender. Drain and return to pot. Add milk, butter and sugar. Season with salt and ground pepper. Using a hand blender, purée until smooth.

When the beef is cooked, cool for a few minutes; then slice on a cutting board.

TO SERVE

Serve slices of beef topped with apple-and-pear gravy and fruit pieces. Place a dollop of smashed yams on each plate.

grilled new york striploin steak salad

SERVES 4 | TOTAL TIME 25 MINUTES | ACTIVE TIME 25 MINUTES

Start spreading the news … I'm pregnant today … You'll be singing along as you prepare this harmonious medley of warm and cool vegetables, topped with thin slices of New York striploin. Wouldn't it be great to go to the Big Apple for a maternity and baby clothes shopping spree?

INGREDIENTS

4 New York striploin steaks (approx 4 to 6 ounces each)

3 tablespoons balsamic vinegar

½ red onion, sliced

1 cup halved mushrooms

¼ cup walnuts

1 firm ripe avocado

1 cup cherry or grape tomatoes

4 cups mixed or spring greens

¼ cup shredded Asiago or cheddar cheese

6 tablespoons olive oil

METHOD

Drizzle 1 tablespoon of balsamic vinegar on both sides of steaks. On a grill or barbecue over medium-high heat, cook steaks to desired doneness. Lightly brush a piece of foil with cooking oil; spread onion and mushrooms on foil. About 6 to 8 minutes before end of cooking time, place on barbecue and cook until mushrooms are browned and onions translucent. (Or sauté in a frying pan with a bit of olive oil if cooking indoors.)

Meanwhile, toast walnuts on a baking sheet in a 375°F oven until fragrant and golden. Peel, pit and thinly slice avocado; arrange along with tomatoes on top of greens on individual plates.

Slice steak into thin strips and arrange on top of greens. Add grilled onion and mushrooms. Sprinkle cheese generously over top. Combine oil and remaining vinegar and drizzle over top.

TO SERVE

Serve with crusty bread.

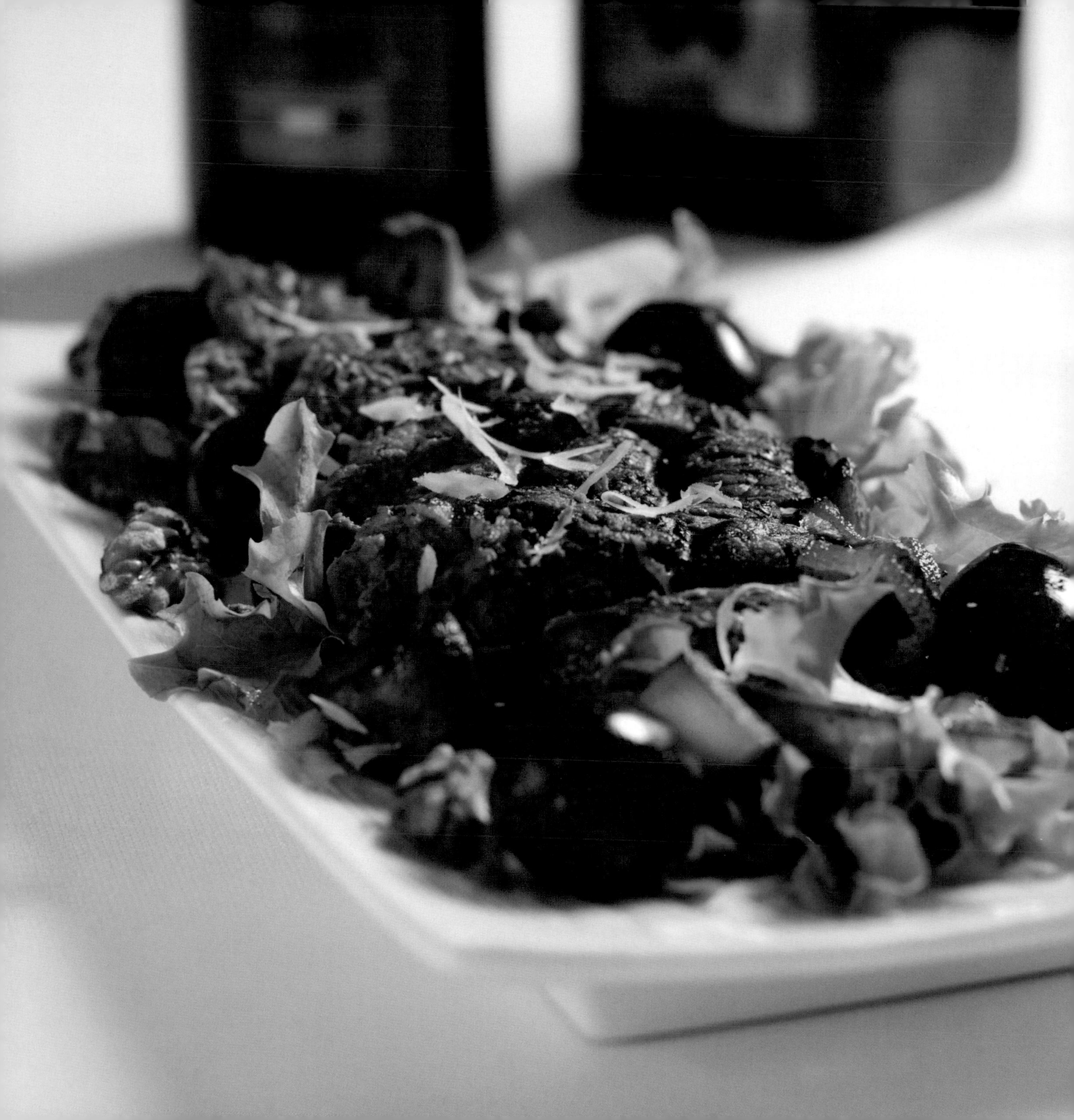

moroccan spiced chicken quesadilla with dried fruits

SERVES 4 | TOTAL TIME 45 MINUTES | ACTIVE TIME 40 MINUTES

Take a quesadilla from pub-style to perfection with this exotic and elegant blend of spices. Adding dried fruit instead of salsa brings it way upscale. Your sweetie will be talking about what a fantastic meal this is long after your baby is born!

INGREDIENTS

2 teaspoons each ground cumin, ground coriander and ground ginger

½ teaspoon each turmeric, cinnamon and chili powder

¼ teaspoon ground cloves

2 tablespoons olive oil

4 boneless, skinless chicken breasts

4 teaspoons butter

1 onion, sliced

2 cloves garlic, minced

¼ cup each dried apricots, blueberries, apple rings and cranberries

⅔ cup cranberry juice

3 tablespoons champagne vinegar

Salt and freshly ground black pepper

4 flour tortillas

1 cup shredded Monterey Jack cheese

4 tablespoons sour cream

Fresh mint leaves, for garnish

METHOD

Preheat oven to 400°F. In a small bowl, combine cumin, coriander, ginger, turmeric, cinnamon, chili powder and cloves. Set aside 2 teaspoons of the spice mixture. Stir in olive oil to remaining spice mixture.

Pat chicken dry with paper towel and rub with spice-oil mixture. Heat 3 teaspoons of the butter in a frying pan over medium heat; cook chicken for about 4 minutes per side. Remove chicken and add onion and garlic to pan. Slice chicken and return to pan to finish cooking.

In a saucepan, combine dried fruit, cranberry juice, vinegar and remaining spice mixture. Season with salt and ground pepper. Bring to a boil; then reduce heat and simmer for 5 minutes.

With the remaining 1 teaspoon of butter, lightly butter tortillas on one side. Sprinkle cheese and chicken mixture on half of each tortilla, dividing evenly. Fold in half and bake for 6 to 8 minutes, until golden.

TO SERVE

Cut tortillas into quarters and serve on individual plates with fruit mixture and a dollop of sour cream on the side. Garnish fruit with mint leaves.

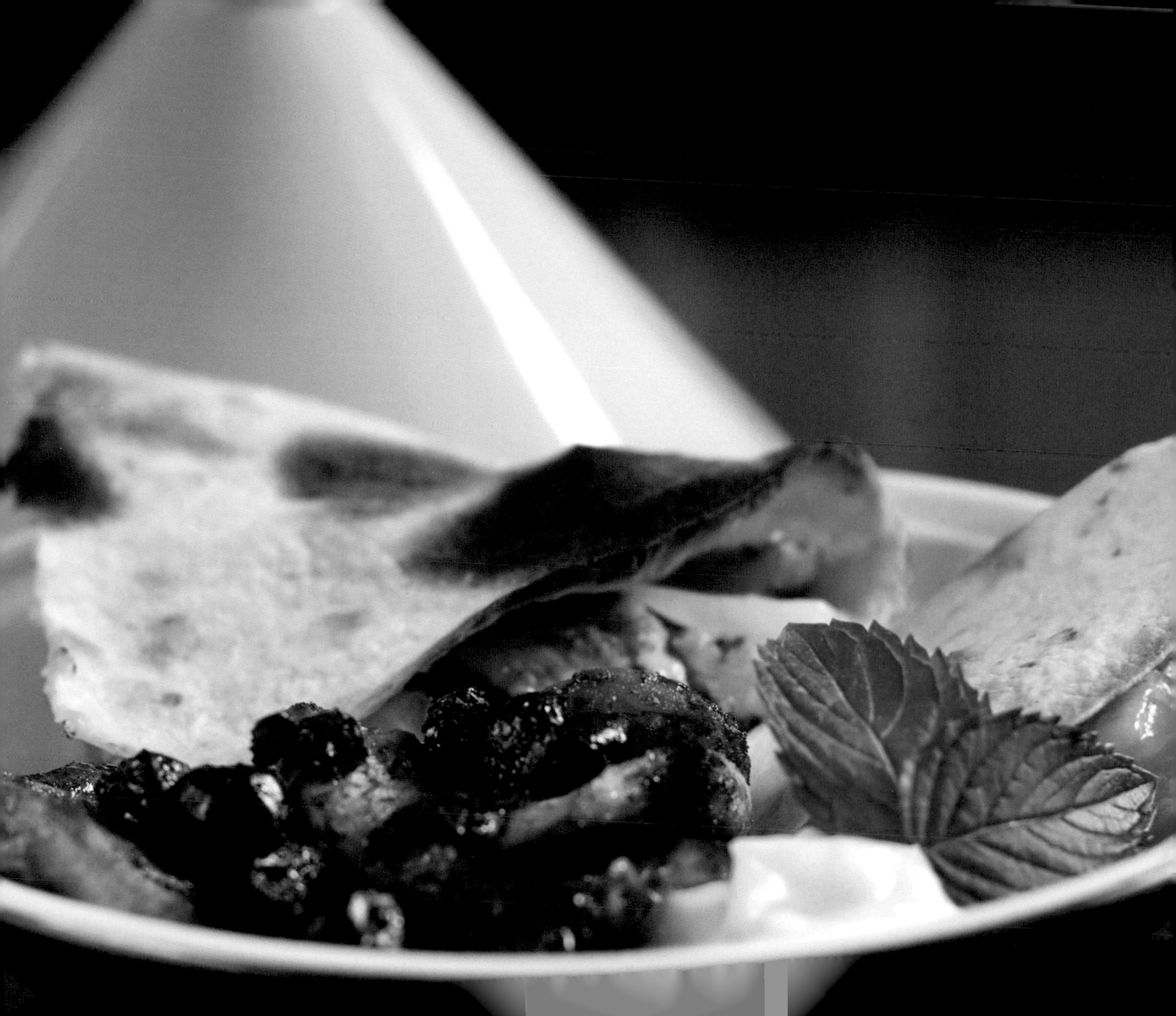

ancho chili chicken and zucchini with garlic roasted potatoes

SERVES 2 | TOTAL TIME 1 HOUR 15 MINUTES | ACTIVE TIME 1 HOUR

Roasted chili peppers provide abundant gentle heat, without the fire of raw chilies. I had lots of cravings for Mexican food while pregnant but quickly tired of regular tacos and burritos. This adventurous dish is spicy, different and so very satisfying.

POTATOES

4 medium red potatoes

1 clove garlic, finely chopped

2 tablespoons olive oil

¼ teaspoon salt

CHICKEN

1 habanero chili pepper

½ teaspoon ground cumin

½ teaspoon ancho chili powder

2 boneless, skinless chicken breasts

2 tablespoons olive oil

1 large zucchini, sliced

½ small onion

2 tablespoons milk

METHOD

Preheat oven to 425°F. Scrub and quarter potatoes. Place the potatoes and garlic in a roasting pan, add 2 tablespoons of olive oil and the salt; toss to coat. Roast for 45 to 60 minutes, tossing occasionally, until potatoes are crisp but still tender inside.

To prepare the chicken, place habanero pepper under broiler set at high. Using tongs, turn the pepper every 5 to 6 minutes, until skin is blistered and blackened on all sides (about 20 minutes in total). Remove from oven and seal in a paper bag for 15 minutes to steam.

In a small bowl, combine cumin and ancho chili, and sprinkle on both sides of chicken breasts. Add olive oil to a heavy-bottomed pan over medium-low heat; brown chicken on both sides. Meanwhile, remove the skin from the roasted pepper. Thinly slice the pepper, discarding all seeds.

Add sliced pepper, zucchini and onion to the pan and cook until onion is translucent. Add milk in the last 1 to 2 minutes of cooking time.

TO SERVE

On individual plates, make a base with the potatoes and place zucchini and chicken on top.

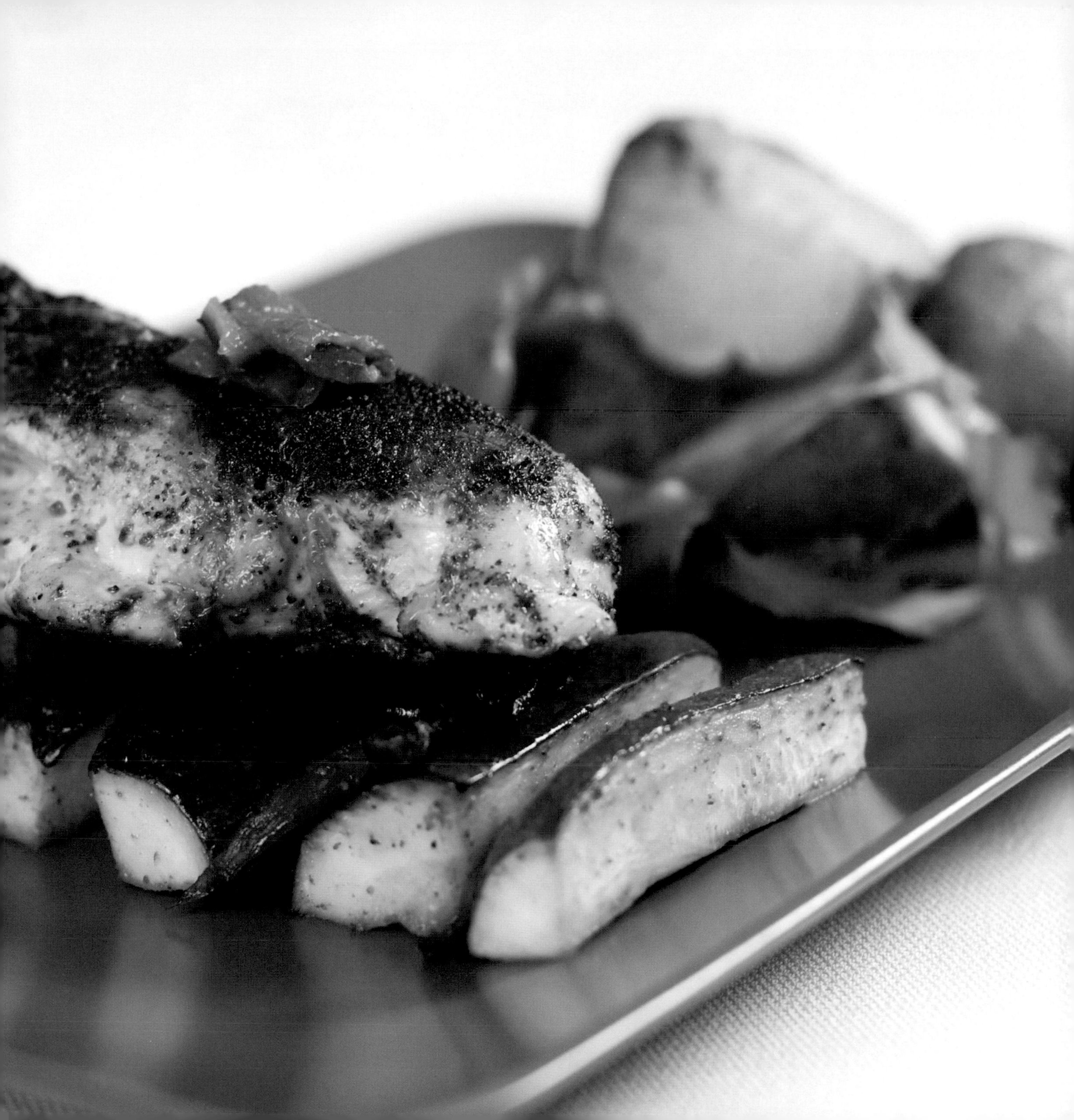

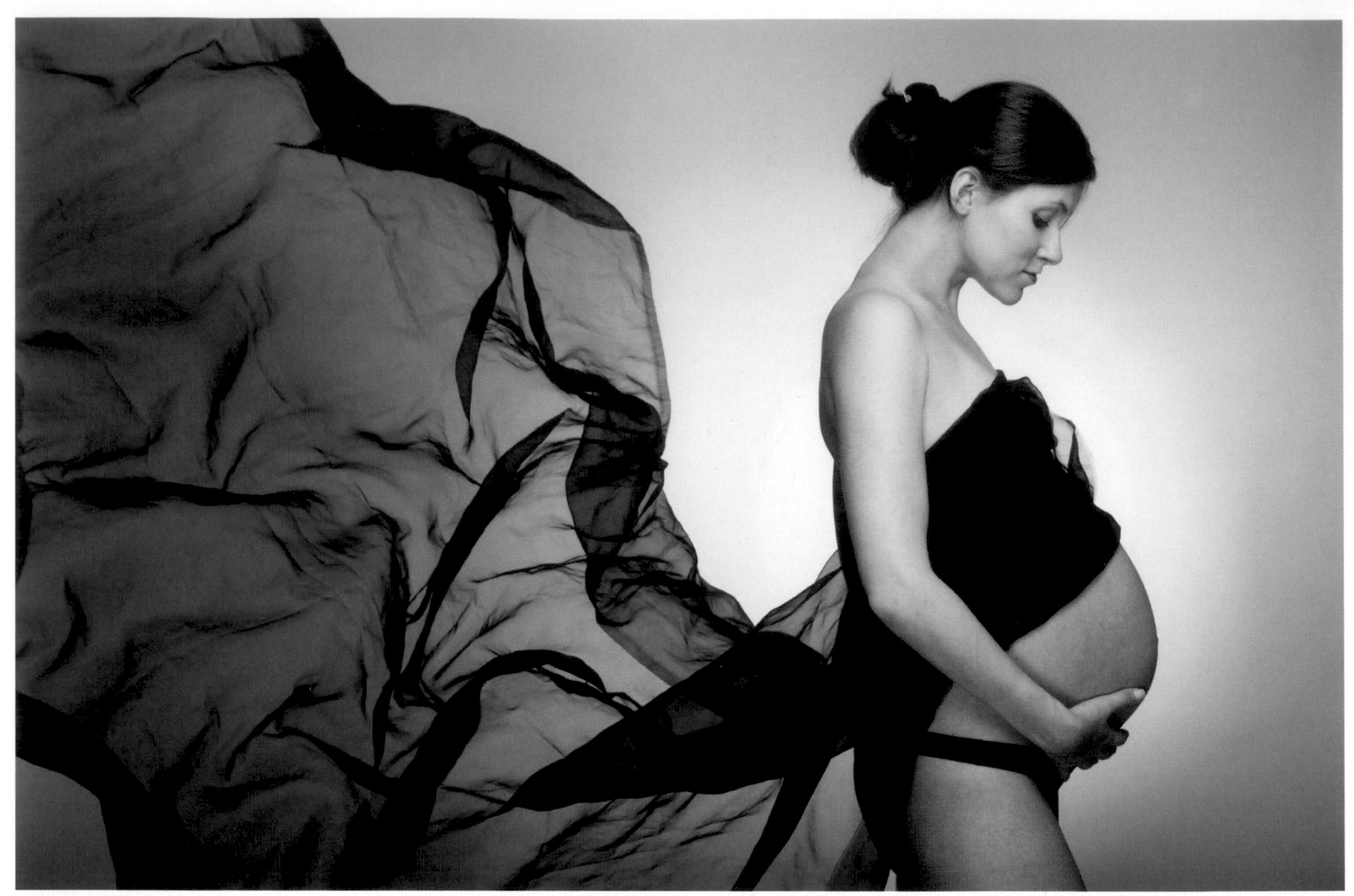

© iStockphoto.com/MariyaL

a bite for you, a bite for baby, a bite for you:

desserts

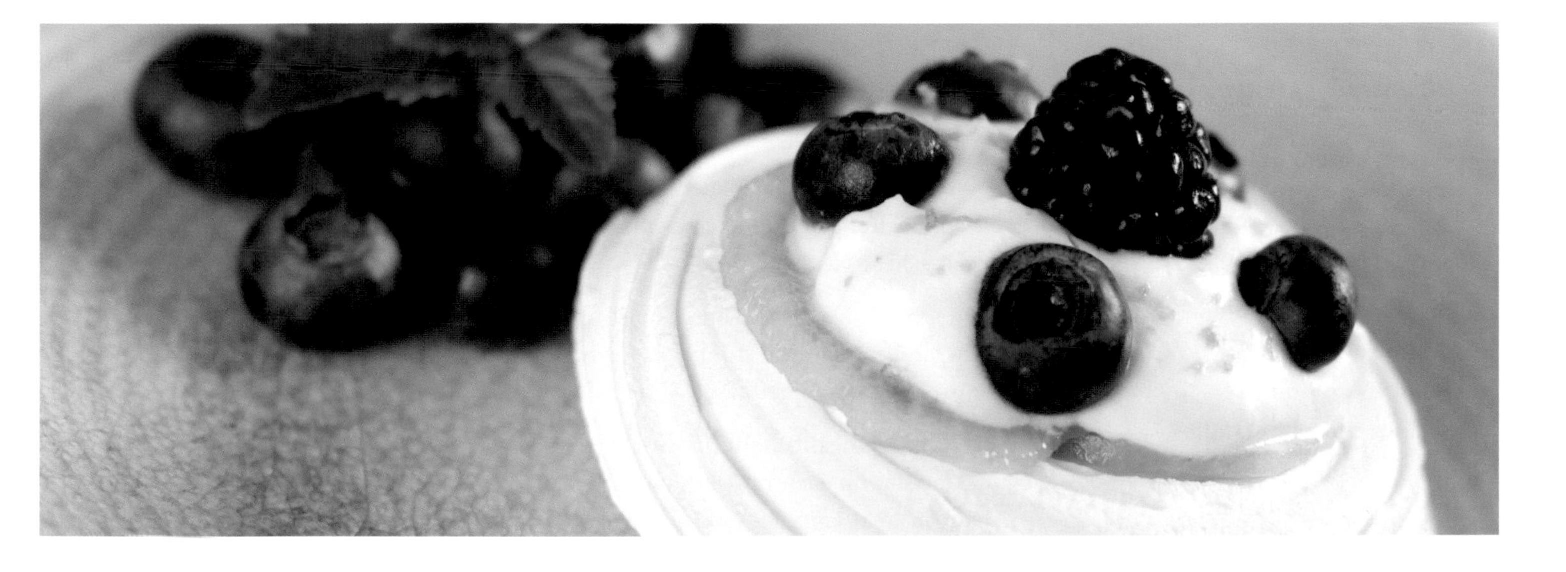

"Ice cream is exquisite.
What a pity it isn't illegal."

~ Voltaire

chocolate truffle soufflés

SERVES 4 | TOTAL TIME ABOUT 1 HOUR | ACTIVE TIME 30 TO 40 MINUTES

There's a naughty little surprise in the centre of these smooth chocolaty soufflés. The first few bites are scrumptious, but the next few bites will take you over the edge. While savouring this dessert, your sweetie will fall in love with you again.

INGREDIENTS

3 tablespoons butter, plus extra for ramekins

6 tablespoons granulated sugar, plus extra for ramekins

1 cup semisweet chocolate, chopped

3 tablespoons whipping cream

1 teaspoon pure vanilla extract

3 large egg yolks

4 large egg whites

4 Lindt chocolate truffles

METHOD

Preheat oven to 400°F. Butter six 7-ounce ramekins. Coat thoroughly with sugar. Chill in the refrigerator until ready to use.

Melt semisweet chocolate in a double boiler. Stir in whipping cream, butter and vanilla. Remove from heat; whisk in 3 tablespoons of the sugar and the egg yolks. Set aside to let cool.

In a bowl, beat eggs whites until frothy. Add in the remaining 3 tablespoons of sugar, beating until stiff peaks form. Fold the egg whites into the chocolate mixture until combined.

Fill the ramekins halfway with the chocolate mixture; then add a truffle to each cup. Top up each ramekin with the remaining chocolate mixture. Bake soufflés for 17 to 20 minutes or until they are firm yet still jiggle when lightly shaken.

TO SERVE

The ramekins will be very hot, so place each on a dessert plate. Serve immediately, before the soufflés fall.

Note: *The mixture can be prepared and poured into ramekins several hours in advance of baking.*

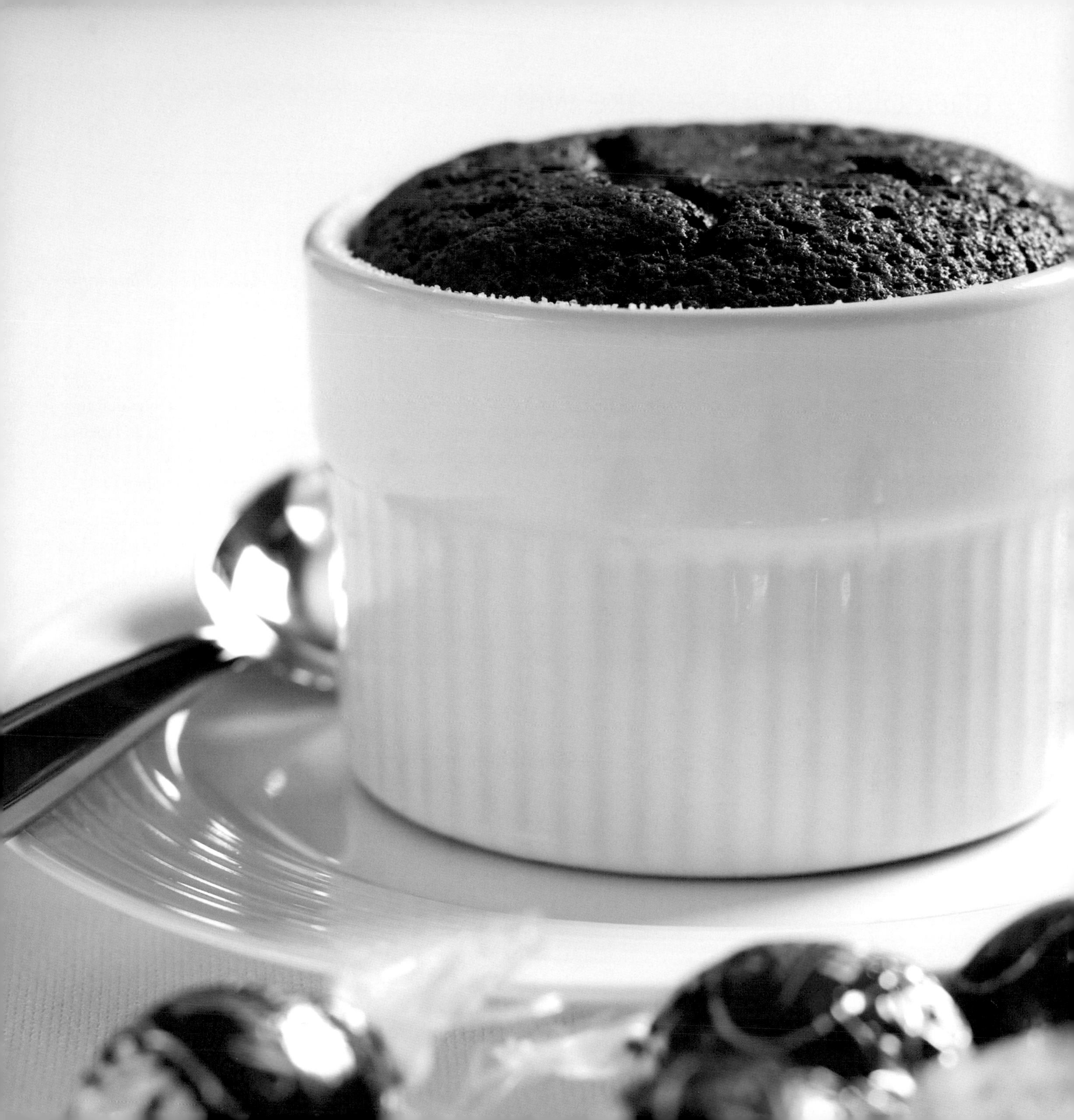

chocolate mousse cake with chocolate cookie toffee crust

SERVES 10 TO 12 | TOTAL TIME 3 HOURS | ACTIVE TIME 30 TO 40 MINUTES

This heavenly chocolate cake is a regular indulgence in my home. I make it every year for my husband's birthday, and he is always sure to show his appreciation! I keep it in the freezer and have an icy cold slice of chocolate toffee richness whenever we feel like eating something wicked.

CRUST

1 pkg chocolate sandwich cookies (with chocolate filling)

⅓ cup Skor bits

¼ cup butter, melted

CHOCOLATE MOUSSE

2 cups semisweet chocolate chips

1 teaspoon pure vanilla extract

3 cups whipping cream

¼ cup granulated sugar

METHOD

Preheat oven to 350°F. To make the crust, grind cookies in a blender to a medium-fine consistency; pour into a large mixing bowl. Add Skor bits and melted butter, stirring to mix well. Press the crust evenly into the bottom of a 9-inch springform pan. Bake for 4 to 5 minutes. Cool crust in pan on a cooling rack.

To make the chocolate mousse, in a large saucepan over low heat, warm chocolate chips, vanilla and 1 cup of the whipping cream, stirring gently until chocolate is melted and mixture is smooth. Transfer to a bowl; let cool in the refrigerator.

In a separate large mixing bowl, add the remaining 2 cups of whipping cream and the sugar. Beat until stiff peaks form. Fold in the cooled chocolate mixture; spread evenly over crust. Let the cake cool in the refrigerator or freezer for at least 2 hours before serving.

TO SERVE

Place wedges of cake on individual dessert plates.

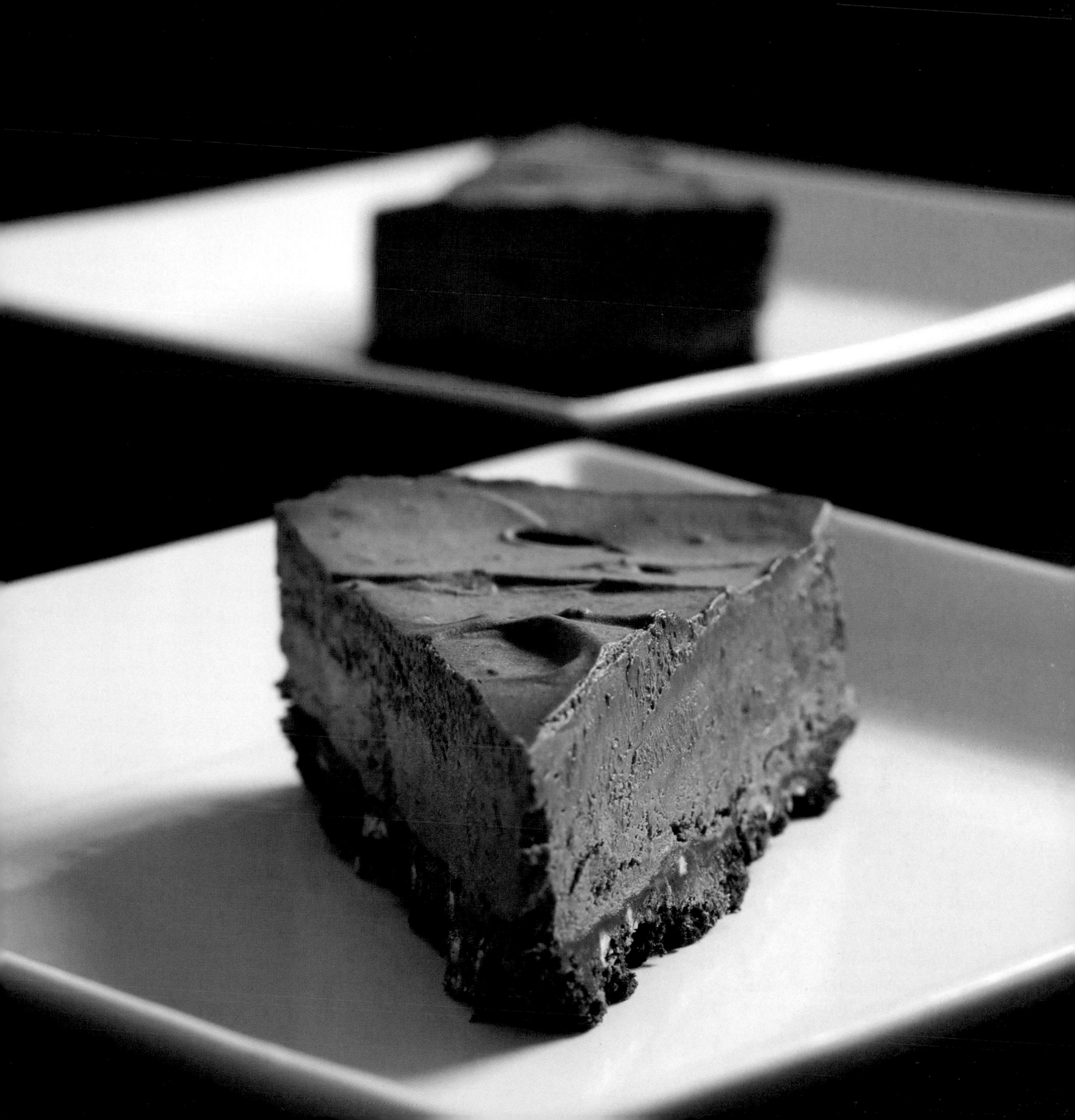

dulce de leche sex in a pan

SERVES 16 TO 20 | TOTAL TIME 2 HOURS | ACTIVE TIME 2 HOURS

We all know how great sex can be. How else would we be in this glorious pregnant state? Try this dessert and see how it compares! It is like the love child of two fabulous things — the traditional "sex in a pan" dessert, and smooth Spanish milk candy, or dulce de leche. It is layered in with cream cheese ganache, a rich crust and fresh whipped cream. Soooo delicious. It takes a bit of time, like all good things, but it sure is worth it in the end.

DULCE DE LECHE

1 vanilla bean

4 cups whole (3.5% MF) milk

1½ cups granulated sugar

1 teaspoon baking soda

1 teaspoon cornstarch stirred in 2 tablespoons water

CRUST

½ cup butter, melted

1½ cups graham cracker crumbs

1 cup pecan pieces

GANACHE

1 cup whipping cream

1 cup semisweet chocolate chips

8 ounces cream cheese, softened and divided into 4

TOPPING

2 cups whipping cream

3 tablespoons icing sugar

1 teaspoon pure vanilla extract

Oreo-type cookie crumbs or chocolate shavings, for garnish (optional)

METHOD

To make dulce de leche (third layer), slice the vanilla bean in half lengthwise. In a large saucepan, combine milk, sugar, vanilla bean halves and baking soda. Warm over medium-high heat, stirring frequently with a wooden spoon, until mixture comes to a gentle boil. Reduce heat to medium, continuing to stir. The mixture will darken and reduce significantly. Being careful not to let the mixture boil over, stir continuously for 30 minutes. (If it starts to bubble up or rise, take the pot off the heat momentarily and/or blow hard on it. You may need to adjust the heat occasionally to keep it at a simmer.) Remove vanilla beans with a fork or tongs. Continue stirring continuously for another 10 to 20 minutes, until mixture is very thick and dark; remove from heat. Stir cornstarch mixture into dulce de leche to thicken it further. Pour dulce de leche into a bowl and refrigerate until ready to use.

To make crust, preheat oven to 350°F. In a bowl, mix melted butter, graham cracker crumbs and pecans. Pat evenly into the bottom of a lightly oiled 13- × 9-inch baking pan. Bake for 20 minutes. Cool crust in pan on a cooling rack.

Meanwhile, to make ganache (second layer), pour chocolate chips in a large mixing bowl. In a large saucepan, bring whipping cream to a boil over medium heat. Whisk hot cream into chocolate chips. Whisk in pieces of cream cheese until smooth. Pour mixture evenly over crust. Remove dulce de leche from refrigerator and spoon evenly over ganache layer.

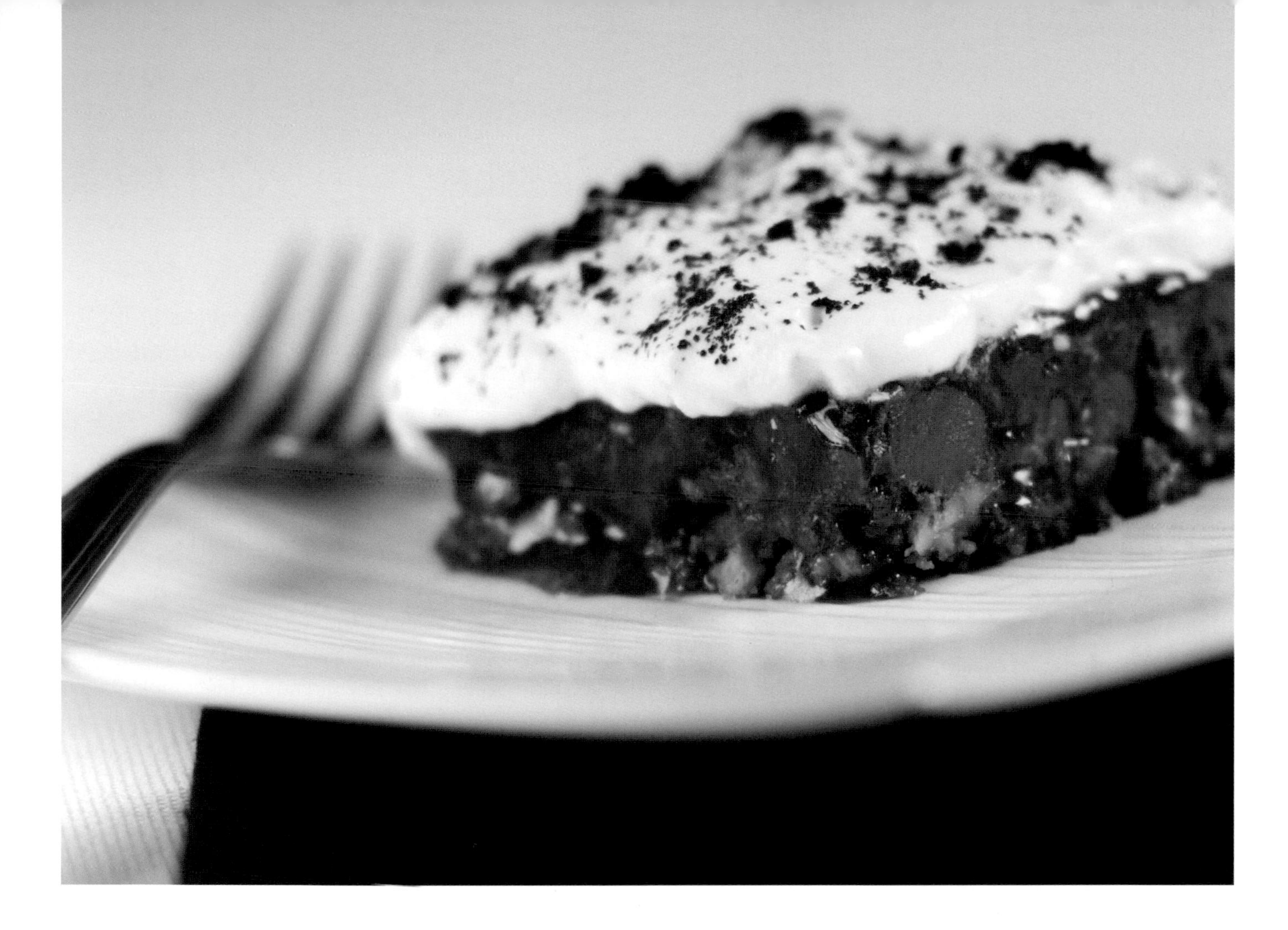

To make topping, pour whipping cream into a large mixing bowl; beat with a hand mixer until soft peaks form. Add sugar and vanilla; continue beating until stiff peaks form, about 8 to 10 minutes. Spread over dulce de leche layer.

TO SERVE

Slice into pieces while still in pan; gently remove each slice with a spatula and place on individual dessert plates. Sprinkle with cookie crumbs or chocolate shavings (if using).

orange ginger pumpkin cheesecake

SERVES 10 TO 12 | TOTAL TIME 2 HOURS | ACTIVE TIME 30 TO 40 MINUTES

This irresistible cheesecake conjures up the scent of falling leaves in autumn and the fresh coolness in the air when trick-or-treating; it'll have you looking forward to all of the fall fun you'll have with your new little baby. The combination of pumpkin, fresh ginger and orange zest makes a distinctly delectable treat.

CRUST

2½ cups ginger snap crumbs

⅔ cup margarine, melted

⅔ cup granulated sugar

FILLING

3 (8-ounce) pkgs cream cheese, softened

¾ cup loosely packed brown sugar

¾ cup granulated sugar

1 tablespoon pure maple syrup

2 tablespoons all-purpose flour

1 teaspoon ground cinnamon

½ teaspoon freshly grated ginger

½ teaspoon ground nutmeg

Zest of 1 large orange

4 eggs

1 (15-ounce) can pumpkin purée

METHOD

Preheat oven to 350°F. To make the crust, in a bowl, combine ginger snap crumbs, margarine and sugar. Press into a greased 9-inch springform pan. Bake for 6 to 8 minutes, until golden. Cool crust in pan on a cooling rack.

To make filling, blend together cream cheese and sugars at low speed until combined. Add maple syrup, flour, cinnamon, ginger, nutmeg and orange zest, stirring to incorporate. Beat in eggs one at a time. Blend in the pumpkin. Pour batter into the crust and bake for 50 to 60 minutes or until centre is almost set. Let stand until cool.

TO SERVE

Serve with whipped cream or sprinkle with cinnamon and garnish with a cinnamon stick.

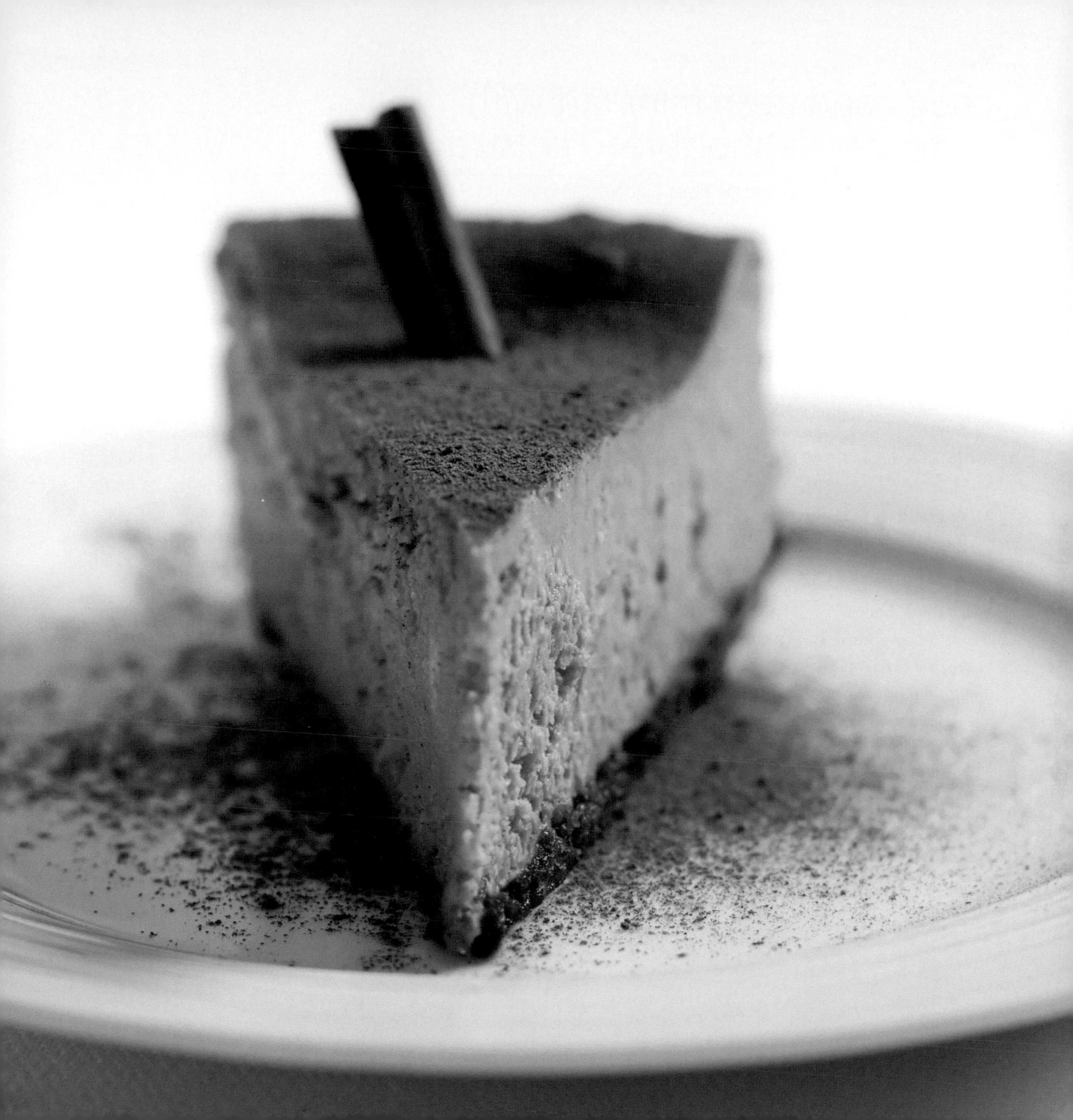

cherry and fresh mint tart with rustic vanilla shortbread crust

SERVES 12 TO 16 | TOTAL TIME ABOUT 1 HOUR | ACTIVE TIME 30 MINUTES

I craved cherries throughout my pregnancy … and I could have eaten this simple and beautiful dessert all day long. It is made with a rich, buttery crust and a sassy, lively fruit topping. The freshness of the cherries makes me smile and shine, and the mint gives me a summery glow any time of the year.

CRUST

1 cup butter

1 teaspoon pure vanilla extract

½ cup icing sugar

1½ cups all-purpose flour

2½ tablespoons cornstarch

FILLING

¼ cup chopped fresh mint leaves

½ cup water, boiled

3 cups cherries, halved and pitted

½ cup granulated sugar

2 tablespoons cornstarch

1 teaspoon pure vanilla extract

Fresh mint sprigs, for garnish

METHOD

Preheat oven to 325°F. To make crust, cream the butter and vanilla. Add sugar and blend well. In a separate bowl, whisk together flour and cornstarch. Add to butter mixture and whip with a hand mixer until well blended. Transfer dough to a parchment-lined baking sheet, and press with hands to make a relatively flat and even 8- × 12-inch rectangle. Roll up the edges to form a rustic-looking crust, about ¾ inch in height. Prick base all over with a fork; bake until just golden, about 15 to 20 minutes. Remove from oven and let cool completely before using.

To make the filling, place mint in a heatproof glass or bowl; pour hot water over top. Muddle the mint with a wooden spoon, crushing it into the water. Let the mint and water stand for 10 minutes. Once the water is cool, pour the mint mixture into a large saucepan. Add the cherries, sugar, cornstarch and vanilla, mixing well. Cook, stirring often, over medium heat until cherries soften and mixture becomes thick and glossy. Spread cherry filling evenly on crust. Let cool completely.

TO SERVE

Cut tart into squares after cooled. Place a sprig of mint on each square.

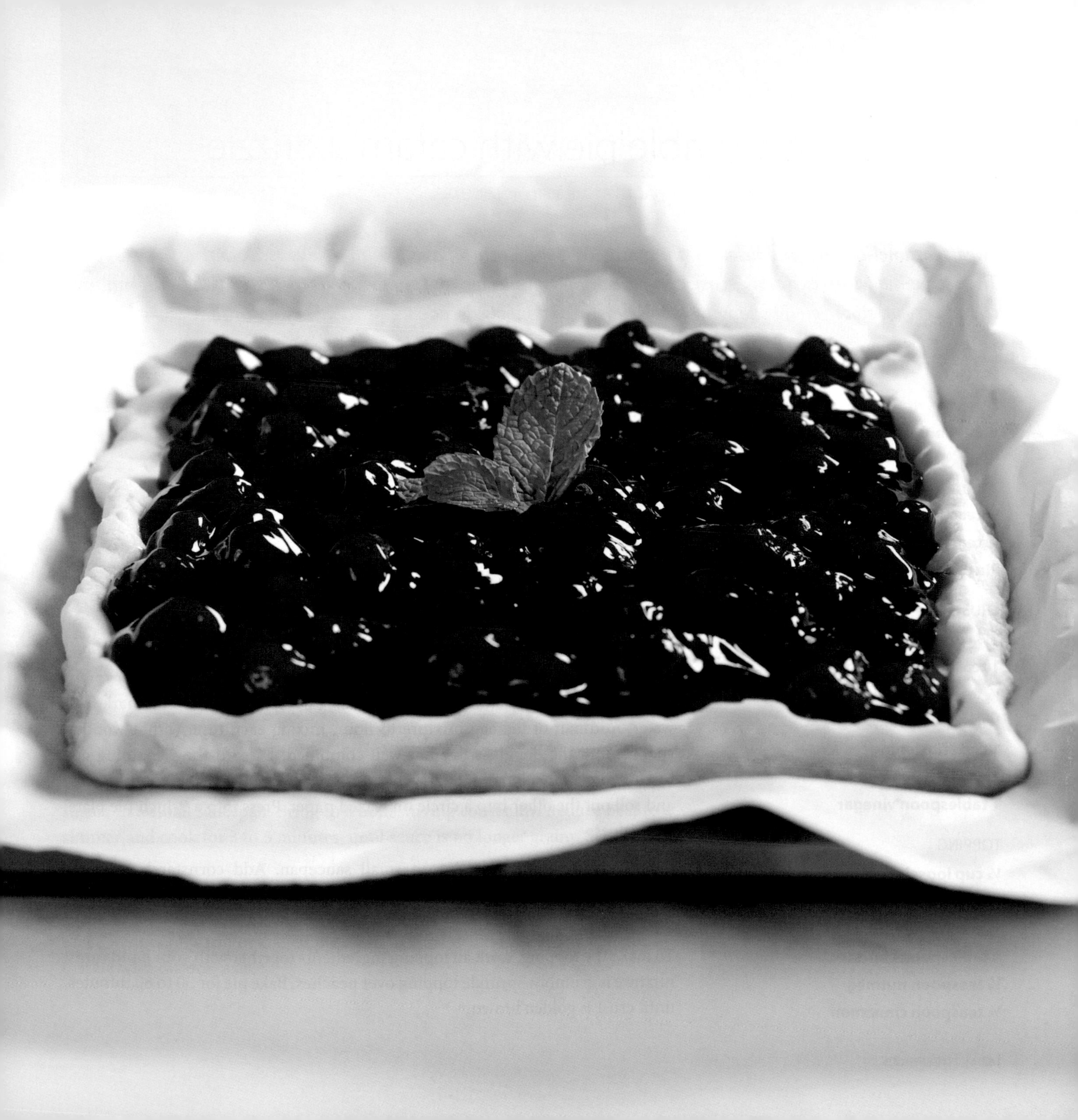

berry kiwi citrus cream meringues

SERVES 4 | TOTAL TIME 20 MINUTES | ACTIVE TIME 20 MINUTES

Light, tart and sweet, this refreshing dessert will melt in your mouth and energize your taste buds. The zesty lemon whipped cream can be used to add a fresh twist to other recipes as well, so don't be shy to experiment. Save yourself some time by using store-bought meringues (you can buy them at any large grocery store, and they taste just as good as homemade).

INGREDIENTS

1 cup whipping cream

2 tablespoons icing sugar

1 tablespoon fresh lemon juice

1 teaspoon lemon zest

2 kiwis, peeled and cut into 12 to 16 slices

4 store-bought meringue nests

¼ cup combination of fresh blueberries and blackberries

METHOD

Beat the whipping cream until stiff peaks form. Beat in the sugar, lemon juice and half of the lemon zest. Set aside.

TO SERVE

Arrange 3 or 4 slices of kiwi on each meringue. Spoon the lemon whipped cream over the kiwi and top with fresh berries. Serve on individual dessert plates, sprinkled with the remaining lemon zest.

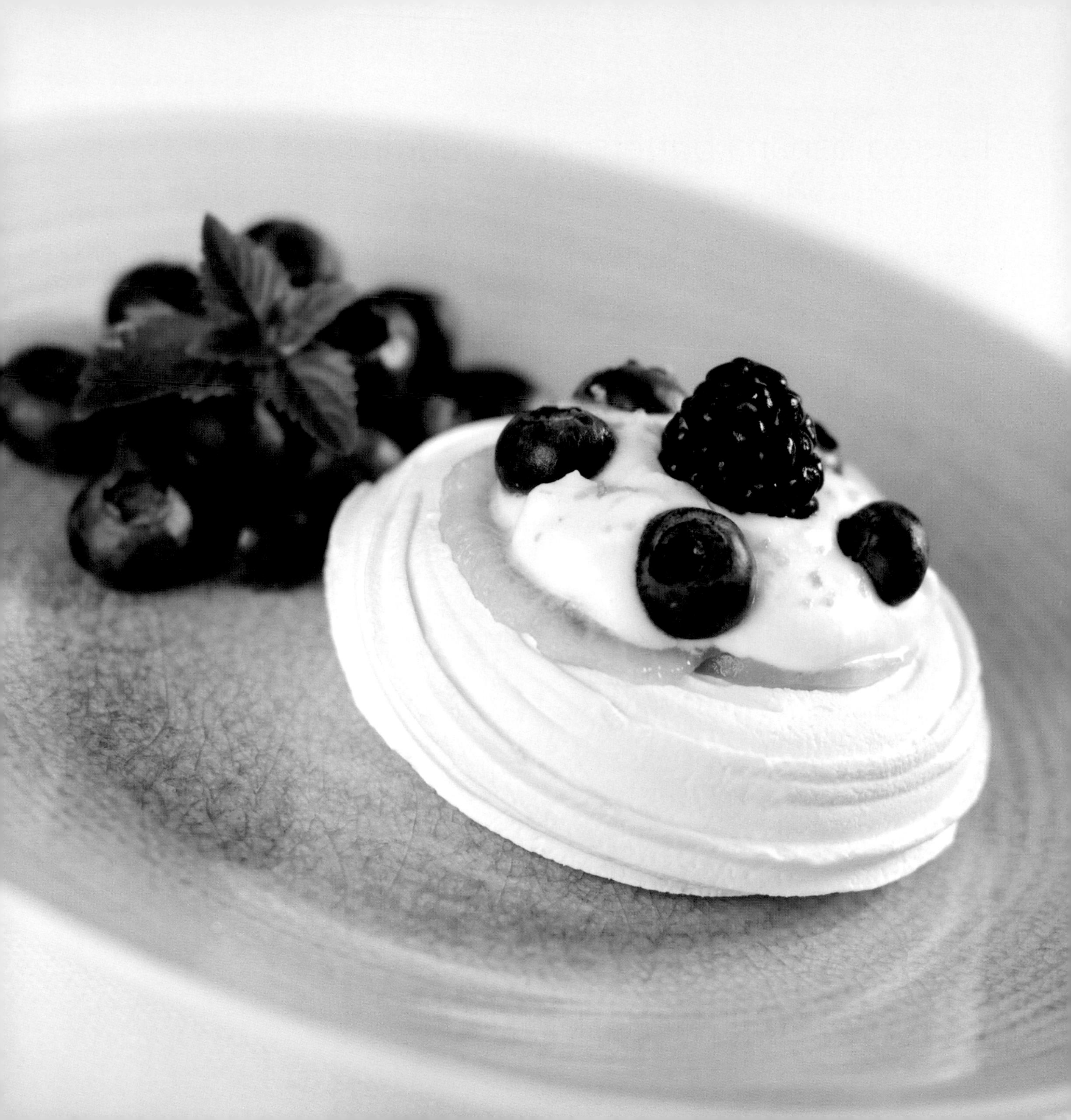

layered banana butterscotch pudding

SERVES 4 | TOTAL TIME 1 HOUR | ACTIVE TIME 30 TO 40 MINUTES

You might as well use those champagne flutes for something, as it'll be a few more months before you can have a sip of bubbly! This sweet, upscale pudding with a kiss of bananas and cream makes for a dramatic and classy presentation. Don't worry — there's no Scotch in butterscotch, despite the name.

PUDDING

4 large egg yolks

¾ cup loosely packed brown sugar

¼ cup cornstarch

⅛ teaspoon salt

2½ cups whole (3.5% MF) milk

¼ cup unsalted butter, cut in small pieces

1 tablespoon pure vanilla extract

1 tablespoon pure maple syrup

TOPPINGS

1 cup whipping cream

1 tablespoon icing sugar

½ teaspoon pure vanilla extract

2 ripe bananas

½ cup graham wafers, crushed

METHOD

In a large heatproof bowl, stir together the egg yolks, sugar, cornstarch and salt. Whisk in ¼ cup of the milk until well combined. Set aside.

In a medium saucepan, bring the remaining milk to a boil, stirring occasionally. Remove from heat and gradually whisk the hot milk into egg mixture until smooth. Transfer to a clean saucepan and, stirring constantly, cook over medium-low heat for about 2 minutes, until mixture thickens. Remove from heat and whisk in butter, vanilla and maple syrup. Pour through a fine strainer to remove any lumps.

Let the pudding cool while preparing the toppings. Beat whipping cream until stiff peaks form; mix in the icing sugar and vanilla. Slice bananas into rounds.

TO SERVE

Fill 4 champagne flutes with pudding to one-third full. Sprinkle evenly with graham wafer crumbs to form thin, even layers. Top with several banana slices. Add more pudding, to three-quarters full. Add another layer of graham crumbs, a generous dollop of whipped cream and a banana slice to each to top them off.

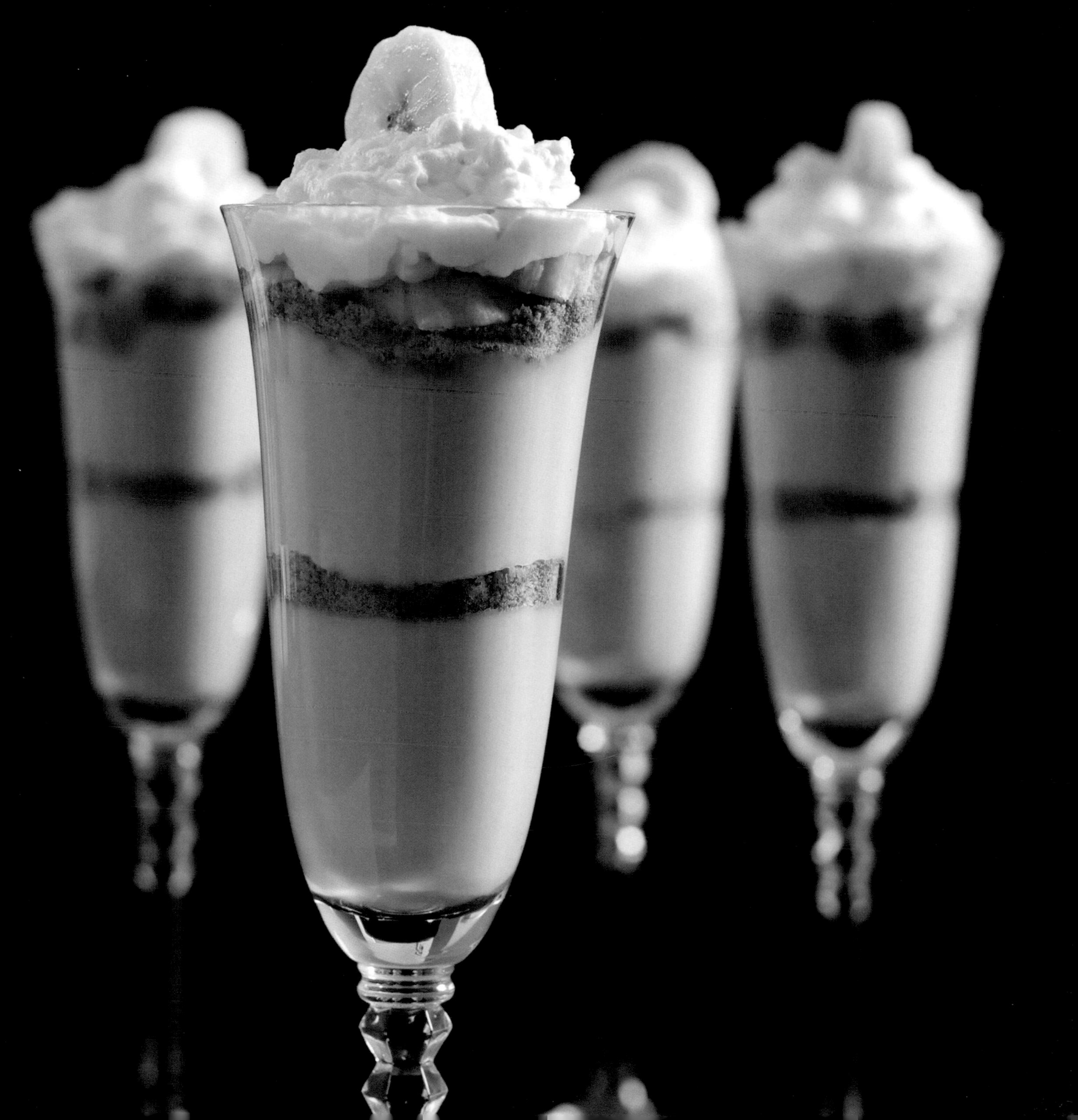

duet of dried cranberry shortbread and candy cane ice creams

SERVES 6 TO 8 | TOTAL TIME 1 HOUR | ACTIVE TIME 40 MINUTES

This may become the holiday treat that everyone can't get enough of. It is a long-standing favourite for our family at Christmastime, and perfectly gorgeous and festive. It can be made ahead and returned to the freezer for entertaining. As an added bonus, shortbread cookies don't include raw eggs — so you pregnant ladies can feel free to nibble on the dough before baking.

TOPPINGS

1 cup butter, softened

2 cups sifted all-purpose flour

¾ cup icing sugar

½ cup dried cranberries, chopped

1½ teaspoon pure vanilla extract

½ teaspoon salt

10 small (or 5 large) candy canes

ICE CREAM

4 cups good-quality vanilla ice cream

6 to 8 fresh mint sprigs, for garnish

METHOD

Preheat oven to 325°F. To make shortbread, cream butter in a large mixing bowl. Add flour, sugar, cranberries, vanilla and salt, stirring to incorporate. In a greased 8-inch square baking pan, press in cookie mixture, distributing evenly. Bake for at least 30 minutes, until golden brown. Remove from pan and place on a cooling rack. Cut into squares when cool.

Place one-quarter of the shortbread into a resealable bag and crush it to a fairly fine consistency. In another resealable bag, crush unwrapped candy canes to a similar consistency. Transfer both to separate bowls.

Let ice cream soften at room temperature for about 5 minutes, then use an ice cream scooper to make round balls and, using your fingers, gently roll alternately in candy cane or cranberry shortbread topping until generously and consistently coated. Refreeze in a shallow container immediately after rolling each ball. Make 1 candy cane ball and 1 cranberry shortbread ball for each person.

TO SERVE

Serve a ball of each on individual dessert plates, garnished with a sprig of mint.

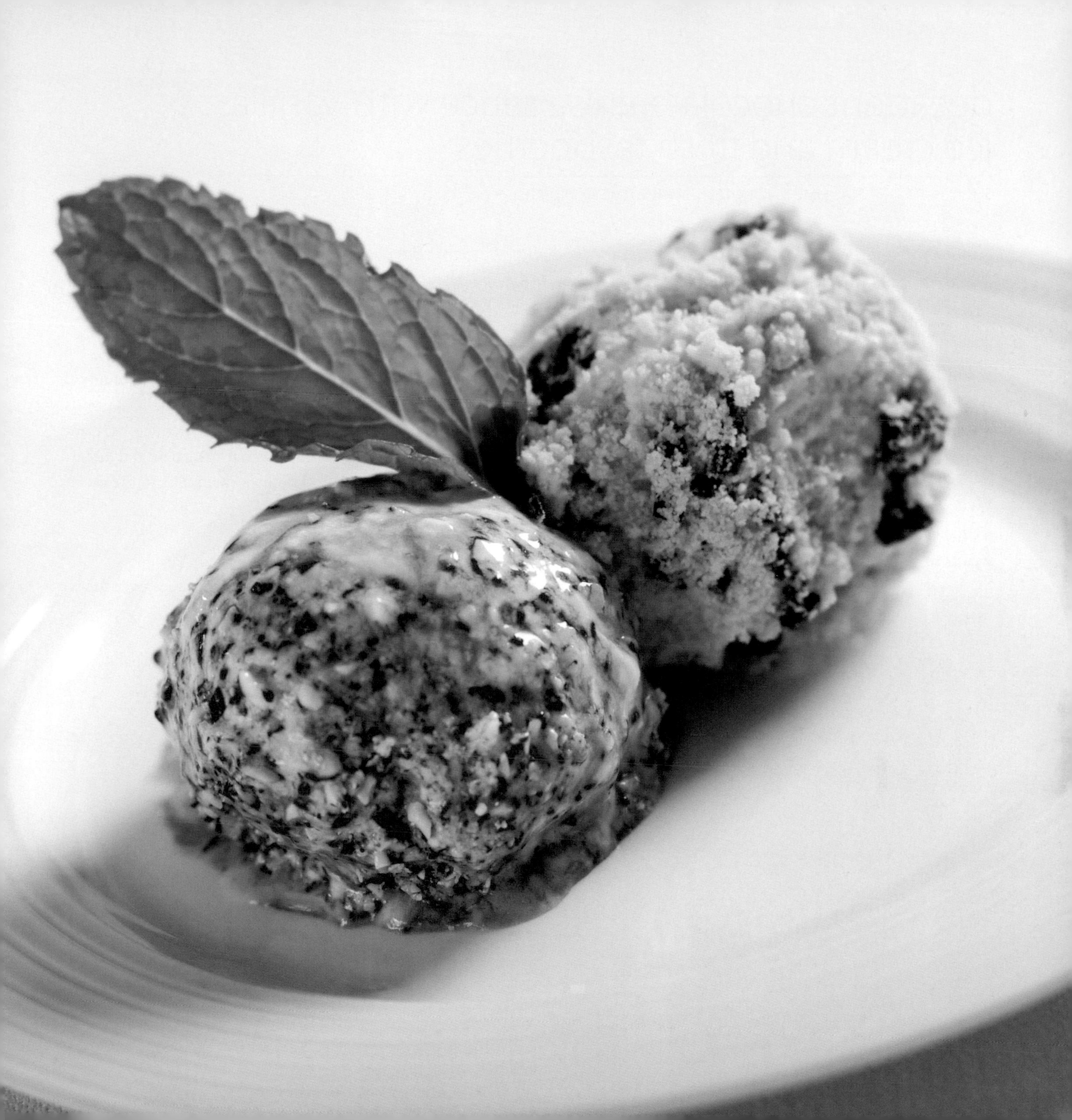

decadent chocolate anise sauce with vanilla ice cream and fresh raspberries

SERVES 6 TO 8 | TOTAL TIME 15 MINUTES | ACTIVE TIME 15 MINUTES

Should you eat more ice cream? Of course! It's for the baby. The exotic flavour of this sauce is splendid with mellow and delicate licorice notes, to add a grown-up touch. It pairs perfectly with sweet fruits such as raspberries.

INGREDIENTS

½ cup water

½ cup icing sugar

4 whole star anise

8 ounces good-quality dark chocolate

½ cup half-and-half cream

4 cups vanilla ice cream

2 cups fresh raspberries

METHOD

Pour water into a small saucepan. Add star anise and sugar and bring to a boil, stirring frequently. If the seeds are missing from some of the star anise pods, don't worry — it's the pods that have the strongest flavour. Reduce heat and continue cooking for 4 minutes, stirring frequently. Remove from heat and discard star anise. Stir in the chocolate until melted and incorporated. Stir in the cream until smooth.

TO SERVE

Scoop vanilla ice cream into individual bowls. Pour the warm sauce over the ice cream and top with fresh raspberries.

cashew brittle frost

SERVES 6 TO 8 | TOTAL TIME ABOUT 1 HOUR | ACTIVE TIME 20 TO 30 MINUTES

Are you craving sweet and salty with delectable ice cream? This splendid mix of textures is sure to please any pregnant palate with its mouth-watering chunky, crunchy taste. I know it is clichéd for pregnant women to crave ice cream — so why resist? Enjoy!

INGREDIENTS

2 tablespoons butter
1 teaspoon pure vanilla extract
1 teaspoon baking soda
¾ cup honey
¼ cup warm water
1 cup raw cashews
4 cups vanilla ice cream

METHOD

To make cashew brittle, pre-measure the butter, vanilla and baking soda; set aside. Butter a baking sheet and set aside — you will not have time to do these steps once the brittle is cooked.

In a heavy-bottomed saucepan over high heat, add honey and water. Once mixture reaches a boil, reduce heat to low; cook for 5 to 8 minutes. Add cashews and simmer, stirring consistently and being careful not to let the mixture burn, until nuts are golden, about 5 minutes. Remove from heat and quickly add butter, vanilla and baking soda. Mix well and pour onto a baking sheet. Let cool for at least 20 minutes. Break into pieces when hard.

Once cashew brittle is hardened, scoop ice cream into a large mixing bowl. Set aside to soften slightly, about 5 minutes. Meanwhile, with a mortar and pestle, crush three-quarters of the brittle into medium-small pieces. Stir into the softened ice cream, mixing well. Return the ice cream to the freezer for later (reserving the remaining brittle) or serve immediately.

TO SERVE

Scoop dessert into individual ice cream bowls. Use the remaining pieces of cashew brittle for garnish.

toffee coffee chocolate chip cookies

MAKES ABOUT 36 COOKIES | TOTAL TIME ABOUT 1 HOUR | ACTIVE TIME 20 MINUTES

The offbeat flavour pairing of melted toffee and robust coffee brings a ridiculously yummy goodness to these cookies. The buttery richness of the shortbread enhances the taste. Use decaf if you prefer a less wide-eyed effect.

INGREDIENTS

1 cup butter, slightly softened

½ cup loosely packed brown sugar

4 teaspoons instant coffee (decaf or regular)

1 tablespoon water

1 teaspoon pure vanilla extract

2 cups all-purpose flour

½ cup Skor bits

½ cup chocolate chips

METHOD

Using a hand mixer, in a large mixing bowl, cream butter until fluffy. Add brown sugar and continue to beat until incorporated. In a small bowl, dissolve instant coffee in the water. Add coffee and vanilla to butter mixture, beating to incorporate. Gradually add flour, ½ cup at a time, continuing to beat. When all the flour has been added, gently fold in the chocolate chips and Skor bits until just blended. Form a ball with the dough and cover with plastic wrap. Refrigerate until firm, about 30 minutes.

Preheat oven to 300°F. On a dry, flour-dusted surface, roll out chilled dough to about ¼-inch thickness. Using cookie cutters, make various sizes or shapes of cookies and place on an ungreased baking sheet. Bake for 18 to 20 minutes. Let cool on a cooling rack before serving.

TO SERVE

Serve in a stack on a large plate for guests to help themselves.

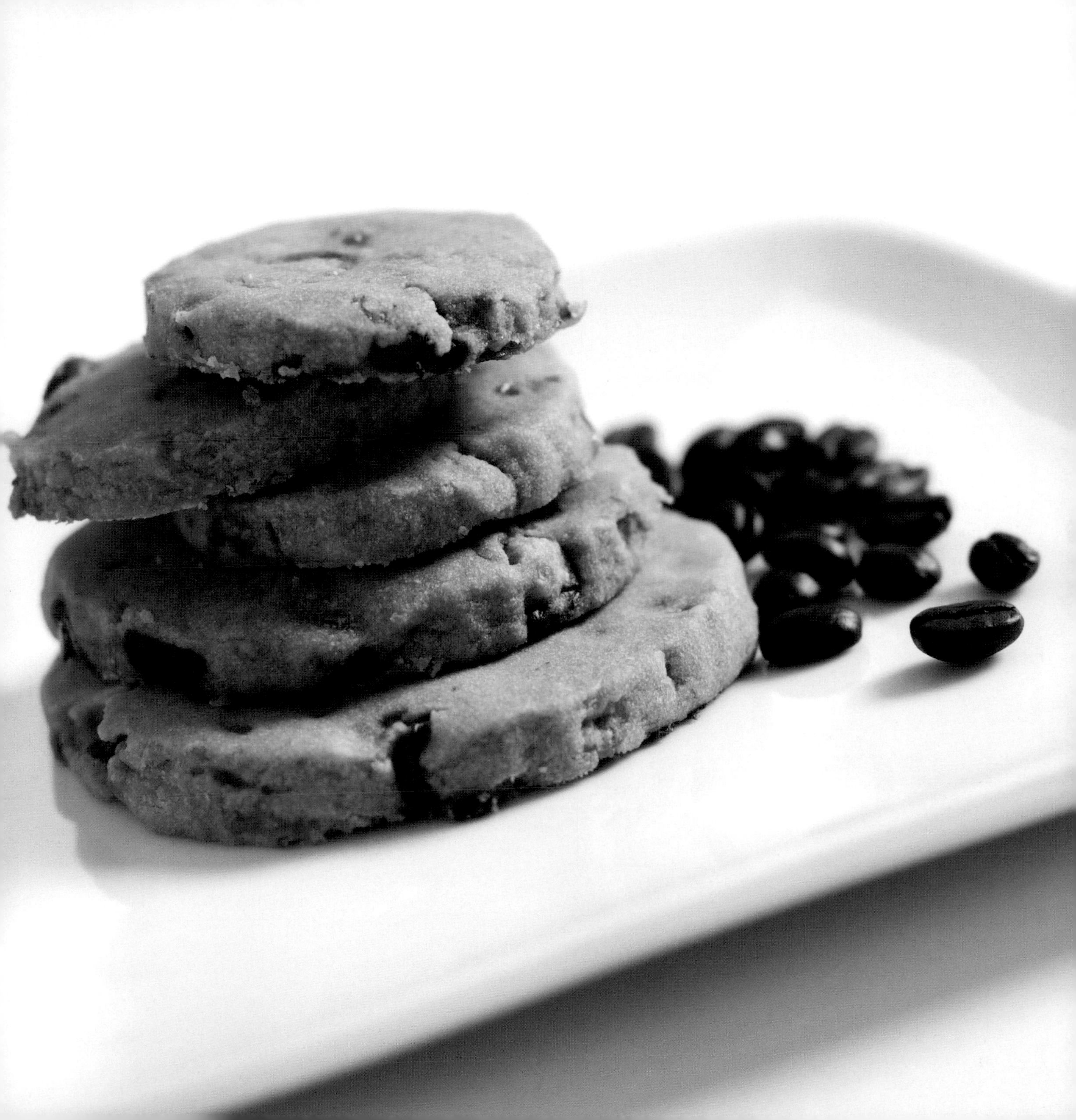

chocolate raspberry fudge

SERVES 12 TO 16 | TOTAL TIME 2 HOURS | ACTIVE TIME 15 MINUTES

Fudge brings back so many memories of simple childhood pleasures, at the beach or fair grounds with family and friends. This spectacularly tasty and quirky version is grown-up, easy and gourmet. I bought the raspberry syrup at a local coffee shop, and it adds a fruity kick to this treat.

INGREDIENTS

2½ cups semisweet chocolate chips

1 (14-ounce) can sweetened condensed milk

2 tablespoons raspberry syrup

1 teaspoon pure vanilla extract

⅛ teaspoon salt

2 cups fresh raspberries (or frozen, thawed and drained)

METHOD

In a saucepan, melt chocolate over medium-low heat. Stir in condensed milk, raspberry syrup, vanilla and salt. Continue to cook, stirring, until smooth. In a greased 8-inch square baking pan, with butter or cooking spray, evenly distribute half of the raspberries. Pour the chocolate fudge over the fruit, pressing it gently into the sides of the pan. Top with the remaining raspberries, pushing slightly into thc fudge. Cover and refrigerate for 1 to 2 hours before serving.

TO SERVE

Serve squares of fudge to guests on individual plates. If pregnant, just eat directly from the refrigerator with your fingers.

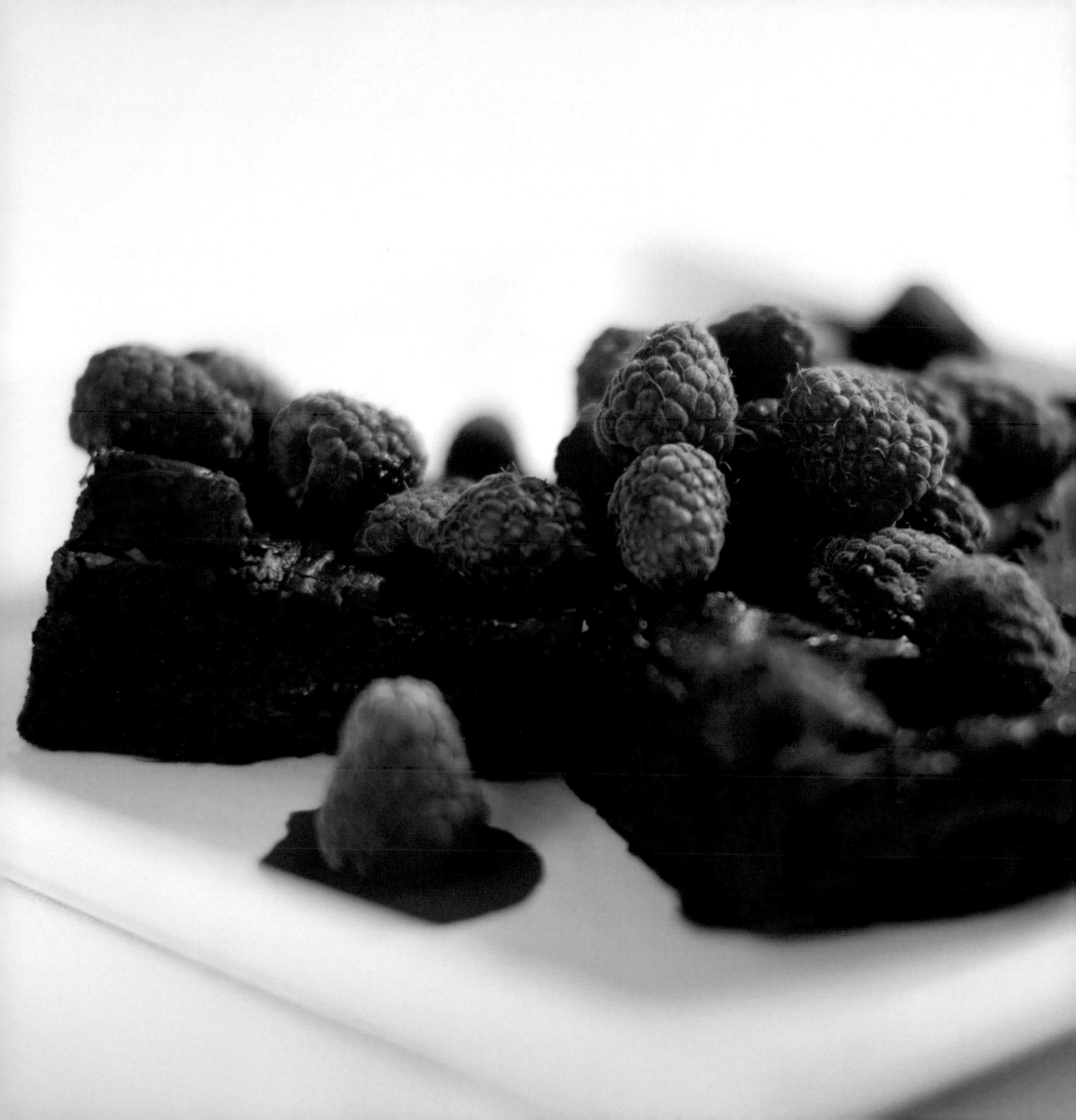

almond mocha nanaimo bars

SERVES 10 TO 12 | TOTAL TIME 2 HOURS | ACTIVE TIME 50 MINUTES

I live only a few hours from Nanaimo, British Columbia, so this smooth and satisfying reinvention of the charming classic has a special place in my heart (and tummy!). The addition of toasted almonds and coffee gives it a divine complexity you are sure to love.

BOTTOM LAYER

¾ cup unsalted butter

½ cup loosely packed brown sugar

2 teaspoons instant coffee granules

1 teaspoon pure vanilla extract

1½ cups graham wafer crumbs

1 cup fine shredded unsweetened coconut

MIDDLE LAYER

2 tablespoons whipping cream

1 tablespoon instant coffee granules

1 teaspoon pure vanilla extract

½ cup unsalted butter

2 cups icing sugar

TOP LAYER

¼ cup finely chopped almonds

¾ cup semisweet chocolate chunks (approx 6 ounces)

3 tablespoons unsalted butter

METHOD

To make the bottom layer, melt butter in a saucepan over medium-low heat. Stir in sugar, coffee and vanilla. Remove from heat and stir in coconut and graham wafer crumbs. Firmly press mixture into a greased 8-inch square baking dish; chill in the refrigerator until the next layer is ready.

To make the middle layer, in a cup, stir together whipping cream, coffee and vanilla until coffee is dissolved. In a bowl, beat together butter, whipping cream mixture and sugar until well combined. Spread evenly over the bottom layer and return the pan to the refrigerator to chill.

To make the top layer, toast almonds lightly on a baking sheet in a 350°F oven; set aside to let cool. Melt chocolate and butter in a double boiler, stirring to combine. Remove from heat and allow to cool but not solidify. Pour over the middle layer and smooth out. Sprinkle with almonds, gently pressing them into the top layer. Chill in refrigerator for at least 1 hour to allow dessert to set.

TO SERVE

Cut into squares and serve on individual plates.

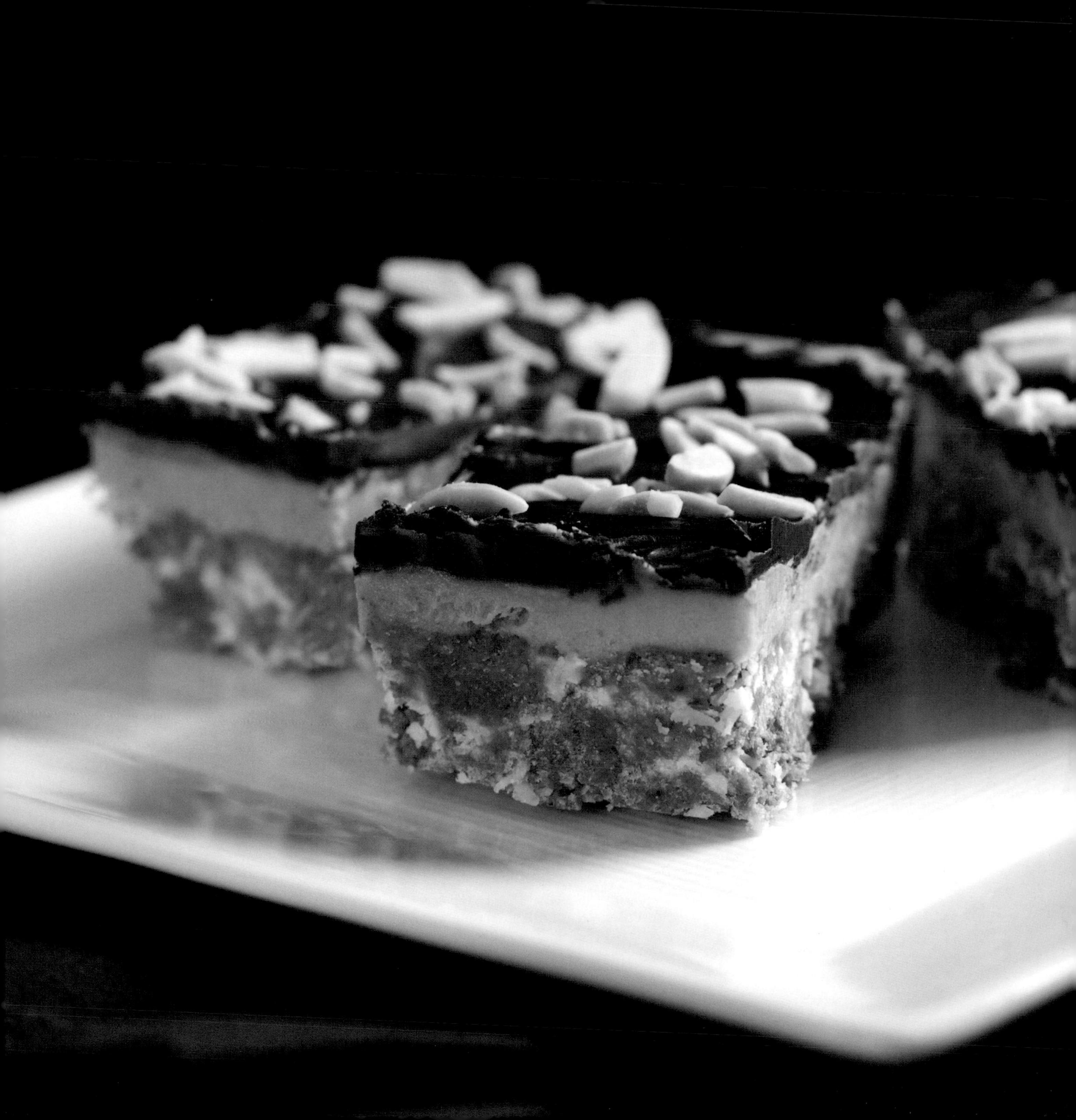

london fog cupcakes

MAKES 18 CUPCAKES | TOTAL TIME ABOUT 1 HOUR | ACTIVE TIME 30 TO 40 MINUTES

After waking from a refreshing nap on a rainy British afternoon, this is the treat you would dreamily indulge in. Its misty and creamy frosting gives a modern, sensuous and romantic feel to a classic indulgent cupcake. Both the cake and the frosting are infused with delicious Earl Gray tea. Use premium tea for the best flavour.

CUPCAKES

1½ cups milk (2% or 3.5% MF)
4 Earl Grey tea bags
½ cup butter
1 cup granulated sugar
3 large eggs
2 teaspoons pure vanilla extract
2 teaspoons baking powder
½ teaspoon salt
2 cups all-purpose flour

FROSTING

1 cup butter
2 teaspoons pure vanilla extract
4 cups icing sugar

METHOD

In a small heavy-bottomed pot, heat milk until scalding. Remove from heat and add the tea bags. Set aside for 20 to 30 minutes to steep.

Preheat oven to 350°F. In a large mixing bowl, using a hand mixer, cream the butter and sugar until fluffy. Add eggs and the vanilla; beat well. Add baking powder and salt. Remove the tea bags from the tea-steeped milk. Add half of the flour and ½ cup of the milk to butter mixture; beat on low. Add the remainder of the flour and another ½ cup of the milk; beat on low.

Line two 9-cup muffin tins with paper cupcake liners; distribute batter evenly, filling to two-thirds full. Bake for 18 to 20 minutes or until a toothpick inserted in the centre comes out clean. Transfer cupcakes to a cooling rack.

To make frosting, in a mixing bowl, beat butter until creamy. Beat in vanilla. Gradually add sugar while continuing to beat. Add 4 tablespoons of the tea-infused milk. Chill frosting in the refrigerator until cupcakes have cooled.

Frost cupcakes using an icing bag with a large tip or with a spatula. The frosting will not form well if it gets too soft from the heat of your hands; if it becomes too runny, return it to the refrigerator to chill slightly.

TO SERVE

Present several cupcakes on a large plate or cake tray.

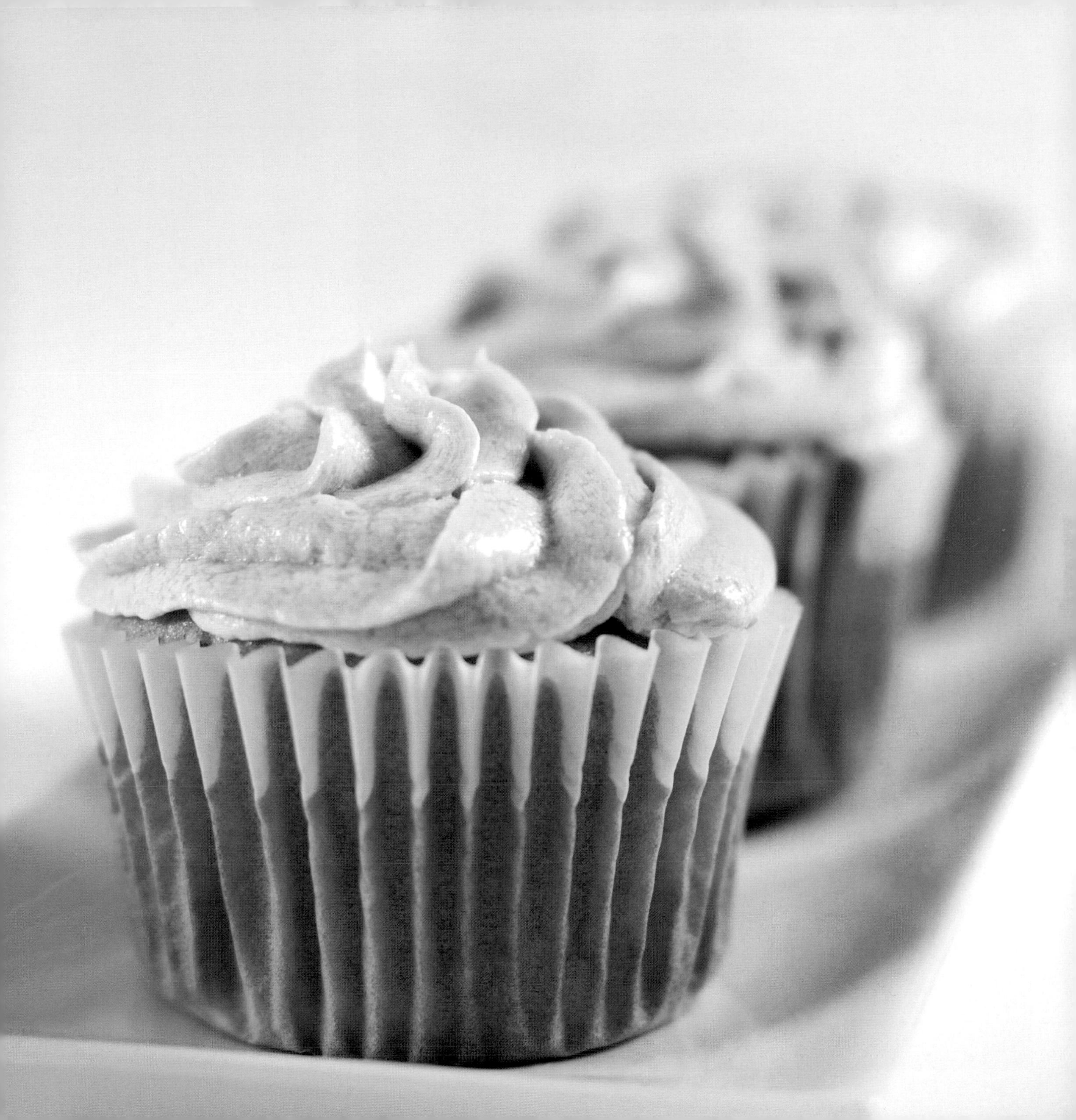

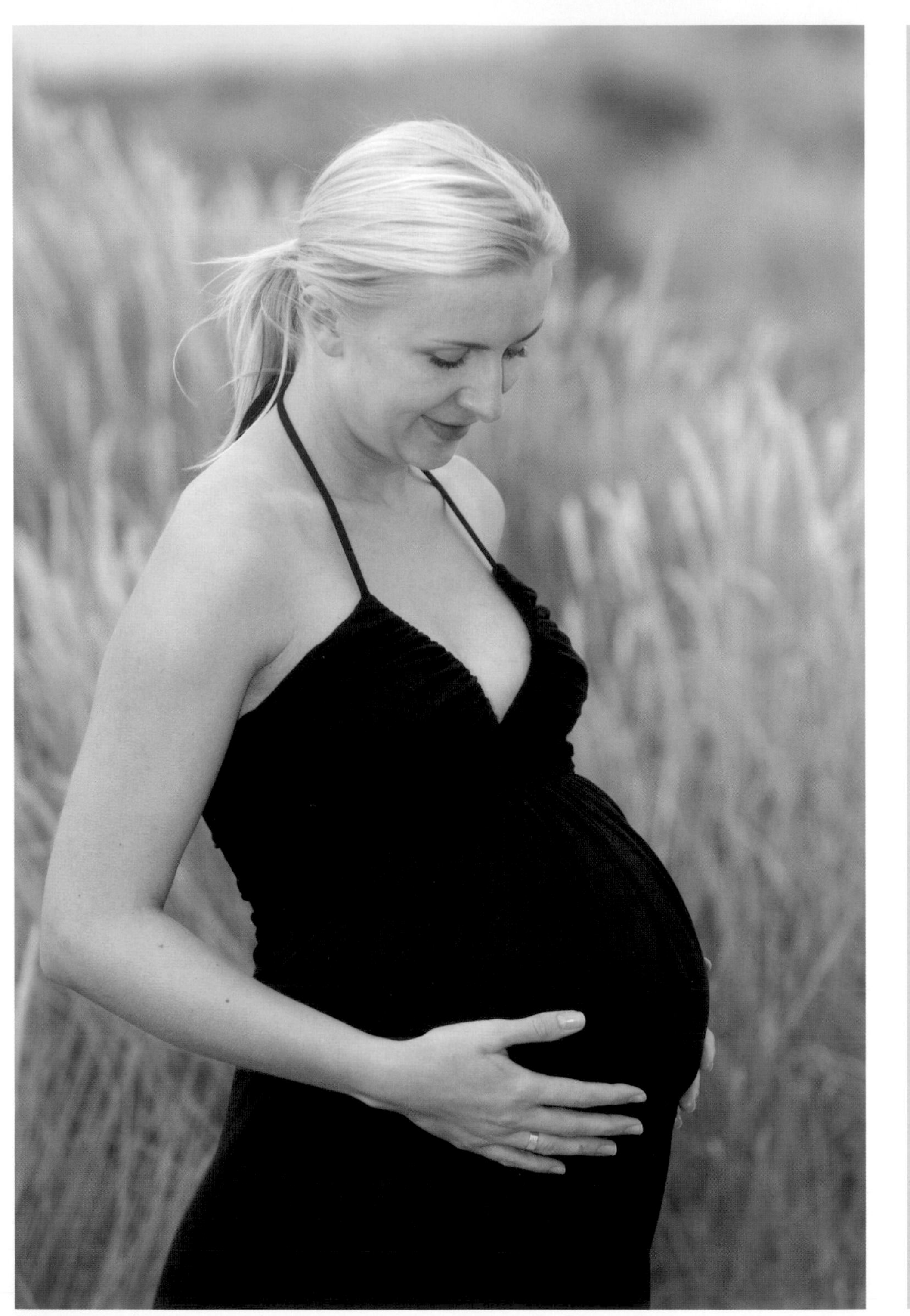

all of the flavour,
none of the booze:

drinks

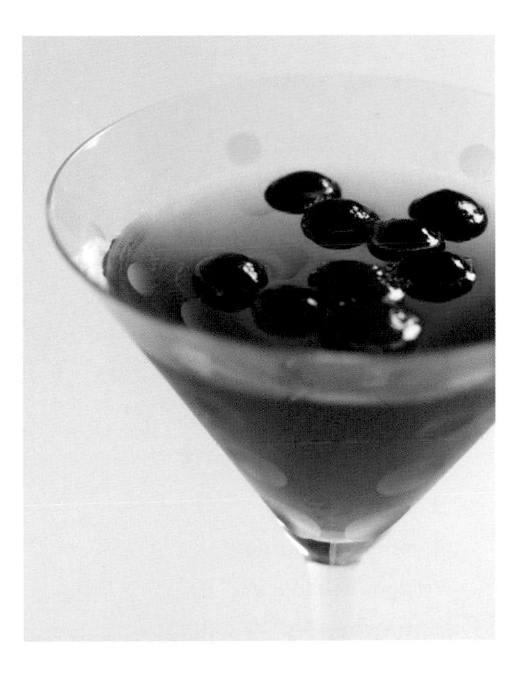

"The highlight of my childhood was making my brother laugh so hard that food came out of his nose."

~ Garrison Keillor

fresh mango strawberry lemonade

SERVES 4 | TOTAL TIME 10 MINUTES | ACTIVE TIME 10 MINUTES

This super-refreshing and colourful drink balances sweet and tart and will quench even that deep pregnancy thirst. Enjoy this on a summer evening on a patio or anytime with girlfriends. Cheers!

INGREDIENTS

2 lemons

1 very ripe mango

1 cup crushed ice

4 strawberries (plus 2, for garnish, if desired)

½ cup granulated sugar

2 cups club soda

METHOD

Place lemons in a bowl of warm water for 5 minutes, to make juicing them easier. Meanwhile, core and dice mango, removing the skin. In a bowl using a fork, mash the mango until smooth. Refrigerate mango until ready to serve the drinks.

Cut lemons in half and squeeze out the juice (should be approximately ½ cup), discarding seeds. Pour lemon juice into a blender over crushed ice. Cut the strawberries in half and toss them in. Add sugar, blending until incorporated. Stir in club soda.

TO SERVE

Spoon about 2 teaspoons of the mashed mango into the bottom of each martini glass, and pour the strawberry lemonade over top. Garnish with sliced strawberries if desired.

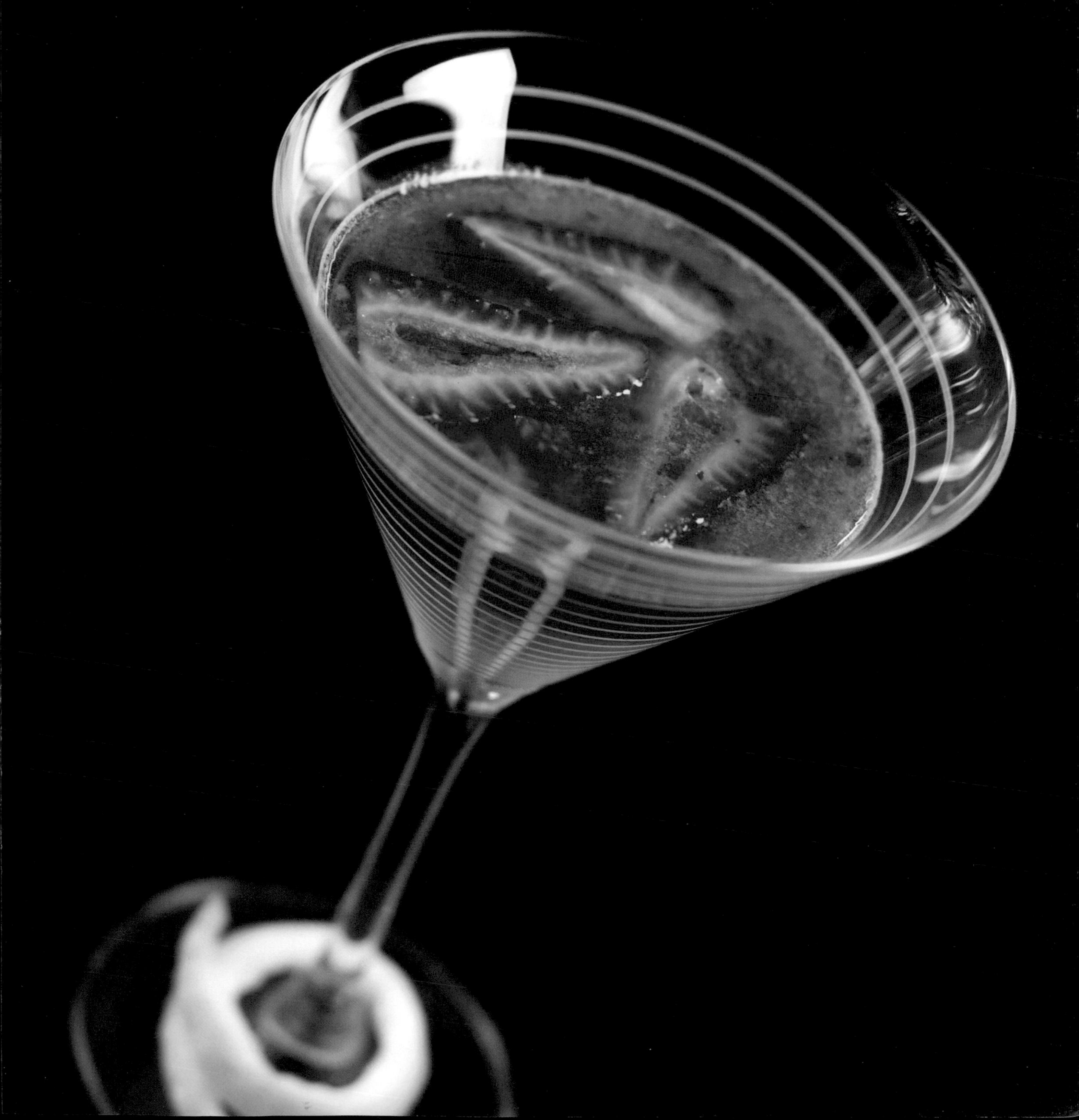

blueberry lychee kiss

SERVES 2 | TOTAL TIME 5 MINUTES | ACTIVE TIME 5 MINUTES

Served in a highball glass, this easy drink is modern and sophisticated, with a retro touch. The pineapple adds a delicate flavour and balances the sweetness of the lychee syrup.

INGREDIENTS

¾ cup blueberry juice

½ cup lychee syrup (from canned lychee fruit)

2 pineapple rings

10 ice cubes

METHOD

Pour blueberry juice and lychee syrup into a pitcher and stir well to blend. Chop pineapple ring into small chunks.

TO SERVE

Divide ice cubes evenly between highball glasses. Pour blueberry-lychee mixture over ice and top with pineapple chunks.

ginger beer no-jito

SERVES 2 | TOTAL TIME 5 MINUTES | ACTIVE TIME 5 MINUTES

If you love mojitos, you'll definitely dig this virgin version, the "no-jito." It has a zippy little kick from the ginger and will liven up any patio party. The flavour is addictive! You may actually find you prefer this recipe to the traditional one.

INGREDIENTS

½ lime

6 fresh mint leaves

1 cup crushed ice

1¼ cups ginger beer

½ teaspoon freshly grated ginger

METHOD

Squeeze lime juice into a pitcher. Add mint leaves and muddle with a wooden spoon. Add the ice, pour in the ginger beer and stir in the ginger.

TO SERVE

Pour into sturdy glasses, and spoon some of the mint into each.

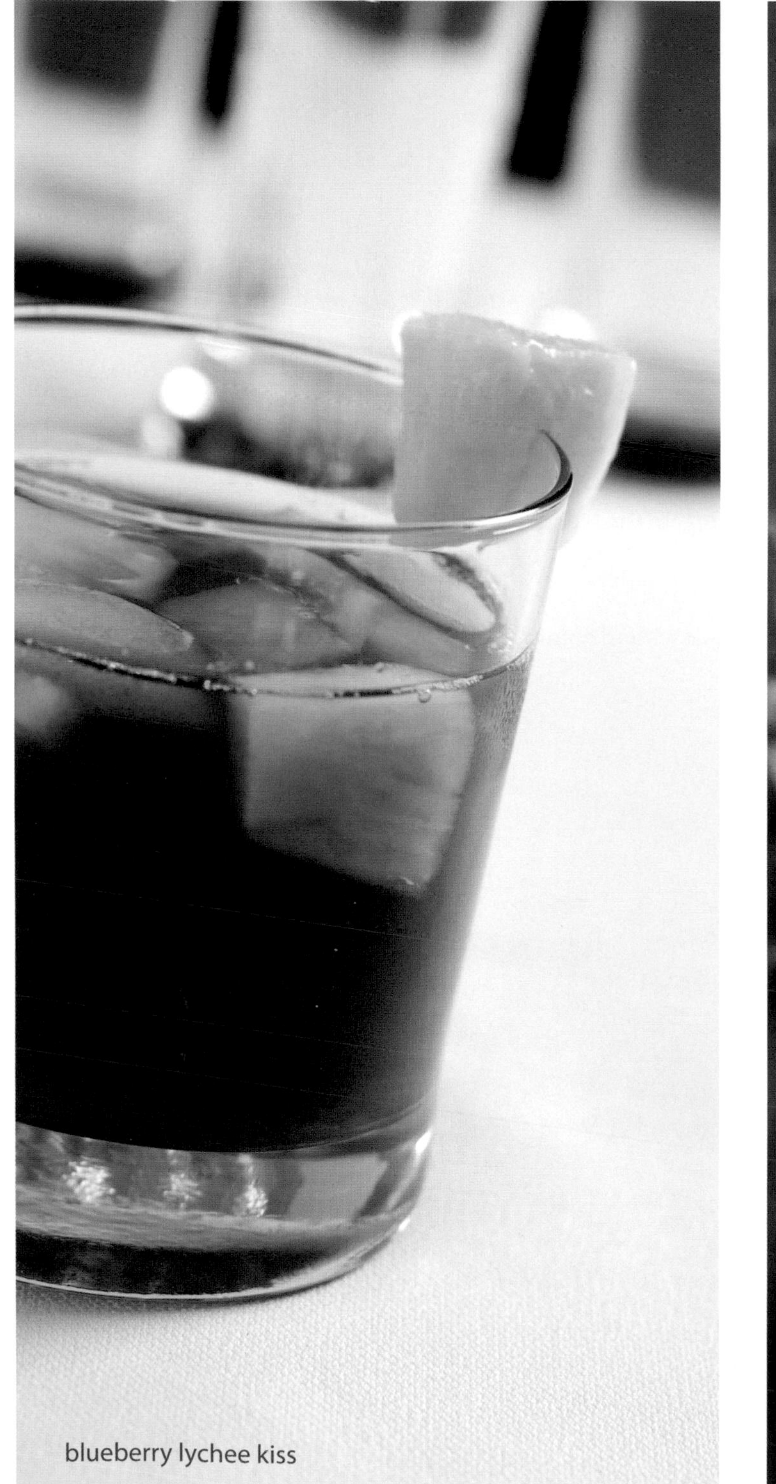

blueberry lychee kiss

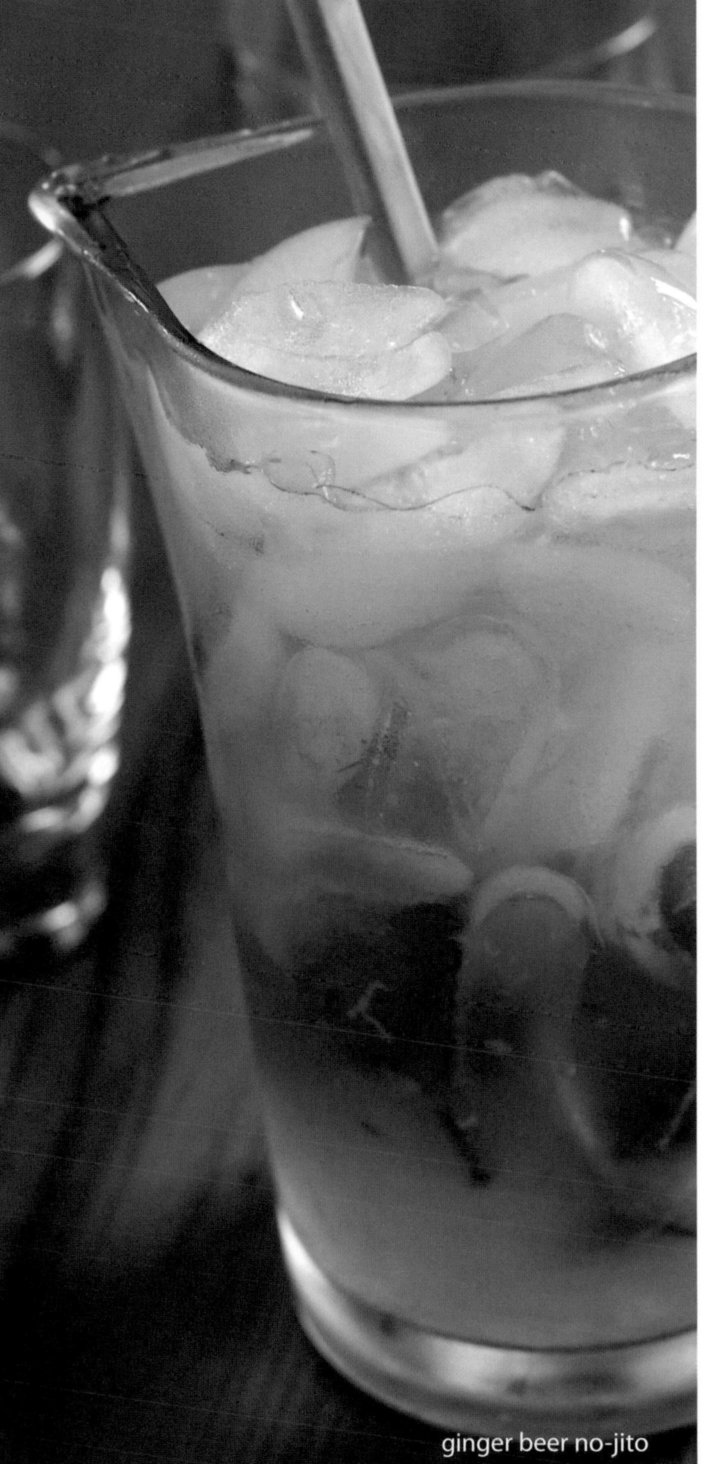

ginger beer no-jito

white peach bellini

SERVES 2 | TOTAL TIME 10 MINUTES | ACTIVE TIME 10 MINUTES

Fresh, juicy peaches add a spectacular quality to this drink. It has just as much flavour as a traditional Bellini and is a delightful indulgence. You can use regular peaches if white are not available.

INGREDIENTS

2 ripe white peaches

Juice of 1 lemon

2 teaspoons grenadine

1 cup crushed ice

1 teaspoon pure orange extract

METHOD

Peel peaches and remove pits. Chop each peach into quarters and place in blender. Add all other ingredients to the blender and blend until smooth.

TO SERVE

Pour into large wine glasses and enjoy.

lemon drop cosmopolitan

SERVES 2 | TOTAL TIME 5 MINUTES | ACTIVE TIME 5 MINUTES

Close your eyes as you sip this drink and you'll easily recall those Sex in the City inspired fun times. This classy drink will get you in the mood for a dynamic evening or party.

INGREDIENTS

1 cup cranberry juice

1 cup white grape juice

¼ teaspoon pure lemon extract

1 cup crushed ice

12 to 15 frozen cranberries

METHOD

To a cocktail shaker, add cranberry and grape juices, lemon extract and crushed ice. Shake vigorously.

TO SERVE

Pour into martini glasses. Top with frozen cranberries.

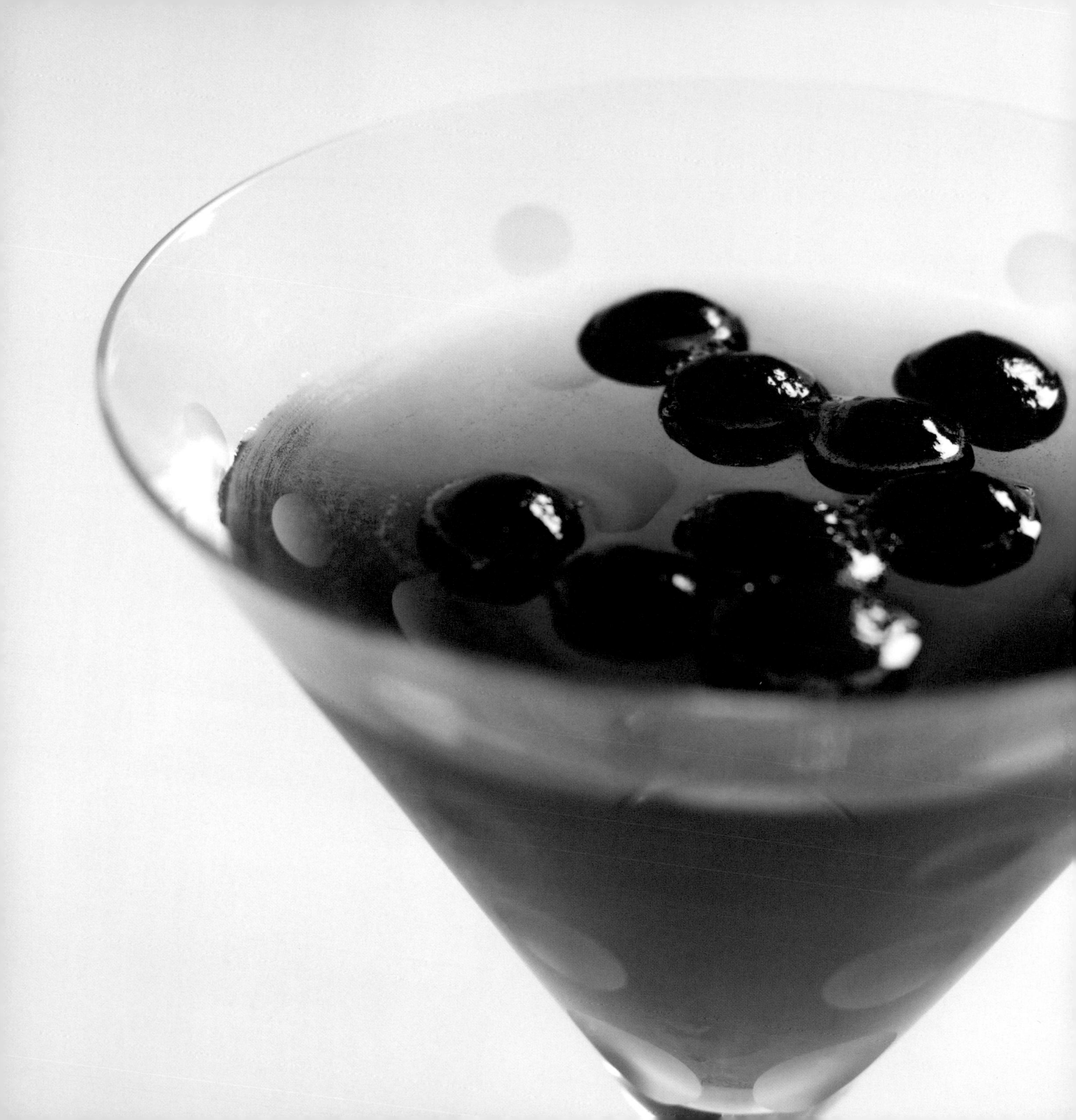

pickled mary

SERVES 2 | TOTAL TIME 5 MINUTES | ACTIVE TIME 5 MINUTES

You may have gotten pickled on Caesars or Bloody Marys in the past, but now that you're pregnant you might just be craving pickles. This zesty drink will amuse your friends and satisfy (some of!) your pregnancy desires.

INGREDIENTS

1 cup crushed ice

2 cups tomato juice

Dash of salt and freshly ground black pepper

4 dashes hot sauce (such as Tabasco)

4 dashes Worcestershire sauce

2 teaspoons fresh lemon juice

4 tablespoons dill pickle juice

2 pickles

Fresh dill sprigs, for garnish

METHOD

To a cocktail shaker add crushed ice, tomato juice, salt and pepper, hot sauce, Worcestershire sauce, and lemon and pickle juices. Shake vigorously.

TO SERVE

Strain into fancy glasses. Garnish with sprigs of dill. Pierce pickles with toothpicks and prop a pickle on the rim of each glass.

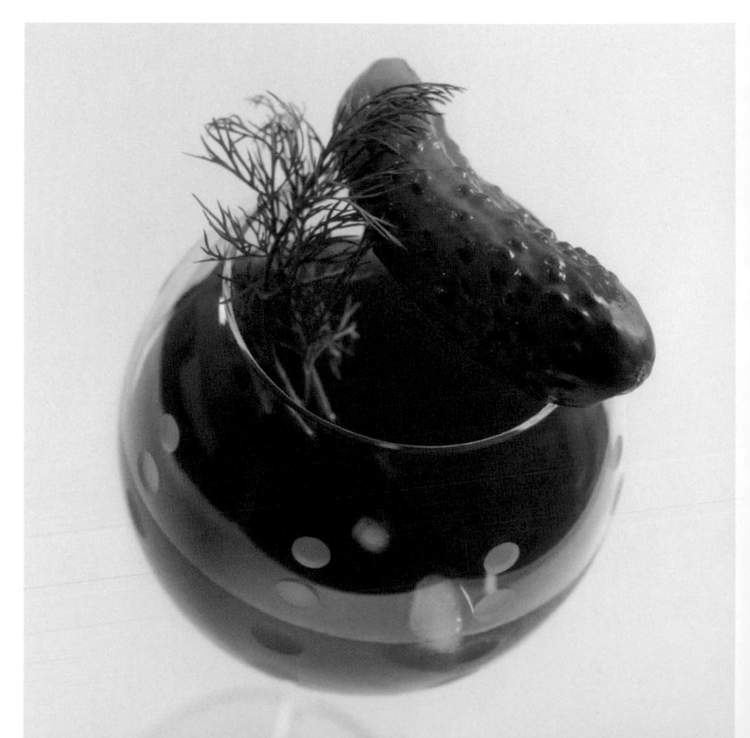

sparkling raspberry float

SERVES 2 | TOTAL TIME 5 MINUTES | ACTIVE TIME 5 MINUTES

Remember the good old days of root beer floats, and the carefree days of childhood summers? This fresh and fruity drink kicks it up a notch but delivers the same nostalgic enjoyment, comfort and refreshment. It is best enjoyed with fresh seasonal raspberries but will work with frozen ones as well.

INGREDIENTS

1 cup raspberries

1 cup club soda

2 tablespoons natural cane sugar

6 ice cubes

2 scoops vanilla ice cream or frozen yogurt

METHOD

Muddle berries and club soda together in a pitcher. Stir in sugar until well combined. Stir in ice cubes.

TO SERVE

Pour raspberry soda into tall glasses, leaving most of the ice cubes in the pitcher. Top each with a scoop of ice cream. Use long spoons to enjoy, or drink directly from the glass.

vanilla rooibos and passion fruit teaser

SERVES 2 | TOTAL TIME 20 MINUTES | ACTIVE TIME 5 MINUTES

Need some passion in your life? This drink delivers. Naturally caffeine-free and not too sweet, this harmonious beverage will get you in the mood for whatever else you fancy.

INGREDIENTS

2 cups fresh boiled water
4 vanilla rooibos tea bags
2 cups crushed ice
1 cup passion fruit juice
2 slices lemon, for garnish

METHOD

In a large cup, pour water over tea bags. Let steep for 5 minutes. Remove tea bags and chill tea in refrigerator for at least 10 minutes. Pour into a pitcher over crushed ice. Stir in passion fruit juice.

TO SERVE

Pour into fancy glasses. Garnish with lemon slices.

iced mint tea with cucumber

SERVES 2 | TOTAL TIME 15 MINUTES | ACTIVE TIME 5 MINUTES

Cucumbers provide a cool and aromatic freshness to this chilled herbal tea. It is perfect for breezy chats with girlfriends, or entertaining your curious in-laws. You'll always keep your cool with a glass of this in hand.

INGREDIENTS

2 cups fresh boiled water
2 mint tea bags
1 cup crushed ice
8 thin slices English cucumber

METHOD

In a large cup, pour water over tea bags. Let steep for 10 minutes. Pour over 1 cup crushed ice in a pitcher; refrigerate until cooled. Slice cucumber.

TO SERVE

Place 4 slices of cucumber in each of 2 glasses. Pour cold tea over top and add ice cubes.

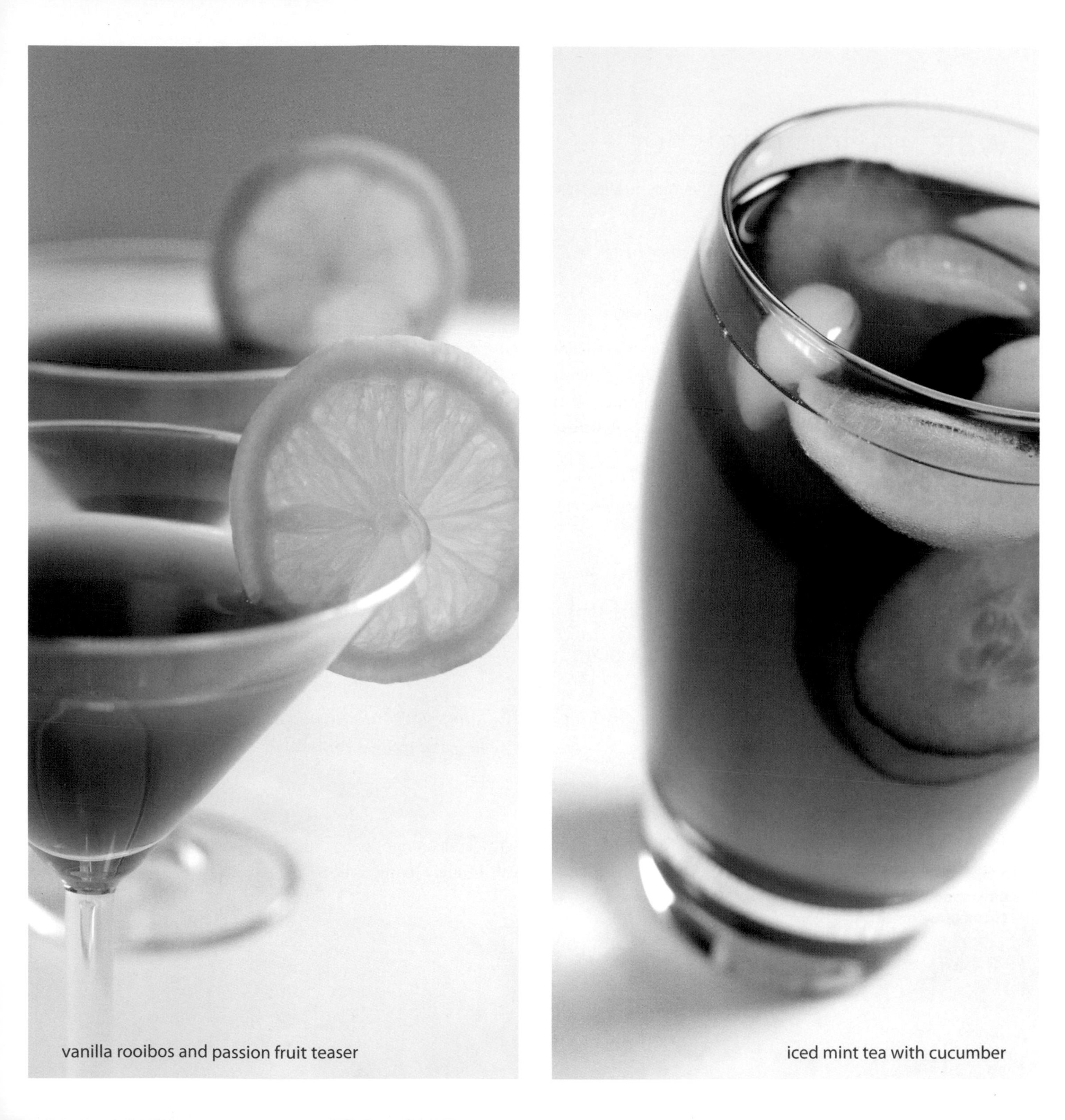

vanilla rooibos and passion fruit teaser

iced mint tea with cucumber

watermelon refresher

SERVES 2 | TOTAL TIME 10 MINUTES | ACTIVE TIME 10 MINUTES

Pure, simple and very refreshing, this juice tastes like liquid summer sunshine. Drink it cold and enjoy.

INGREDIENTS

1 seedless watermelon

1 to 2 limes

10 ice cubes

METHOD

Slice watermelon, remove rind and cut the flesh into chunks. Crush watermelon through a sieve, collecting juice in a bowl. Strain juice to remove any seeds or pulp. Juice limes; stir in 2 teaspoons of lime juice per 1 cup watermelon juice. Pour watermelon juice into a pitcher and refrigerate until ready to serve.

TO SERVE

Pour watermelon mixture over ice in highball glasses.

good morning, sunshine!

SERVES 2 | TOTAL TIME 5 MINUTES | ACTIVE TIME 5 MINUTES

This sassy and energizing drink is delicious any time of day. It does have an unusual colour, but the taste more than makes up for it — and pregnancy is a great opportunity to learn to love things new and unusual!

INGREDIENTS

1 cup vanilla-flavoured yogurt

2 cups orange juice

4 teaspoons unsweetened cocoa powder, sifted

METHOD

To a pitcher, add yogurt and orange juice; mix well with a wooden spoon. Add cocoa 1 teaspoon at a time, mixing well.

TO SERVE

Pour into juice glasses.

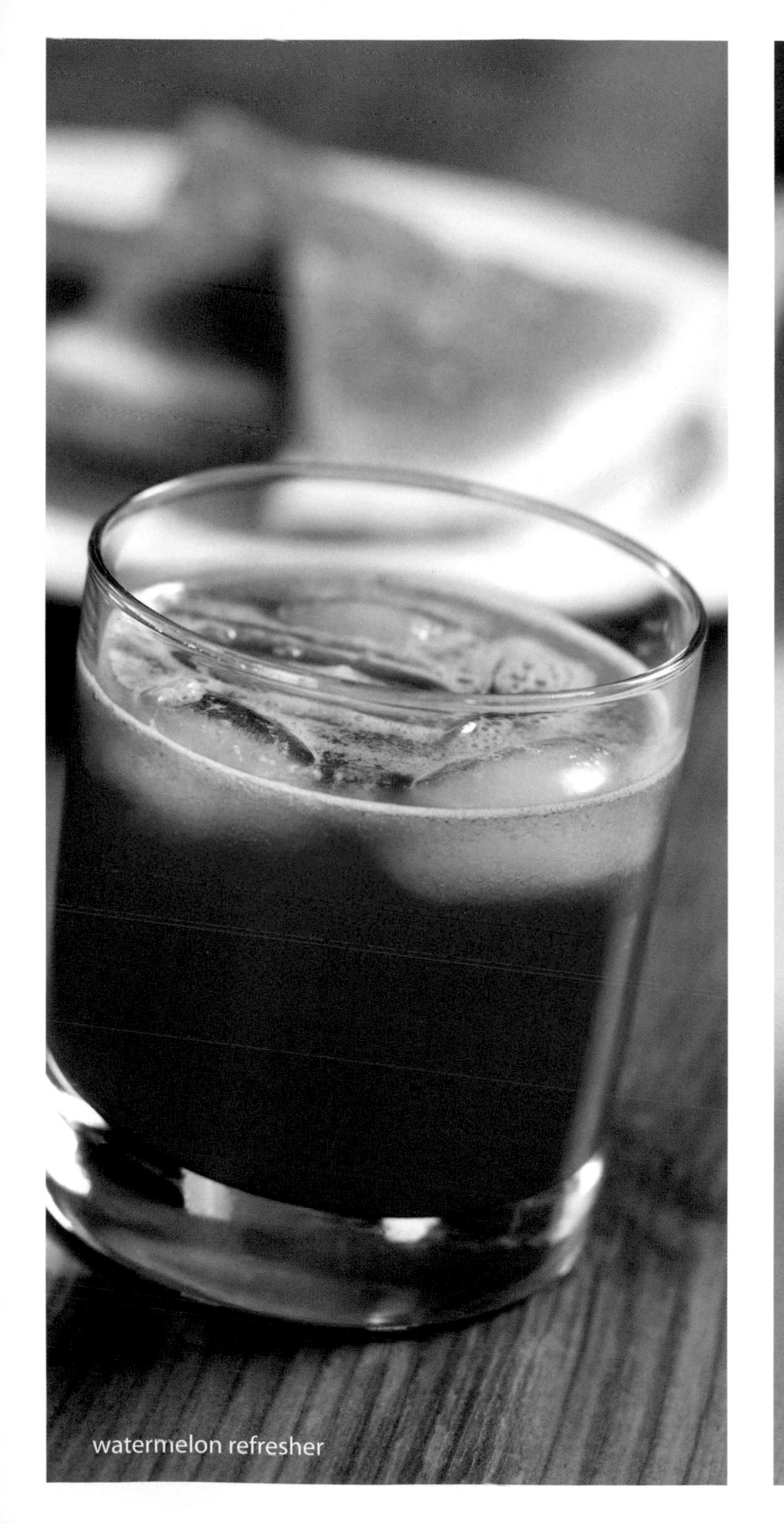

watermelon refresher

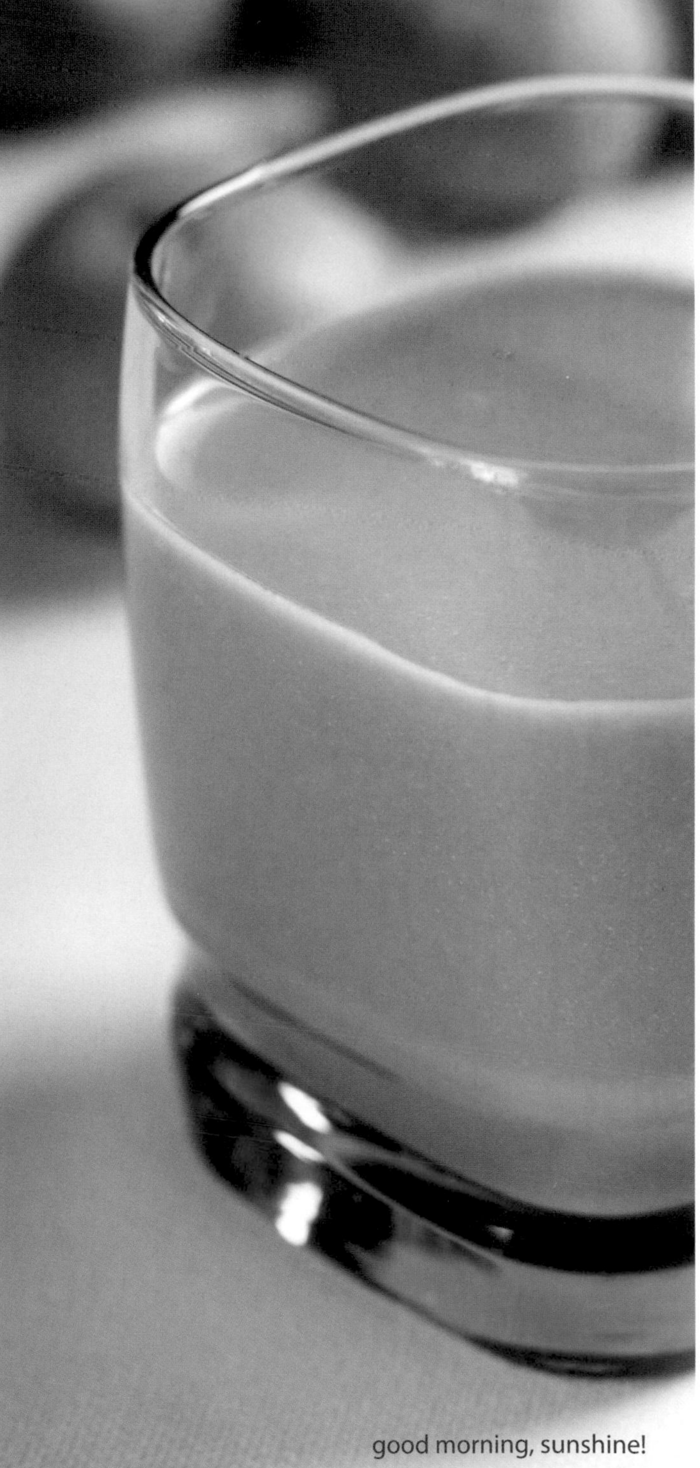

good morning, sunshine!

blueberry coconut smoothie

SERVES 2 | TOTAL TIME 5 MINUTES | ACTIVE TIME 5 MINUTES

The offbeat pairing of coconut and blueberry makes this cheerful drink creamy, tasty and invigorating. It is fantastic first thing in the morning or with a snack, and so simple to make. You can use fresh or frozen blueberries.

INGREDIENTS

1 cup crushed ice

1 cup blueberry juice

1 cup plain yogurt

⅓ cup coconut milk

⅓ cup blueberries

METHOD

Pour all ingredients into a blender. Mix on low-medium until smooth.

TO SERVE

Pour into tall glasses.

chocolate chai white tea

SERVES 2 | TOTAL TIME 15 MINUTES | ACTIVE TIME 10 MINUTES

Mmm … chai tea with rich milk and chocolate is sweet and comforting. White tea offers a gourmet twist on this classic but exotic hot drink. The complex notes make this a charming choice for times to relax and unwind.

INGREDIENTS

2 cups fresh boiled water

2 white chai tea bags

1 cup milk

1 tablespoon unsweetened cocoa powder

2 tablespoons granulated sugar

⅛ teaspoon pure vanilla extract

2 tablespoons pure maple syrup

METHOD

In a large cup, pour water over tea bags. Set aside to steep for 5 to 7 minutes. Heat milk in a saucepan over medium heat until scalding. Remove from heat; add cocoa, sugar, vanilla and maple syrup. Stir in tea.

TO SERVE

Pour into large mugs.

vanilla cinnamon latte

SERVES 2 | TOTAL TIME 5 MINUTES | ACTIVE TIME 5 MINUTES

This unique latte offers separate flavours in the milk and coffee. Your first sip of frothy milk delivers soothing vanilla, while the coffee combines it with cinnamon for a melodic finish. Decaf coffee works equally well, if you prefer to indulge at the dreamy end of the day.

INGREDIENTS

1 cup milk

2 teaspoons granulated sugar

½ teaspoon pure vanilla extract

⅛ teaspoon pure cinnamon extract

2 cups brewed coffee

METHOD

Divide milk, sugar and vanilla evenly between 2 large mugs. Using a milk frother, make stiff, bubbly foam in each. Stir cinnamon extract into the coffee.

TO SERVE

Pour coffee into the milk in the mugs.

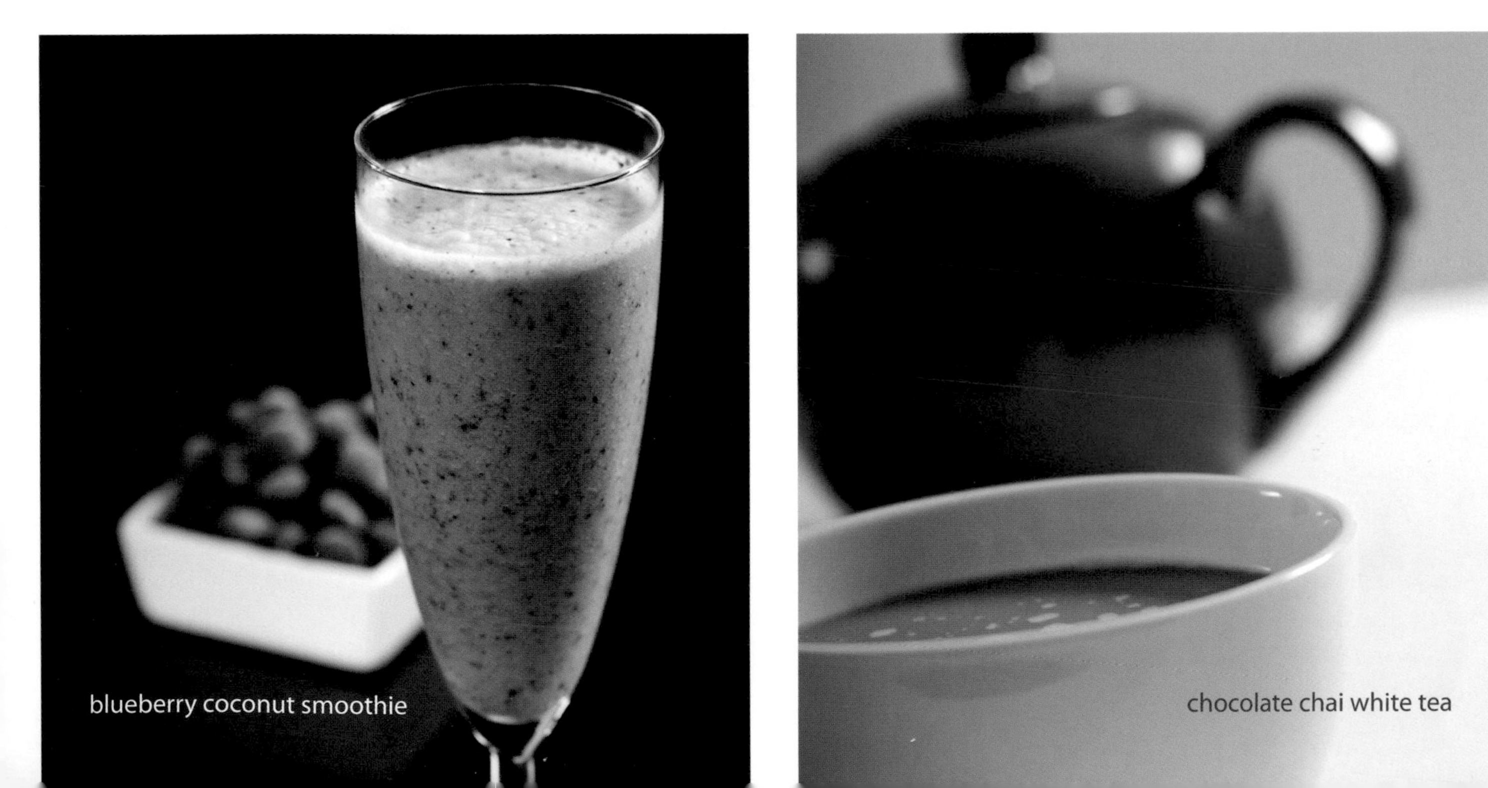

blueberry coconut smoothie

chocolate chai white tea

rich hazelnut hot cocoa

SERVES 2 | TOTAL TIME 10 MINUTES | ACTIVE TIME 10 MINUTES

Snuggle up with your sweetheart to enjoy a mug of this rich hot cocoa. It will keep you toasty warm on chilly autumn or winter evenings. It will also heat up your (and your sweetie's) hands — so be sure to ask for a foot rub when the mug is empty!

INGREDIENTS

4 cups milk

6 tablespoons granulated sugar

4 tablespoons unsweetened cocoa powder

1 teaspoon hazelnut syrup

½ teaspoon pure vanilla extract

12 to 16 mini marshmallows, for garnish

METHOD

In a saucepan, heat milk until scalding. Remove from heat; stir in sugar and cocoa until well combined. Add hazelnut syrup and vanilla, stirring well.

TO SERVE

Pour into large mugs and top with mini marshmallows.

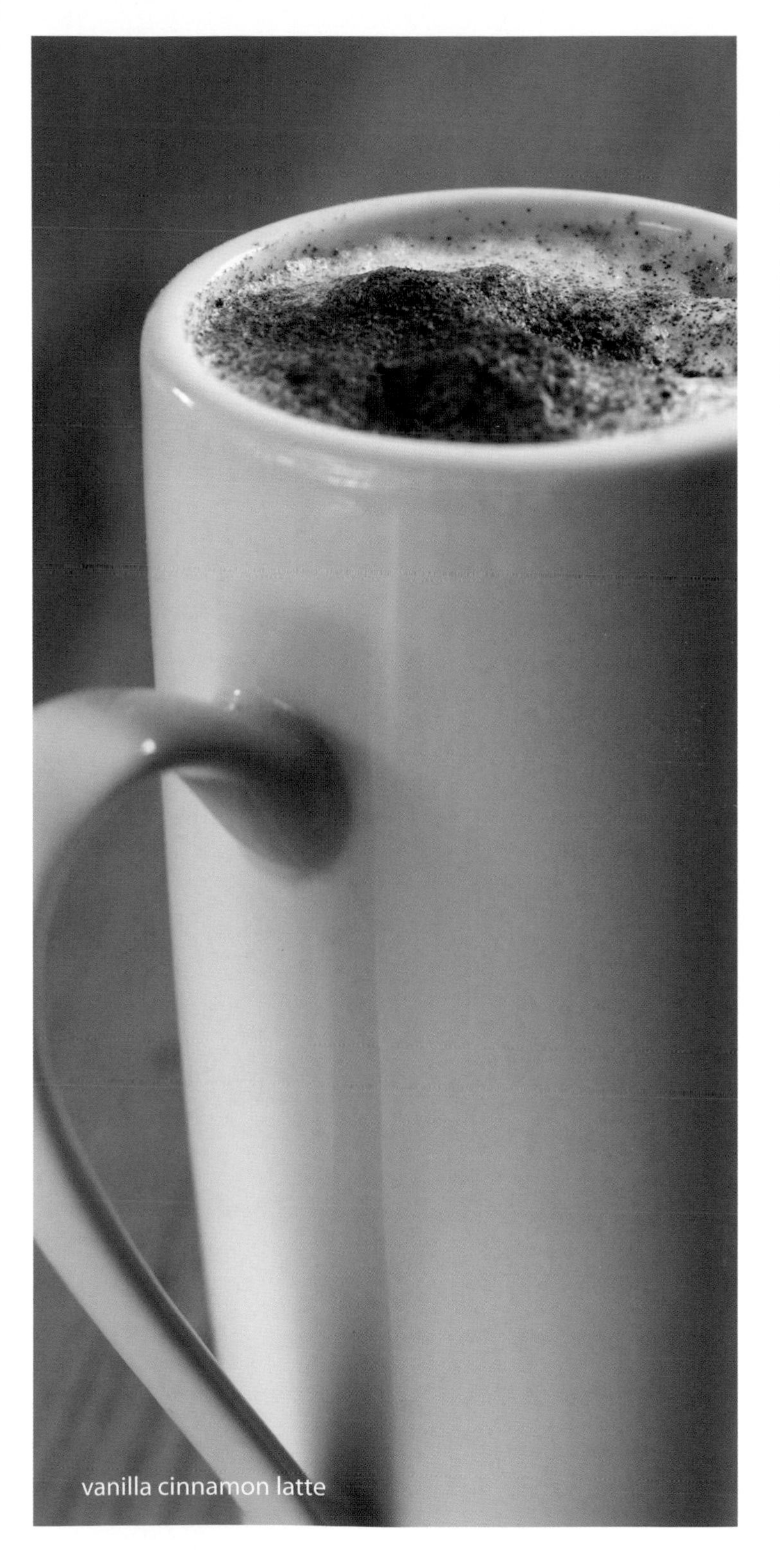
vanilla cinnamon latte

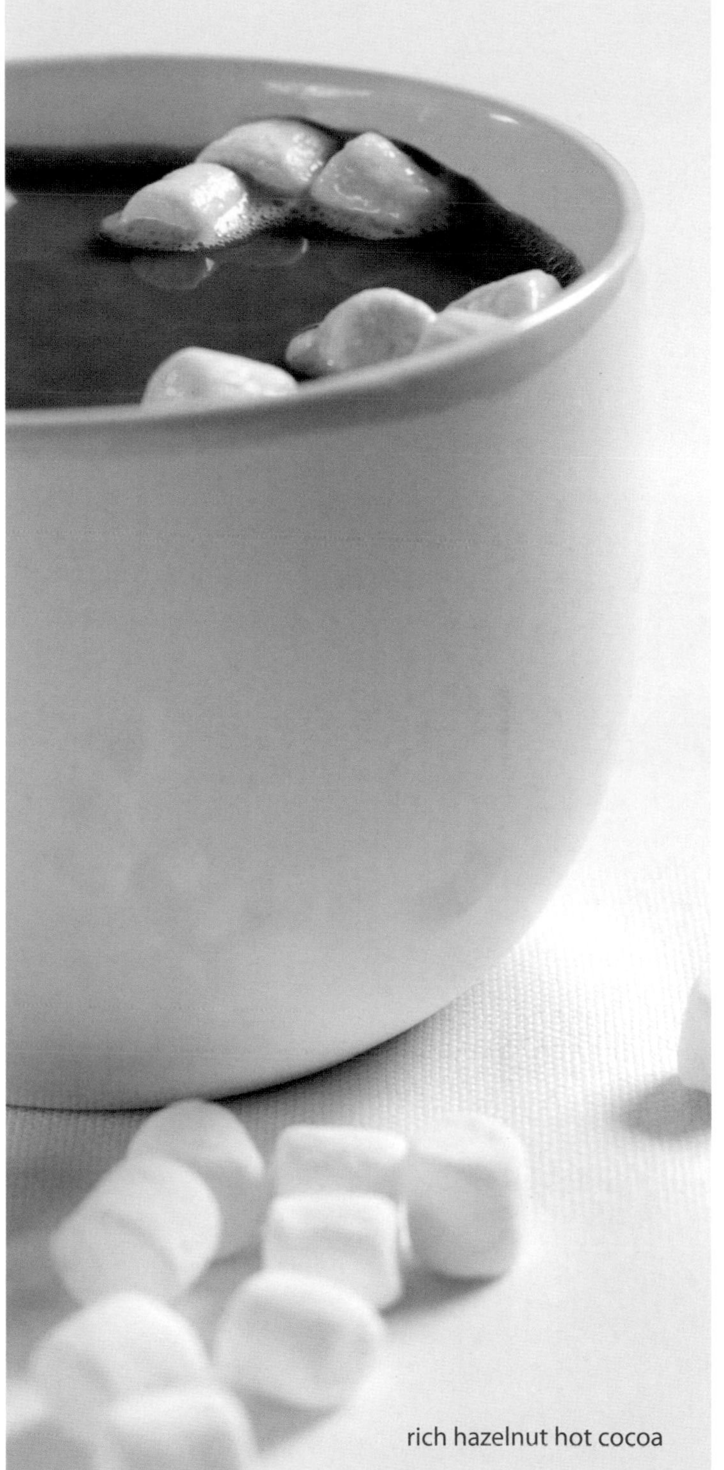
rich hazelnut hot cocoa

menus

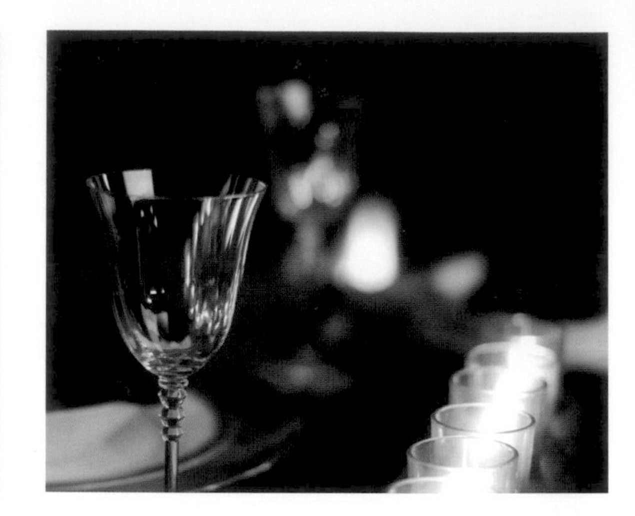

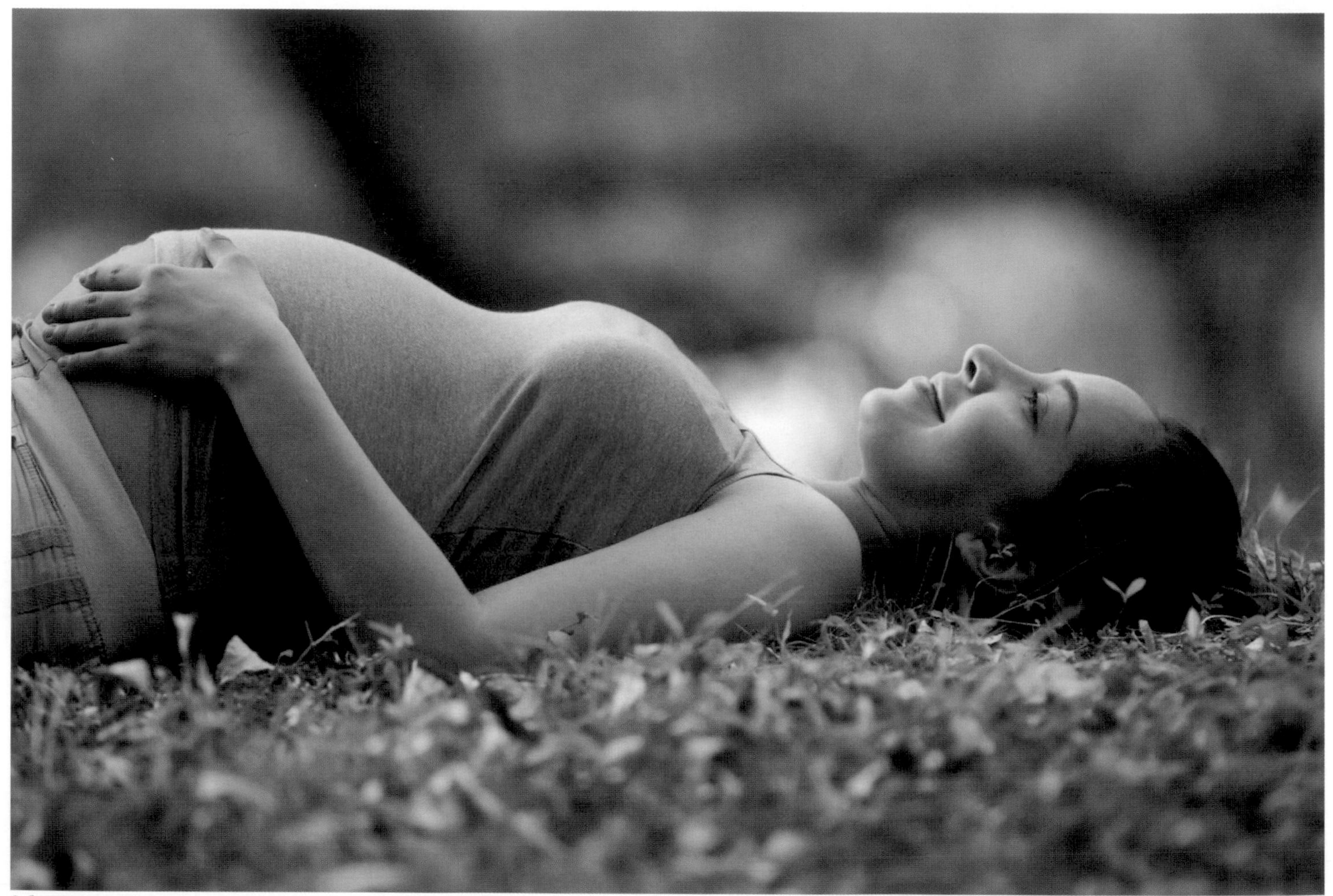

ARE YOU PLANNING to host a friend's baby shower, or invite your friends over for a fun brunch to show off your awesome cooking skills? Perhaps you want to have a gourmet restaurant experience at your home with a fine dining evening, or a romantic picnic for you and your sweetie? Try one of these specially designed menus for the ultimate in pleasurable dining experiences.

romantic picnic

SERVES 2

- Mango Cilantro Salsa
- Rustic Sesame Vegetable Tart (bring 2 to 4 slices)
- Apple Slices, Belgian Endive, Flatbreads and Portobello Mushroom Pâté
- Butternut Squash and Carrot Ginger Soup with Crème Fraîche (bring in a Thermos)
- Chocolate Raspberry Fudge (wrap individual pieces in wax paper)
- Fresh Mango Strawberry Lemonade

baby shower

SERVES 6 TO 8

- Exotic Fruit Salad with Sweet Citrus Guacamole
- Sushi Vegetables with Asian and Wasabi Yogurt Dipping Sauces
- Caramelized Onion and Balsamic Cherry Jam
- Tempura Dill Pickles with Sambal Oelek Dip
- Ham and Grilled Pineapple Bagel with Honey Mustard Cream Cheese (adjust the recipe to half a bagel per guest)
- Eggplant and Spinach Lasagna with Béchamel Sauce
- Maple Walnut Caramel Corn
- London Fog Cupcakes
- Iced Mint Tea with Cucumber

fine dining

SERVES 4

- Bacon-Wrapped Dried Plums Stuffed with Maple Roasted Pecans
- Meyer Lemon and Blueberry Salad in Parmesan Baskets
- Sautéed Sablefish with Eggplant Caviar
- Orange Ginger Pumpkin Cheesecake
- Blueberry Lychee Kiss (serve before or with dinner)
- Chocolate Chai White Tea (serve with dessert)

girlfriends' brunch

SERVES 4

- Herbed Cream Cheese Eggs Benedict
- Sourdough French Toast with Blueberry Crème
- Grilled Peaches with Pink Grapefruit and Mint
- Almond Mocha Nanaimo Bars
- Lemon Drop Cosmopolitan

imperial/metric conversions

IF YOU ARE NOT YET FAMILIAR with weight and volume conversions, this is a good time to learn — in addition to cooking, you'll have to weigh and measure your baby, and breast milk or formula, baby food, and so on, in a few months! Wherever you live, you may encounter various systems of measurement and these tables are very handy to have.

Conversions are approximate and have been rounded up or down.

Weight

Imperial	Metric
½ oz	15 g
1 oz	25 g
2 oz	50 g
3 oz	75 g
4 oz (¼ lb)	100 g
5 oz	150 g
6 oz (⅓ lb)	175 g
7 oz	200 g
8 oz (½ lb)	225 g
9 oz	250 g
10 oz	275 g
11 oz	300 g
12 oz (¾ lb)	350 g
13 oz	375 g
14 oz	400 g
15 oz	425 g
16 oz (1 lb)	450 g
18 oz (1½ lb)	675 g
32 oz (2 lb)	900 g
35 oz (2.2 lb)	1,000 g (1 kg)

Volume

Imperial	Metric
¼ tsp	1 mL
½ tsp	2 mL
¾ tsp	4 mL
1 tsp	5 mL
2 tsp	10 mL
1 tbsp	15 mL
4 tsp	20 mL
2 tbsp	25 mL
3 tbsp	45 mL
¼ cup	50 mL
⅓ cup	75 mL
½ cup	125 mL
⅔ cup	150 mL
¾ cup	175 mL
1 cup	250 mL
4 cups	1 L
6 cups	1.5 L
8 cups	2 L

Common Package Sizes (Volume)

Imperial	Metric
6 oz	170 mL
10 oz	284 mL
14 oz	398 mL
19 oz	540 mL
28 oz	796 mL

Baking Dishes

Imperial	Metric
8-inch square	2 L
9-inch square	2.5 L
10-inch square	3 L
9-inch springform	2.5 L
10-inch springform	3 L
13- × 9-inch baking dish	3.5 L

Measurements

Imperial	Metric
¼ inch	5 mm
⅓ inch	8 mm
½ inch	1 cm
¾ inch	2 cm
1 inch	2.5 cm
1½ inches	4 cm
2 inches	5 cm
3 inches	8 cm
4 inches	10 cm
5 inches	12 cm
6 inches	15 cm

Temperature

Fahrenheit (F) (rounded to nearest tenth)	Celsius (C)
225°	105°
250°	120°
275°	140°
300°	150°
325°	160°
350°	180°
375°	190°
400°	200°
425°	220°
450°	230°
475°	240°
500°	260°

index

A

aioli
- garlic, with vegetable panini, 112
- truffle, with sweet potato fries, 48

alcohol, 7
allspice, corn with spiced maple butter, 50
almonds
- bacon and leek risotto, 144
- chocolate chip cookies, 64
- granola bars, 60
- mocha Nanaimo bars, 182
- mushroom pâté, 90

ancho chili powder
- chicken, 154
- in mixed nuts, 44

anise chocolate sauce, 176
Anjou pears with slow-cooked beef, 149
appetizers, 70–96
apples
- bacon, lettuce, tomato, cheddar, avocado sandwich, 26
- cornbread, 56
- dried, Moroccan chicken quesadilla, 152
- fruit muffins, 36
- with mushroom pâté, 90
- slow-cooked beef, 149

apricots, dried
- chicken in grape leaves, 76
- fruit muffins, 36
- Moroccan chicken quesadilla, 152

arborio rice, bacon, leek and almond risotto, 144
artichoke hearts, seven-layer dip, 82
artificial sweeteners, 7
arugula with scallops, 134
Asiago cheese
- olive and Italian sausage omelet, 20
- steak salad, 150
- tomato, olive and tuna zucchini rounds, 78

asparagus
- salmon and pea salad, 104
- with truffle oil and pine nuts, 42

avocados
- bacon, apple, lettuce, tomato, cheddar sandwich, 26
- cashew, cabbage and noodle salad, 108
- citrus guacamole, 37
- crostinis, 88
- ginger wasabi sliders, 118
- mango salsa, 54
- seven-layer dip, 82
- steak salad, 150

B

baby greens, lemon and blueberry salad in Parmesan baskets, 92
baby shower menu, 205
bacon
- apple, lettuce, tomato, cheddar, avocado sandwich, 26
- bacon-wrapped dried plums, 74
- chicken wrap, 116
- cravings, 9
- leek and almond risotto, 144
- savoury crêpes, 32

bagels, ham and pineapple, 16
baguettes, crostinis, 88
baked beans, savoury crêpes, 32
balsamic vinegar
- caramelized onion and balsamic cherry jam, 80
- fig brown butter sauce, 138
- French onion soup, 100
- pear compote, 96
- steak salad, 150
- vegetable panini, 112

bananas
- butterscotch pudding, 172
- sweet crêpes, 32
- yogurt and juice popsicles, 67

basil
- cilantro honey pesto, 134
- eggplant caviar, 128
- grilled pear sandwich, 114
- tomato bocconcini skewers, 94

beans
- baked, savoury crêpes, 32

black, scrambled eggs and, 22
refried, seven-layer dip, 82
béchamel sauce, 140
beef
cravings, 9
ground, eggplant and spinach lasagna, 140
ground, ginger wasabi sliders, 118
ground, meatball skewers, 84
roast, rosemary garlic, 146
roast, with apples and pears, 149
steak salad, 150
beets, tempura, 148
Belgian endive with mushroom pâté, 90
bell peppers
crab cakes, 122
olive and Italian sausage omelet, 20
panini, 112
roasted sweet potatoes and eggs, 25
seven-layer dip, 82
stuffed mushrooms, 124
tiger prawn and chickpea salad, 106
vegetable frittata, 24
vegetable sushi, 70
vegetable tart, 86
bellini, white peach, 192
berries. See specific type of berry
biscotti, chocolate, ginger and orange, 62
biscuits, chorizo, chive and buttermilk, 28
black beans with scrambled eggs, 22
black olives
Italian sausage omelet, 20
tomato tuna zucchini rounds, 78
blackberries, meringues, 170
BLT (bacon, lettuce, tomato) sandwich, 26
blueberries
banana, yogurt and juice popsicles, 67
dried, chocolate chip cookies, 64
dried, Moroccan chicken quesadilla, 152
french toast with blueberry crème, 34
and lemon salad, 92
and lychee drink, 190
meringues, 170
smoothie, 200
bocconcini, tomato basil skewers, 94
bread
cornbread, 56
dill onion, 115
breakfast, 14–37
brittle, cashew, 177
broccoli with salmon, 130
brunch, 14–37
brunch menu, 205
burgers
cravings, 9
ginger wasabi, 118
buttermilk biscuits, 28
butternut squash
ravioli with fig brown butter sauce, 138
roasted with green curry drizzle, 72
soup, 102
butterscotch and banana pudding, 172

C

cabbage, cashew noodle salad, 108
caffeine, 7
cakes, London fog cupcakes, 184
candy
candy cane ice cream, 174
cravings, 11
caramel corn, 66
caramel drizzle, peach crumble pie and, 168
carrots
butternut squash soup, 102
cashew, cabbage and noodle salad, 108
salmon, asparagus and pea salad, 104
tangerine muffins, 58
vegetable sushi, 70
cashews
brittle, 177
cabbage noodle salad, 108
cauliflower, caramelized, and pecan salad, 110
caviar, eggplant, 128
celery, vegetable sushi, 70
chai tea, chocolate, 200
cheddar cheese
bacon, apple, lettuce, tomato, avocado sandwich, 26
chorizo, chive, buttermilk biscuits, 28
grilled pear sandwich, 114
with pear compote, 96
savoury crêpes, 32
steak salad, 150
toasted cheese sandwich, 115
cheesecake, orange, ginger, pumpkin, 164
cheeses
See also specific type of cheese
avoidance of, 7
toasted sandwich, 115
cherries
dried, fruit muffins, 36
dried, jam, 80
mint tart, 166
chicken
chili, 154
curried pizza, 120
in grape leaves with apricots and rice, 76
quesadilla, 152
rosemary horseradish wrap, 116
chickpeas
with olives and nuts, 44
and tiger prawn salad, 106
chili pepper, chicken, 154

chili sauce, peanut chili dip, 46
chips, pita with peanut chili dip, 46
chives and chorizo biscuits, 28
chocolate
 anise sauce, 176
 biscotti, 62
 chai white tea, 200
 cravings, 8
 ganache, 162
 granola bars, 60
 hazelnut hot cocoa, 202
 mousse cake, 160
 Nanaimo bars, 182
 orange yogurt drink, 198
 raspberry fudge, 180
 with salmon, 130
 sweet crêpes, 32
 truffle soufflés, 158
chocolate chips
 blueberry almond cookies, 64
 toffee coffee cookies, 178
chorizo sausage
 buttermilk biscuits, 28
 savoury crêpes, 32
cilantro
 eggplant caviar, 128
 pesto, 134
 salsa, 22, 54
 seven-layer dip, 82
 tiger prawn and chickpea salad, 106
cinnamon
 corn with spiced maple butter, 50
 french toast with blueberry crème, 34
 peanut butter sandwich, 30
 vanilla latte, 201
cloves, corn with spiced maple butter, 50
cocoa
 biscotti, 62
 chai white tea, 200
 hot, with hazelnut, 202
 orange yogurt drink, 198
coconut, tangerine muffins, 58
coconut milk
 butternut squash soup, 102
 curry cream sauce, 132
 green curry drizzle, 72
 smoothie, 200
coffee
 cravings, 10
 Nanaimo bars, 182
 toffee chocolate chip cookies, 178
 vanilla cinnamon latte, 201
cookies
 chocolate chip blueberry almond, 64
 dried cranberry shortbread, 174
 toffee coffee chocolate chip, 178
corn
 cornbread, 56
 popping, caramel, 66
 salmon and zucchini latkes, 18
 with spiced maple butter, 50
cornbread, with apples, 56
cosmopolitan, lemon, 192
crab cakes, 122
cranberries
 banana, yogurt and juice popsicles, 67
 dried, Moroccan chicken quesadilla, 152
 dried, shortbread, 174
 lemon cosmopolitan, 192
 tangerine muffins, 58
cravings, 8–11
cream
 with banana butterscotch pudding, 172
 crème fraîche and butternut squash soup, 102
 french toast with blueberry crème, 34
 lemon, 170
 sex in a pan, 162
cream cheese
 cheesecake, 164
 eggs benedict, 14
 ganache, 162
 ham and pineapple bagel, 16
 mushroom pâté, 90
 peanut chili dip, 46
crème fraîche and butternut squash soup, 102
cremini mushrooms in scrambled eggs with black beans, 22
crêpes, sweet or savoury, 32
crostinis, hazelnut and avocado, 88
croutons, French onion soup, 100
crumble pie, white peach, 168
cucumbers, iced mint tea, 196
cupcakes, London fog, 184
curry
 butternut squash soup, 102
 cauliflower pecan salad, 110
 chicken pizza, 120
 coconut cream sauce, 132
 green curry drizzle, 72

D

deli meats, 7
dessert crêpes, 32
desserts, 158–184
diet
 balanced, 5
 off-limit foods, 7
Dijon mustard
 crab cakes, 122
 ham and pineapple bagel, 16
 lemon and blueberry salad in Parmesan baskets, 92
dill
 eggplant caviar, 128
 eggs benedict, 14
 onion bread, 115
 salmon, asparagus and pea salad, 104
 sour cream, 18

dill pickles
Pickled Mary drink, 194
tempura-style with dip, 40
dinner menu, 205
dips
caramelized onion and balsamic cherry jam, 80
eggplant caviar, 128
garlic aioli, 112
peanut chili, 46
sambal oelek, 40
seven-layer, 82
truffle aioli, 48
wasabi yogurt, 70
drinks, 188–202
drizzles
caramel, 168
green curry, 72
dulce de leche, 162

E

Earl Grey tea, cupcakes, 184
egg noodles, cashew and cabbage salad, 108
eggplants
caviar with sablefish, 128
panini, 112
spinach lasagna, 140
eggs
avoidance of, 7
eggs benedict, 14
french toast with blueberry crème, 34
olive and Italian sausage omelet, 20
roasted sweet potatoes and, 25
scrambled with black beans and salsa, 22
vegetable frittata, 24
endive with mushroom pâté, 90
English muffins, eggs benedict, 14
entrées, 128–154

F

feta cheese
garlic shrimp and linguine, 136
vegetable frittata, 24
fig balsamic vinegar
brown butter sauce, 138
pear compote, 96
fish
avoidance of, 7
sablefish, 128
salmon, asparagus and pea salad, 104
salmon, chocolate sesame, 130
salmon, zucchini and corn latkes, 18
tilapia with coconut curry cream sauce, 132
tuna with olives and tomato zucchini rounds, 78
flatbreads
with mushroom pâté, 90
vegetable panini, 112
floats, raspberry, 195
French bread, vegetable panini, 112
French onion soup, 100
french toast, 34
fries, sweet potatoes, 48
frittatas, vegetable, 24
fruits
See also specific type of fruit
cravings, 11
dried, chicken quesadilla, 152
grilled, 16, 52, 114
muffins, 36
popsicles, 67
safety, 7
salad, 37, 92
fudge, chocolate raspberry, 180

G

ganache, 162
garlic
aioli, 112
hazelnut and avocado crostinis, 88
meatball, pita skewers, 84
roasted potatoes, 154
rosemary roast beef, 146
ginger
biscotti, 62
butternut squash soup, 102
chocolate sesame salmon, 130
ginger beer no-jito, 190
orange pumpkin cheesecake, 164
stuffed mushrooms, 124
wasabi dipping sauce, 70
wasabi sliders, 118
ginger beer no-jito, 190
gnocchi with truffle butter sauce, 142
granola bars, M&M, 60
grape juice, lemon cosmopolitan, 192
grape leaves, chicken, apricots and rice, 76
grapefruit, grilled peaches and, 52
green olives, with chickpeas and nuts, 44
green peppers
panini, 112
roasted sweet potatoes and eggs, 25
greens
lemon and blueberry salad in Parmesan baskets, 92
salmon, asparagus and pea salad, 104
steak salad, 150
ground beef
eggplant and spinach lasagna, 140
ginger wasabi sliders, 118
meatball skewers, 84
Gruyère cheese, seven-layer dip, 82
guacamole, citrus, 37

H

habanero chili peppers and chicken, 154
ham
cravings, 9
and pineapple bagel, 16

hamburgers, ginger wasabi sliders, 118
hazelnuts
  crostinis, 88
  hot cocoa, 202
  peanut butter sandwich, 30
healthy diet, 5
herbal teas, 7
honey
  cilantro pesto, 134
  cornbread, 56
  granola bars, 60
  ham and pineapple bagel, 16
  peanut butter sandwich, 30
  roasted squash with green curry drizzle, 72
  wasabi dipping sauce, 70
horseradish, in chicken wrap, 116

I

ice, cravings, 8
ice cream
  candy cane, 174
  with cashew brittle, 177
  cravings, 8
  with raspberries and chocolate anise sauce, 176
  raspberry float, 195
Italian omelet, 20

J

jalapeño peppers, salsa, 22
jams
  caramelized onion and balsamic cherry, 80
  sweet crêpes, 32
Japanese bread crumbs, 118, 122, 124
juice
  avoidance of, 7
  banana and yogurt popsicles, 67
  blueberry and lychee, 190
  cosmopolitan, 192
  lemonade, 188
  orange chocolate, 198
  passion fruit and rooibos, 196
  Pickled Mary drink, 194
  smoothie, 200
  watermelon, 198

K

kale, vegetable frittata, 24
kiwis
  fruit salad, 37
  meringues, 170

L

lasagna, eggplant and spinach, 140
latkes, salmon, zucchini and corn, 18
lattes, vanilla cinnamon, 201
leeks
  bacon and almond risotto, 144
  gnocchi with truffle butter sauce, 142
lemonade, mango strawberry, 188
lemongrass, tiger prawn and chickpea salad, 106
lemons
  and blueberry salad, 92
  citrus guacamole, 37
  mango strawberry lemonade, 188
  tomato, basil and bocconcini skewers, 94
  whipped cream, 170
lettuce, bacon, apple, tomato, cheddar, avocado sandwich, 26
licorice, cravings, 11
light meals, 100–124
limes
  dill sour cream, 18
  ginger beer no-jito, 190
  roasted squash with green curry drizzle, 72
  salsa, 22
  watermelon juice, 198
linguine, garlic shrimp and, 136
liver, 7
lychees
  and blueberry drink, 190
  fruit salad, 37

M

M&M granola bars, 60
mangos
  fruit salad, 37
  salsa, 54
  strawberry lemonade, 188
maple syrup
  bacon-wrapped dried plums, 74
  caramel corn, 66
  corn with spiced maple butter, 50
mayonnaise
  garlic aioli, 112
  safety, 7
  sambal oelek dip, 40
  truffle aioli, 48
meals, light, 100–124
meat
  See also beef
  avoidance of, 7
  cravings, 9
meatballs, garlic pita skewers, 84
menus, 205
mercury, 7
meringues, berry kiwi citrus cream, 170
Mexican seven-layer dip, 82
Meyer lemons and blueberry salad in Parmesan baskets, 92
milk and milk products, avoidance of, 7
mint
  and cherry tart, 166
  crab cakes, 122
  fruit salad, 37
  ginger beer no-jito, 190
  grilled peaches and, 52
  iced tea with cucumber, 196
  lemon and blueberry salad in Parmesan baskets, 92

mocha almond Nanaimo bars, 182
mojitos, ginger beer no-jito, 190
Monterey Jack cheese
  chicken pizza, 120
  chicken wrap, 116
  Moroccan chicken quesadilla, 152
mousse, chocolate, 160
mozzarella cheese
  eggplant and spinach lasagna, 140
  tomato, basil and bocconcini skewers, 94
  vegetable panini, 112
muffins
  fruit, 36
  tangerine, 58
mushrooms
  panini, 112
  pâté, 90
  scrambled eggs with black beans, 22
  steak salad, 150
  stuffed grilled, 124
  tempura, 148
  vegetable frittata, 24

N

naan, chicken pizza, 120
Nanaimo bars, almond mocha, 182
New York striploin steak, 150
noodles, egg, cashew and cabbage salad, 108
nori, vegetable sushi, 70
Nutella, sweet crêpes, 32
nuts
  See also specific type of nut
  mixed, with green olives and chickpeas, 44

O

oats, granola bars, 60
olive oil, lemon, 94
olives
  with chickpeas and nuts, 44
  cravings, 11
  Italian sausage omelet, 20
  tomato tuna zucchini rounds, 78
omelets, olive and Italian sausage, 20
onions
  caramelized, and balsamic cherry jam, 80
  dill bread, 115
  panini, 112
  savoury crêpes, 32
  soup, 100
  tempura, 148
  vegetable tart, 86
oranges
  biscotti, 62
  citrus guacamole, 37
  fruit salad, 37
  ginger pumpkin cheesecake, 164
  juice, banana and yogurt popsicles, 67
  juice, chocolate yogurt drink, 198

P

panini, roasted balsamic vegetable, 112
panko
  crab cakes, 122
  ginger wasabi sliders, 118
  stuffed mushrooms, 124
papayas, fruit salad, 37
Parmesan cheese
  baskets, with lemon and blueberry salad, 92
  cilantro honey pesto, 134
  toasted cheese sandwich, 115
  vegetable frittata, 24
passion fruit juice, rooibos and, 196
pasta
  butternut squash ravioli, 138
  eggplant and spinach lasagna, 140
  garlic shrimp and linguine, 136
  gnocchi with truffle butter sauce, 142
  roasted vegetables and, 112
pâté
  avoidance of, 7
  mushroom, 90
PCBs, 7
peaches
  bellini, 192
  crumble pie, 168
  with grapefruit and mint, 52
peanut butter
  cravings, 9
  pita chips with peanut chili dip, 46
  sandwich, 30
pears
  compote with cheddar, 96
  slow-cooked beef, 149
  Thai basil sandwich, 114
peas
  salmon, asparagus salad, 104
  vegetable sushi, 70
pecans
  bacon-wrapped dried plums, 74
  candied, and cauliflower salad, 110
  crust, sex in a pan, 162
  with olives and chickpeas, 44
peppers, bell
  crab cakes, 122
  olive and Italian sausage omelet, 20
  panini, 112
  roasted sweet potatoes and eggs, 25
  seven-layer dip, 82
  stuffed mushrooms, 124
  tiger prawn and chickpea salad, 106
  vegetable frittata, 24
  vegetable sushi, 70
  vegetable tart, 86
peppers, habanero chili, chicken, 154
peppers, jalapeño, salsa, 22
pesto, cilantro honey, 134
pickles
  cravings, 11
  Pickled Mary drink, 194
  tempura-style with dip, 40

picnic menu, 205
pies, peach crumble, 168
pine nuts
asparagus and truffle oil, 42
cilantro honey pesto, 134
with olives and chickpeas, 44
salmon, asparagus and pea salad, 104
pineapples
banana, yogurt and juice popsicles, 67
blueberry and lychee drink, 190
fruit salad, 37
and ham bagel, 16
pitas
chips with peanut chili dip, 46
garlic, meatball skewers, 84
plums, dried, bacon-wrapped, 74
popping corn, caramel, 66
poppy seeds, tangerine muffins, 58
popsicles, banana, yogurt and juice, 67
Portobello mushrooms
pâté, 90
stuffed grilled, 124
potatoes
garlic roasted, 154
gnocchi with truffle butter sauce, 142
prawns and chickpea salad, 106
puddings, banana butterscotch, 172
pumpkin, orange ginger cheesecake, 164

Q

quesadillas, Moroccan chicken, 152

R

raisins, tangerine muffins, 58
raspberries
with chocolate anise sauce, 176
chocolate fudge, 180
float, 195
jam, sweet crêpes, 32
red cabbage, cashew noodle salad, 108
red meat, cravings, 9
red peppers
crab cakes, 122
panini, 112
roasted sweet potatoes and eggs, 25
seven-layer dip, 82
stuffed mushrooms, 124
tiger prawn and chickpea salad, 106
vegetable frittata, 24
vegetable sushi, 70
vegetable tart, 86
refried beans, seven-layer dip, 82
rice
bacon, leek and almond risotto, 144
chicken and apricots, 76
ricotta cheese
eggplant and spinach lasagna, 140
stuffed mushrooms, 124
risotto, bacon, leek and almond, 144
roast beef
with apples and pears, 149
rosemary garlic, 146
Romano cheese, cilantro honey pesto, 134
rooibos and passion fruit drink, 196
rosemary
chicken wrap, 116
garlic roast beef, 146

S

salads
cabbage noodle salad, 108
cauliflower pecan, 110
fruit salad, 37
lemon and blueberry, 92
prepared, 7
roasted vegetables, 112
salmon, asparagus and pea, 104
scallops with cilantro honey pesto, 134
steak, 150
tiger prawn and chickpea, 106
salmon
asparagus and pea salad, 104
chocolate sesame, 130
zucchini and corn latkes, 18
salsa
mango cilantro, 54
tomato, 22
salty snacks, cravings, 8
sambal oelek dip, 40
sandwiches
apple, lettuce, tomato, cheddar, avocado, 26
chicken wrap, 116
grilled pear and Thai basil, 114
peanut butter, 30
toasted cheese, 115
vegetable panini, 112
sauces
avoidance of, 7
béchamel, 140
caramel drizzle, 168
chocolate anise, 176
chocolate sesame, 130
coconut curry, 132
fig brown butter, 138
green curry, 72
tarragon sour cream, 122
tomato feta, 136
truffle butter, 142
wasabi yogurt, 70
sausage
chorizo, buttermilk biscuits, 28
chorizo, savoury crêpes, 32
cravings, 9
Italian, and olive omelet, 20
scallops, with cilantro honey pesto, 134
seafood
avoidance of, 7
crab cakes, 122
cravings, 11

sablefish, 128
salmon, asparagus and pea salad, 104
salmon, chocolate sesame, 130
salmon, zucchini and corn latkes, 18
scallops with cilantro honey pesto, 134
shrimp and feta linguine, 136
tiger prawns and chickpea salad, 106
tilapia with coconut curry cream sauce, 132
tuna with olives and tomato zucchini rounds, 78
seaweed, vegetable sushi, 70
sesame oil, chocolate salmon, 130
sesame seeds
cashew, cabbage and noodle salad, 108
vegetable tart, 86
sex in a pan, 162
shallots
dill sour cream, 18
lemon and blueberry salad in Parmesan baskets, 92
shortbread
crust, cherry mint tart, 166
dried cranberry, 174
shrimp, feta linguine, 136
sirloin
garlic, meatball and pita skewers, 84
ginger wasabi sliders, 118
skewers
garlic, meatball and pita, 84
tomato, basil and bocconcini, 94
sliders, ginger wasabi, 118
Slurpee, cravings, 8
smoked meats, avoidance of, 7
smoothies, blueberry coconut, 200
snacks, 40–67
soufflés, chocolate truffle, 158
soups
butternut squash, 102
French onion, 100
sour cherries, fruit muffins, 36
sour cream
chicken wrap, 116
crème fraîche and butternut squash soup, 102
dill, 18
seven-layer dip, 82
tarragon sauce, 122
sourdough bread
French onion soup, 100
french toast, 34
grilled pear sandwich, 114
spicy foods, cravings, 9
spinach
cashew, cabbage and noodle salad, 108
cauliflower pecan salad, 110
chicken pizza, 120
chicken wrap, 116
eggplant lasagna, 140
scrambled eggs with black beans, 22
stuffed mushrooms, 124
vegetable frittata, 24
sprouts, 7
squash
butternut ravioli, 138
butternut soup, 102
pumpkin cheesecake, 164
steak
cravings, 9
salad, 150
strawberries
fruit salad, 37
mango lemonade, 188
sweet crêpes, 32
sugar peas, vegetable sushi, 70
sumac, chicken, apricots and rice, 76
sun-dried olives, zucchini tomato rounds, 78
sun-dried tomatoes, olive and tuna zucchini rounds, 78
sunflower seeds, tangerine muffins, 58
sushi
avoidance of, 7
cravings, 11
vegetable, 70
sweet potatoes
butternut squash soup, 102
fries, 48
roasted with eggs, 25
sweeteners, 7
Swiss cheese
French onion soup, 100
savoury crêpes, 32
seven-layer dip, 82
toasted cheese sandwich, 115

T

tangerines, muffins, 58
tangy foods, cravings, 9
tarragon sour cream sauce, 122
tart foods, cravings, 9
tarts
cherry mint, 166
vegetables, 86
teas
chocolate chai, 200
herbal, 7
iced, mint with cucumber, 196
London fog cupcakes, 184
rooibos and passion fruit drink, 196
tempura
beets, mushrooms, onions, 148
dill pickles, 40
Thai basil, grilled pear sandwich, 114
Thai sweet red chili sauce, peanut chili dip, 46
tiger prawns and chickpea salad, 106
tilapia with coconut curry cream sauce, 132

toffee
coffee chocolate chip cookies, 178
crust, chocolate mousse cake, 160
tomato juice, Pickled Mary drink, 194
tomatoes
bacon, apple, lettuce, cheddar, avocado sandwich, 26
basil bocconcini skewers, 94
cashew, cabbage and noodle salad, 108
chicken wrap, 116
coconut curry cream sauce, 132
olive and tuna zucchini rounds, 78
salsa, 22
shrimp and feta linguine, 136
steak salad, 150
tortillas
chicken quesadilla, 152
chicken wrap, 116
truffle oil
aioli, 48
asparagus and pine nuts, 42
butter sauce, 142
truffles, chocolate soufflé, 158
tuna, zucchini rounds with olives and tomatoes, 78

V

vanilla cinnamon latte, 201
vegetables
See also specific type of vegetable
cravings, 10
panini, 112
safety, 7
savoury crêpes, 32
sushi, 70
tart, 86

W

walnuts
caramel corn, 66
fruit muffins, 36
with olives and chickpeas, 44
peach crumble pie, 168
pear compote, 96
steak salad, 150
tangerine muffins, 58
wasabi
dipping sauce, 70
ginger sliders, 118
watermelon juice, 198
whipping cream
with banana butterscotch pudding, 172
french toast with blueberry crème, 34
lemon, 170
sex in a pan, 162
white asparagus, salmon and pea salad, 104
white cheddar cheese
grilled pear sandwich, 114
with pear compote, 96
white grape juice, lemon cosmopolitan, 192
white peaches
bellini, 192
crumble pie, 168
wraps
chicken, 116
roasted vegetables, 112

Y

yams, smashed, 149
yellow peppers
olive and Italian sausage omelet, 20
vegetable sushi, 70
yogurt
chocolate orange drink, 198
coconut curry cream sauce, 132
frozen, raspberry float, 195
fruit muffins, 36
popsicles, 67
salmon, asparagus and pea salad, 104
smoothie, 200
wasabi dipping sauce, 70

Z

zucchini
chili chicken, 154
panini, 112
rounds, with olives, tomatoes and tuna, 78
salmon and corn latkes, 18
tiger prawn and chickpea salad, 106
vegetable sushi, 70
vegetable tart, 86